Cardiovascular Risk Factors and Intervention Strategies for the Prevention of Cardiovascular Disease

Cardiovascular Risk Factors and Intervention Strategies for the Prevention of Cardiovascular Disease

Editor

Paolo Palatini

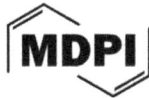

Basel • Beijing • Wuhan • Barcelona • Belgrade • Novi Sad • Cluj • Manchester

Editor
Paolo Palatini
Department of Medicine
University of Padova
Padua
Italy

Editorial Office
MDPI AG
Grosspeteranlage 5
4052 Basel, Switzerland

This is a reprint of articles from the Special Issue published online in the open access journal *Journal of Clinical Medicine* (ISSN 2077-0383) (available at: https://www.mdpi.com/journal/jcm/special_issues/L3VU56J8OY).

For citation purposes, cite each article independently as indicated on the article page online and as indicated below:

Lastname, A.A.; Lastname, B.B. Article Title. *Journal Name* **Year**, *Volume Number*, Page Range.

ISBN 978-3-7258-1789-4 (Hbk)
ISBN 978-3-7258-1790-0 (PDF)
doi.org/10.3390/books978-3-7258-1790-0

© 2024 by the authors. Articles in this book are Open Access and distributed under the Creative Commons Attribution (CC BY) license. The book as a whole is distributed by MDPI under the terms and conditions of the Creative Commons Attribution-NonCommercial-NoDerivs (CC BY-NC-ND) license.

Contents

About the Editor vii

Paolo Palatini, Lucio Mos, Francesca Saladini, Olga Vriz, Claudio Fania, Andrea Ermolao, et al.
Both Moderate and Heavy Alcohol Use Amplify the Adverse Cardiovascular Effects of Smoking in Young Patients with Hypertension
Reprinted from: *J. Clin. Med.* **2023**, *12*, 2792, https://doi.org/10.3390/jcm12082792 1

Milan Radovanovic, Janko Jankovic, Stefan Mandic-Rajcevic, Igor Dumic, Richard D. Hanna and Charles W. Nordstrom
Ideal Cardiovascular Health and Risk of Cardiovascular Events or Mortality: A Systematic Review and Meta-Analysis of Prospective Studies
Reprinted from: *J. Clin. Med.* **2023**, *12*, 4417, https://doi.org/10.3390/jcm12134417 12

Rebeca Lorca, Andrea Aparicio, María Salgado, Rut Álvarez-Velasco, Isaac Pascual, Juan Gomez, et al.
Chromosome Y Haplogroup R Was Associated with the Risk of Premature Myocardial Infarction with ST-Elevation: Data from the CholeSTEMI Registry
Reprinted from: *J. Clin. Med.* **2023**, *12*, 4812, https://doi.org/10.3390/jcm12144812 29

Damiano Rizzoni, Claudia Agabiti-Rosei, Gianluca E. M. Boari, Maria Lorenza Muiesan and Carolina De Ciuceis
Microcirculation in Hypertension: A Therapeutic Target to Prevent Cardiovascular Disease?
Reprinted from: *J. Clin. Med.* **2023**, *12*, 4892, https://doi.org/10.3390/jcm12154892 38

Fabiola Atzeni, Laura La Corte, Mariateresa Cirillo, Manuela Giallanza, James Galloway and Javier Rodríguez-Carrio
Metabolic Syndrome and Its Components Have a Different Presentation and Impact as Cardiovascular Risk Factors in Psoriatic and Rheumatoid Arthritis
Reprinted from: *J. Clin. Med.* **2023**, *12*, 5031, https://doi.org/10.3390/jcm12155031 52

Antonio da Silva Menezes Junior, Vinícius Martins Rodrigues Oliveira, Izadora Caiado Oliveira, André Maroccolo de Sousa, Ana Júlia Prego Santana, Davi Peixoto Craveiro Carvalho, et al.
Dual PPR$\alpha\gamma$ Agonists for the Management of Dyslipidemia: A Systematic Review and Meta-Analysis of Randomized Clinical Trials
Reprinted from: *J. Clin. Med.* **2023**, *12*, 5674, https://doi.org/10.3390/jcm12175674 64

Simona Giubilato, Fabiana Lucà, Maurizio Giuseppe Abrignani, Laura Gatto, Carmelo Massimiliano Rao, Nadia Ingianni, et al.
Management of Residual Risk in Chronic Coronary Syndromes. Clinical Pathways for a Quality-Based Secondary Prevention
Reprinted from: *J. Clin. Med.* **2023**, *12*, 5989, https://doi.org/10.3390/jcm12185989 77

Alejandro de la Sierra
Blood Pressure Variability as a Risk Factor for Cardiovascular Disease: Which Antihypertensive Agents Are More Effective?
Reprinted from: *J. Clin. Med.* **2023**, *12*, 6167, https://doi.org/10.3390/jcm12196167 101

Keisuke Narita, Satoshi Hoshide and Kazuomi Kario
Polypill Therapy for Cardiovascular Disease Prevention and Combination Medication Therapy for Hypertension Management
Reprinted from: *J. Clin. Med.* **2023**, *12*, 7226, https://doi.org/10.3390/jcm12237226 108

Francesca Saladini
Effects of Different Kinds of Physical Activity on Vascular Function
Reprinted from: *J. Clin. Med.* **2024**, *13*, 152, https://doi.org/10.3390/jcm13010152 . . . . **121**

Lanfranco D'Elia and Pasquale Strazzullo
Dietary Salt Restriction and Adherence to the Mediterranean Diet: A Single Way to Reduce Cardiovascular Risk?
Reprinted from: *J. Clin. Med.* **2024**, *13*, 486, https://doi.org/10.3390/jcm13020486 . . . . **132**

About the Editor

Paolo Palatini

Paolo Palatini is a Professor of Medicine and Senior Scholar of the Studium Patavinum at the Department of Medicine, University of Padova, Padua, Italy. He is the former Head of Vascular Medicine at the Department of Medicine of Azienda Ospedaliera and the University of Padova. He was Secretary of the Italian Hypertension League and Member of the Boards of the Italian Society of Hypertension, Italian Society of Sports Cardiology, and the Italian Society of Nephrocardiology. He is Chairman of the ESH Working Group on ABPM and BP Variability. Prof Palatini completed his medical education at the University of Padova, Italy. He worked for 5 years in the Laboratory of Professor Stevo Julius at the University of Michigan (USA), where he received local honours. He was appointed as a lecturer in 2009 by the Belgian Hypertension Society and by the Indian Society of Cardiology. Prof Palatini has coordinated several international and national studies of hypertension and clinical pharmacology. He has served as an Editorial Board Member of several International Journals including Hypertension and the Journal of Hypertension. He has published over 500 original articles and reviews in international journals and his present H-index is 91, with over 40,000 citations according to Google Scholar. He has also received the Alberto Zanchetti Life Achievement Award and the Talal Zein Award of the European Society of Hypertension. Professor Palatini's main areas of research include the pathophysiology of the autonomic nervous system, blood pressure and heart rate variability, exercise hemodynamics, heart rate as a cardiovascular risk factor, epidemiology and the prognostic significance of lifestyle factors, the genetics of hypertension and cardiovascular disease, the pathophysiology of renal hemodynamics in hypertension and myocardial infarction, the assessment and prognostic significance of hypertension mediated organ damage in hypertension, and blood pressure measurement techniques.

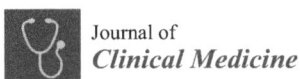

Article

Both Moderate and Heavy Alcohol Use Amplify the Adverse Cardiovascular Effects of Smoking in Young Patients with Hypertension

Paolo Palatini [1,*], Lucio Mos [2], Francesca Saladini [3], Olga Vriz [2], Claudio Fania [4], Andrea Ermolao [1], Francesca Battista [1], Mattia Canevari [2] and Marcello Rattazzi [1]

1. Department of Medicine, University of Padova, 35128 Padova, Italy; francesca.battista@unipd.it (F.B.)
2. San Antonio Hospital, 33038 San Daniele del Friuli, Italy; luciomos@libero.it (L.M.); olgavriz@yahoo.com (O.V.)
3. Cittadella Town Hospital, 35013 Cittadella, Italy; saladinifrancesca@gmail.com
4. Villa Maria Hospital, 35138 Padova, Italy; faniaclaudio@gmail.com
* Correspondence: palatini@unipd.it; Tel.: +39-328-4617036; Fax: +39-049-8754179

Abstract: Aim: To evaluate the association of alcohol and smoking combined with cardiovascular and renal events and investigate whether moderate and heavy alcohol consumption have a different impact on this association. Methods: The study was conducted in 1208 young-to-middle-age stage 1 hypertensive patients. Subjects were classified into three categories of cigarette smoking and alcohol use, and the risk of adverse outcomes was assessed over a 17.4-year follow-up. Results: In multivariable Cox models, smoking showed a different prognostic impact on alcohol drinkers and abstainers. In the former, an increase in the risk of cardiovascular and renal events was observed compared to nonsmokers (hazard ratio, 2.6, 95% CI, 1.5–4.3, $p < 0.001$), whereas in the latter, the risk did not achieve the level of statistical significance ($p = 0.27$) with a significant interaction between smoking and alcohol use ($p < 0.001$). Among the heavy smokers who also drank alcoholic beverages, the hazard ratio from the fully adjusted model was 4.3 (95% CI, 2.3–8.0, $p < 0.0001$). In the subjects with moderate alcohol consumption, the risk of smoking and alcohol combined was similar to that found in the whole population (hazard ratio, 2.7; 95% CI, 1.5–3.9, $p < 0.001$). Among the subjects with heavy alcohol consumption, the hazard ratio was 3.4 (95% CI, 1.3–8.6, $p = 0.011$). Conclusion: These findings indicate that the detrimental cardiovascular effects of smoking can be worsened by concomitant alcohol use. This synergistic effect occurs not only for heavy alcohol consumption but also for moderate use. Smokers should be aware of the increased risk associated with concomitant alcohol consumption.

Keywords: alcohol; smoking; cardiovascular; risk; hypertension

Citation: Palatini, P.; Mos, L.; Saladini, F.; Vriz, O.; Fania, C.; Ermolao, A.; Battista, F.; Canevari, M.; Rattazzi, M. Both Moderate and Heavy Alcohol Use Amplify the Adverse Cardiovascular Effects of Smoking in Young Patients with Hypertension. *J. Clin. Med.* 2023, *12*, 2792. https://doi.org/10.3390/jcm12082792

Academic Editor: Bernhard Rauch

Received: 17 March 2023
Revised: 1 April 2023
Accepted: 8 April 2023
Published: 9 April 2023

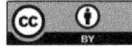

Copyright: © 2023 by the authors. Licensee MDPI, Basel, Switzerland. This article is an open access article distributed under the terms and conditions of the Creative Commons Attribution (CC BY) license (https://creativecommons.org/licenses/by/4.0/).

1. Introduction

The unhealthy effects of smoking, including an increased risk for several types of cancer, chronic obstructive pulmonary disease, coronary heart disease, and cardiovascular disease in general, have been well documented since the publication of the seminal Framingham studies [1–4]. Tobacco use remains the leading cause of morbidity and mortality in the United States [5] and is estimated to cause approximately 8 million deaths per year throughout the world [6]. Conversely, quitting smoking is associated with a significant reduction in the risk of coronary heart disease and stroke [7].

Alcohol use has also been found to increase the risk of developing serious diseases, including cancer, liver cirrhosis, hypertension, and hemorrhagic stroke [8,9]. However, the relationship between alcohol intake and cardiovascular disease is controversial because the results of the literature have been inconsistent. Although epidemiological studies have shown that excessive drinking is harmful to humans, evidence shows that mild-to-moderate alcohol consumption may even reduce cardiovascular risk [10–14]. Indeed, meta-analysis studies have advocated the health benefit of light to moderate alcohol consumption related to cardiovascular disease [15,16].

Epidemiological data suggest that smokers are at a higher risk of greater alcohol use patterns, including greater consumption and higher binge-like alcohol use [17,18]. Indeed, daily smokers have been shown to be more likely to meet the criteria for hazardous drinking and other alcohol-related diagnoses [19,20]. A body of evidence indicates that the detrimental effects seen with the singular abuse of smoking or alcohol use also increase substantially as a result of their co-use [21]. A strong synergistic effect between smoking and alcohol has been found in the induction of several types of cancer [22,23]. The ominous multiplicative consequences of concurrent use extend to other clinical conditions, such as liver cirrhosis, pancreatitis, and psychiatric co-morbidity [24–26]. Recent research has also documented a significant increase in hypertension risk due to tobacco–alcohol interaction [27,28].

However, little is known about the combined effect of alcohol and smoking on cardiovascular events, especially in young individuals, despite emerging concerns about the cardiovascular health of this segment of the population. Recent data indicate that treatment and control of major risk factors for cardiovascular disease among young adults are far from optimal and suggest that cardiovascular disease may now be increasing in this population [29–31].

In a previous analysis of the HARVEST population, we observed an interactive effect of alcohol and smoking on the risk of cardiovascular events in 18- to 45-year-old individuals [32]. The aim of the present analysis was to evaluate the association of alcohol and smoking combined with cardiovascular and renal events over a longer follow-up and investigate whether moderate and heavy alcohol consumption have a different impact on this association.

2. Methods

2.1. Subjects

The HARVEST is a multicenter prospective observational study conducted in 17 hypertension units in Italy that began on 1 April 1990 [33–35]. The study participants are 18- to 45-year-old never-treated patients screened for stage 1 hypertension (systolic blood pressure (BP) $\geq$ 140 mmHg and/or diastolic BP $\geq$ 90 mmHg). Subjects with diabetes, nephropathy, cardiovascular disease, neoplastic diseases, and any other serious clinical condition were excluded [33–35]. Consecutive patients with the above-mentioned clinical characteristics were eligible for recruitment and were sent to the referral centers by their general practitioners. Participants were recruited for five years after the beginning of the study. A total of 1208 participants who had at least 6 months of follow-up were included in this analysis. Patient data and blood and urine samples were periodically sent to the coordinating center in Padova, Italy, where they were processed.

2.2. Data Collection

The questionnaire captured data pertaining to the participants' demographics, personal and family health, medical history, and lifestyle habits, which included information about smoking, alcohol intake, coffee consumption, and physical activity. Participants were classified into three categories according to the daily number of cigarettes smoked: nonsmokers, 1–10 cigarettes/day, and >10 cigarettes/day. They were also divided into three categories of alcohol use: 0 g/day, <50 g/day, and $\geq$50 g/day. Coffee consumption was defined according to the number of caffeine-containing coffees drunk per day. For the present analysis, participants were divided into two categories: coffee drinkers and nondrinkers. Information on physical activity was collected using a previously published classification [33,34]. A family history of cardiovascular disease was defined as stroke, myocardial infarction, or sudden death before the age of 60 in a first-degree relative. More details about the interview and lifestyle assessment have been reported elsewhere [32–35]. All subjects underwent physical examination, anthropometry, blood chemistry, and urine analysis. Body mass index (BMI) was considered as an index of adiposity (weight divided by height squared). BP was measured in the office using the auscultatory method, and the mean of six readings obtained during two visits performed 2 weeks apart was considered as the baseline office BP. Twenty-four-hour ambulatory BP monitoring was performed using the A&D TM-2420 model 7 (Tokyo, Japan) or the ICR Spacelabs 90207 (Redmond, WA, USA). Measurements were taken every 10 min during the day (06.00–23.00 h) and every 30 min during the night (23.00–06.00 h). The procedures followed were in accordance with institutional guidelines, and the study was approved by the Ethics Committee of the HARVEST and by the Department of Clinical and Experimental Medicine of the University of Padova. Written informed consent was given by the participants.

2.3. Follow-up and Outcomes

During the follow-up, visits were scheduled every 6 months. Antihypertensive treatment was started following the recommendations of international guidelines available at the time of the visit (see Supplementary Materials). Then, treated and untreated subjects continued to be checked at 6-month intervals. For survivors who were lost to follow-up, the date of the last available visit was considered. Survival time was defined as the period from the date of the first visit to the date of first adverse event. Detailed information on the follow-up procedures has been reported elsewhere [32–35].

Cardiovascular events included fatal and nonfatal strokes, fatal and nonfatal ST-elevated acute myocardial infarction, non ST-elevated acute coronary syndromes, any myocardial revascularization procedure, heart failure needing hospitalization, any aortic or lower limb revascularization procedure, and development of permanent atrial fibrillation. Renal events were defined as chronic kidney disease at stage 3 or higher (estimated glomerular filtration rate < 60 mL/min/1.73 m^2). We ascertained vital status and the incidence of fatal and nonfatal events from medical records and interviews with attending physicians and patients' families.

2.4. Data Analysis

Quantitative variables were reported as mean ± SD unless specified. For follow-up duration, the median and interquartile range (IQR) were calculated. Categorical variables were reported as percentages and differences in the distribution were tested by χ^2 test. Differences in the distribution of continuous variables across groups were tested by ANCOVA test adjusting for age and sex. Lifestyle factors were modeled as time-dependent categorical variables in Cox proportional hazards regressions adjusting for age and sex. Subsequently, coffee consumption (yes/no), physical activity (yes/no), parental history of cardiovascular disease, BMI, total cholesterol, average 24 h systolic and diastolic BPs, and incident hypertension needing antihypertensive treatment diagnosed during the follow-up were also included. No violations to the proportional hazards assumption were detected by inspection of survival curves. Hazard ratios and corresponding two-sided 95% confidence intervals were derived from the regression coefficients in the Cox models. Tests for interaction effects were conducted in multivariate regression analyses by adding the product of smoking and alcohol in the models. A two-tailed probability value ≤0.05 was considered significant. Analyses were performed using Systat version 12 (SPSS Inc., Evanston, IL, USA) and MedCalc version 20.218 (MedCalc Software Ltd., Ostend, Belgium).

3. Results

Clinical characteristics of the subjects stratified by smoking and alcohol use are reported in Table 1. Compared with nonsmokers who abstained from alcohol consumption, participants who smoke and drank alcohol were slightly older, were more frequently male, and had higher 24 h systolic BP.

Table 1. Characteristics of the participants grouped according to smoking and alcohol use (yes/no).

Variable	Alcohol No Smoking No (N = 525)		Alcohol Yes Smoking No (N = 429)		Alcohol No Smoking Yes (N = 112)		Alcohol Yes Smoking Yes (N = 142)		
	Mean	SD	Mean	SD	Mean	SD	Mean	SD	p-Value
Age, years	30.8	8.8	35.4 *	7.7	32.4	8.0	34.8 *	7.9	<0.001
BMI, kg/m^2	25.0	3.7	25.6	2.9	25.7	3.4	25.4	3.1	0.07
Office SBP, mmHg	145.9	10.7	145.6	10.0	144.5	10.7	144.5	11.2	0.37
Office DBP, mmHg	92.9	6.1	94.4	5.1	93.3	5.4	93.3	6.1	0.26
Heart rate, bpm	75.7	9.6	73.4	9.1	75.3	9.6	73.1	9.7	0.13
Cholesterol, mg/dL	193.4	36.7	201.2	39.0	197.2	38.2	200.2	39.9	0.92
24-h SBP, mmHg	130.3	10.9	131.2	10.2	131.4	12.5	133.8 †	10.6	0.014
24-h DBP, mmHg	81.7	8.2	81.8	8.0	81.3	8.4	82.3	8.1	0.60
Sex, male %	64.8	–	81.2	–	60.7	–	85.2	–	<0.001
Coffee use, yes %	62.7	–	83.5	–	70.5	–	88.7	–	<0.001
Physical activity, yes %	43.0	–	35.7	–	29.5	–	39.4	–	0.02
MACE, yes %	6.3	–	8.6	–	9.8	–	18.3	–	<0.001

* $p < 0.001$ versus alcohol no/smoking no and † $p < 0.01$ versus alcohol no/smoking no, according to a Bonferroni-corrected post hoc test. MACE indicates major adverse cardiovascular and renal events.

3.1. Relationship between Lifestyle Factors

Smokers were more frequently alcohol drinkers than nonsmokers. Alcohol consumption was proportional to the number of cigarettes smoked per day (Figure 1). Coffee consumption was more frequent in alcohol drinkers than nondrinkers and in smokers than nonsmokers (Figure 2). The highest rate of coffee drinkers was found in the group of smokers who also drank alcohol (Table 1). Nonsmokers who abstained from alcohol were more physically active than the other three groups (Table 1).

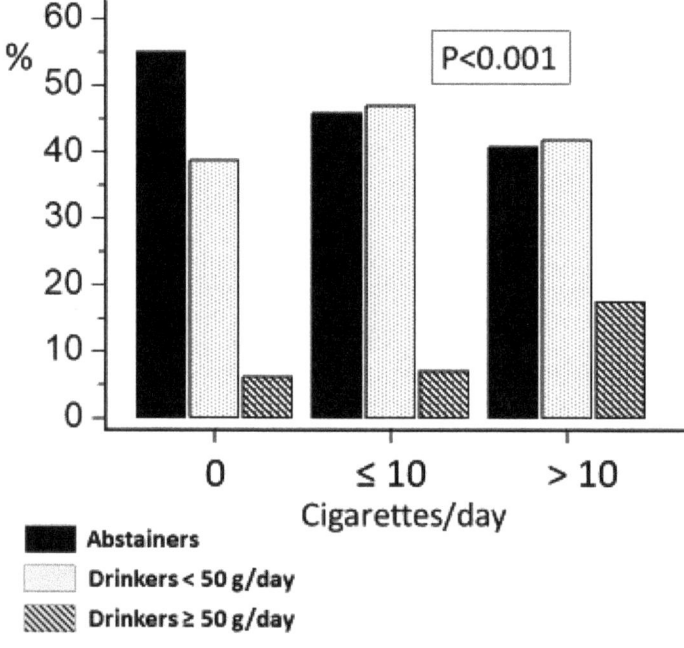

Figure 1. Frequency of alcohol abstainers, moderate alcohol drinkers (<50 g/day), and heavy alcohol drinkers (≥50 g/day) according to smoking category in 1208 participants from the HARVEST study.

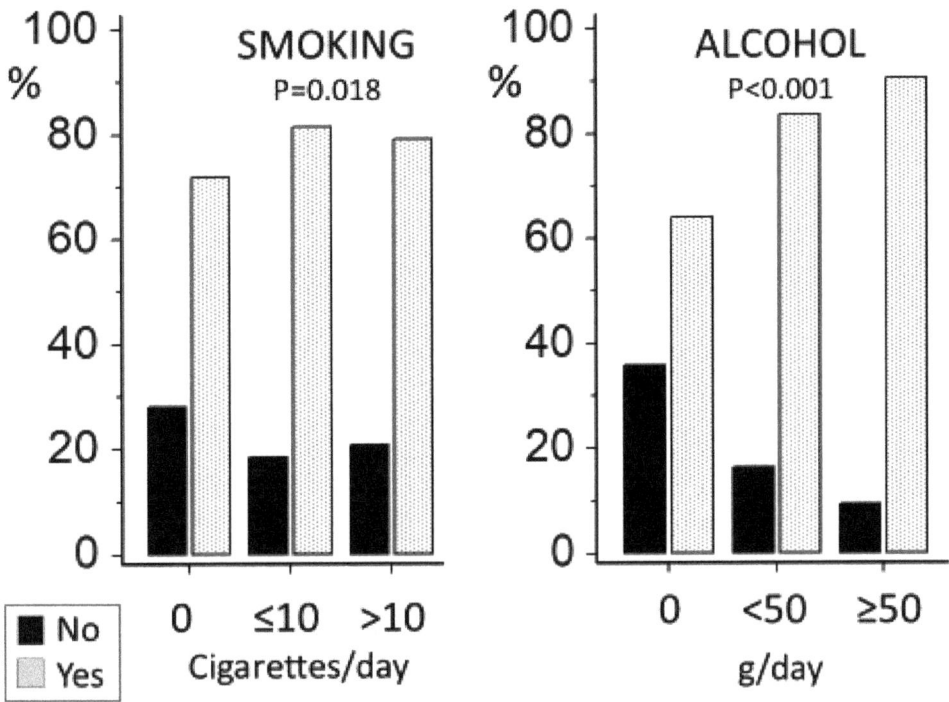

Figure 2. Frequency of coffee users (yes/no) according to alcohol and smoking category in 1208 participants from the HARVEST study.

3.2. Association with Cardiovascular and Renal Events

During a median follow-up of 17.4 (IQR 8.9–23.0) years, there were 108 adverse events (8.9%). Of these, 96 were fatal and nonfatal cardiovascular events (7.9%), and 12 were renal events (1.0%). The rate of total events was higher among the 879 men (N = 88; 10.0%) than the 329 women (N = 20; 6.1%) (chi^2 4.5; $p = 0.033$). The most common events were acute coronary syndromes (n = 50; 4.1%), with 4.9% among men and 2.1% among women (chi^2 4.6; $p = 0.032$).

The risk of cardiovascular and renal events from a multivariable Cox model including age, gender, BMI, parental history for cardiovascular disease, coffee consumption (yes/no), physical activity (yes/no), total cholesterol, mean 24 h systolic and diastolic BPs, and incident hypertension in the subjects stratified by smoking and alcohol drinking is reported in Figure 3. The risk was slightly higher in alcohol drinkers than abstainers but was not statistically significant. Among the smokers, the risk was increased compared to nonsmokers and was proportional to the number of cigarettes smoked per day (Figure 3). However, smoking showed a different prognostic impact on alcohol drinkers and abstainers. In the former, a clear increase in risk was observed compared to nonsmokers (hazard ratio, 2.6, 95% CI, 1.5–4.3, $p < 0.001$). In the latter, the risk did not achieve the level of statistical significance (hazard ratio, 1.5; 95% CI, 0.7–3.0, $p = 0.27$) with a significant interaction between smoking and alcohol use ($p < 0.001$) (Figure 4). Among the heavy smokers (>10 cigarettes/day) who also drank alcoholic beverages, the hazard ratio from the fully adjusted model was 4.3 (95% CI, 2.3–8.0, $p < 0.0001$).

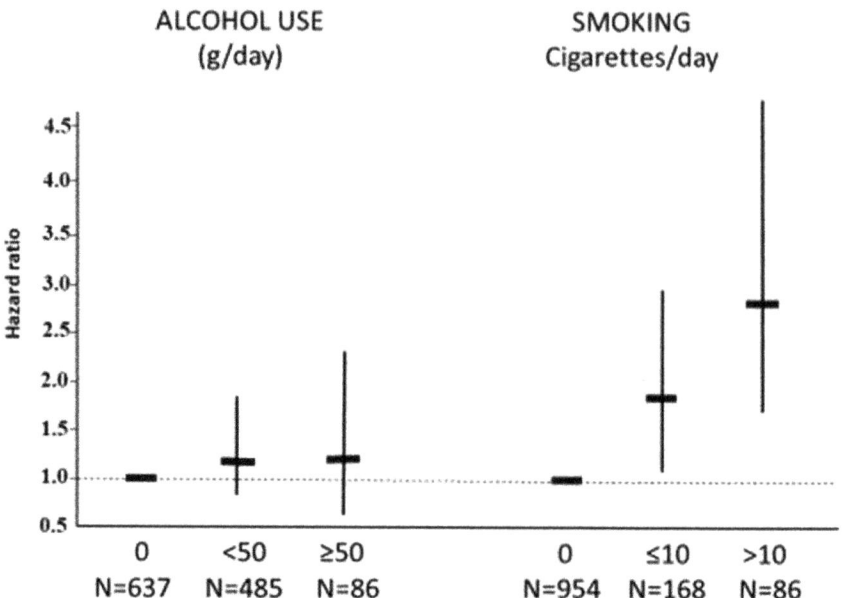

Figure 3. Hazard ratios (95% confidence intervals) for cardiovascular and renal events from multivariable Cox models in the HARVEST participants stratified by tobacco and alcohol categories.

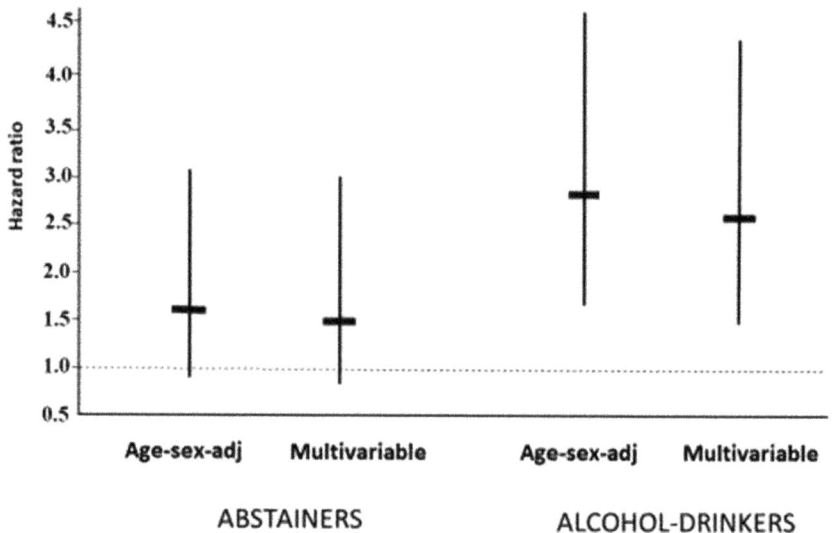

Figure 4. Hazard ratios (95% confidence intervals) for cardiovascular and renal events from multivariable Cox models in the HARVEST participants stratified according to whether they were alcohol drinkers or abstainers. Within each alcohol group, the hazard ratios represent the risk for smokers versus nonsmokers.

The survival curves for the participants stratified according to smoking and alcohol combined are reported in Figure 5. Taking the group of nonsmokers/nonalcohol drinkers as the reference, a clear increase in the risk of adverse outcomes was observed in smokers who drank alcoholic beverages. No increase in risk was observed for the group of alcohol drinkers who did not smoke. The inclusion of incident hypertension in the survival models did not attenuate the synergistic effect of smoking and alcohol on the risk of events.

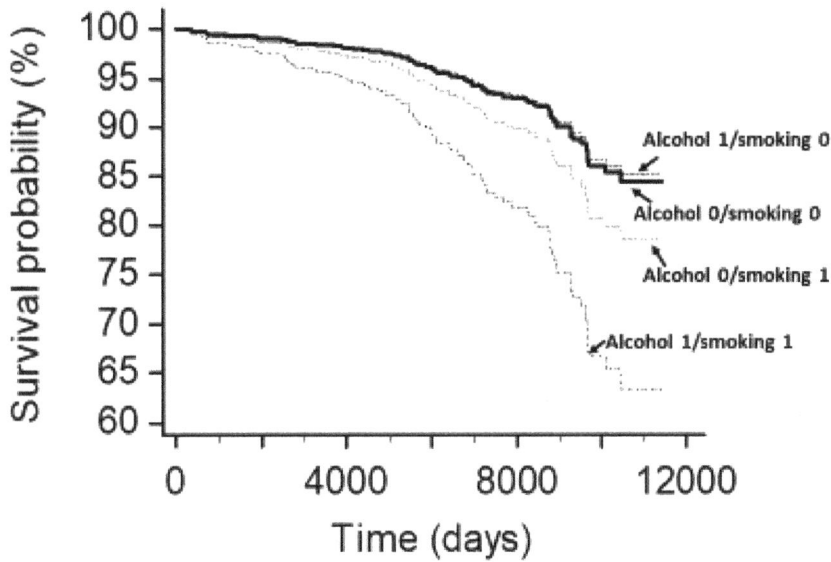

Figure 5. Adjusted survival curves from the Cox multivariable model for the HARVEST participants stratified according to smoking (yes/no) and alcohol use (yes/no). Major adverse cardiovascular and renal events were considered as the outcome variables.

3.3. Risk in Smokers by Level of Alcohol Consumption

The rate of cardiovascular and renal events was 6.3% in nonsmokers/nonalcohol drinkers, 17.4% in the group of smokers with moderate alcohol consumption (<50 g/day), and 22.2% in the smokers with heavy alcohol consumption ($\geq$50 g/day). In a sensitivity Cox analysis, the risk of smoking and alcohol combined in the subjects with moderate alcohol consumption (N = 1121, number of events = 93) was similar to that found in the whole population (hazard ratio, 2.7; 95% CI, 1.5–3.9, $p < 0.001$) (Supplementary Figure S1). Among the subjects with heavy alcohol consumption (N = 723, number of events = 58), the hazard ratio was 3.4 (95% CI, 1.3–8.6, $p = 0.011$) (Supplementary Figure S2).

4. Discussion

In this prospective cohort study of young-to-middle-aged subjects with stage 1 hypertension followed for over 17 years, we observed that the detrimental effects of smoking on cardiovascular health were worsened by concomitant alcohol use confirming our previous findings that smoking and drinking can act synergistically to increase cardiovascular risk [32]. In addition, the present results show that this synergistic effect occurs not only for heavy alcohol consumption but also for moderate use.

Tobacco consumption is widely recognized as an important risk factor for cardiovascular disease and multiple chronic noncommunicable diseases [1–6] and is the leading cause of death among middle-aged and older men [36]. Thus, there is a need to implement actionable interventions to reduce smoking-related cardiovascular risk. In addition to promoting smoking cessation, identifying risk factors that amplify the detrimental effect of smoking may be of help to reduce the burden of tobacco use on public health.

According to the American Heart Association, ideal cardiovascular health should include the combination of the 7 factors that compose the so-called "Life's Simple 7": not smoking, having a healthy diet pattern, adequate physical activity, healthy body weight, and healthy BP, cholesterol, and blood glucose in the absence of pharmacological treatment [37]. Alcohol was not included in this list because findings reported in the literature were often inconsistent across studies.

A strong synergistic effect between smoking and alcohol has been found in several clinical conditions, including some types of cancer [22–24], liver cirrhosis, pancreatitis, and psychiatric co-morbidity [24–26]. Two recent studies have documented a significant increase in the risk of hypertension due to the joint effect of tobacco and alcohol [27,28], emphasizing the importance of controlling the concurrence of smoking and alcohol consumption to prevent hypertension. However, little is known about the combined effect of these two risk factors on cardiovascular events. In a cohort of Korean adults aged 20–65 years with elevated BP, smoking and alcohol consumption, independently and jointly, were found to be associated with the risk of cardiovascular disease, but the interactive effect of these two lifestyle factors was not tested [38].

A J-shaped relationship between alcohol use and cardiovascular mortality has been described in several studies and meta-analyses, suggesting an increase in risk among heavy drinkers and a protective effect among light users [9–13]. However, recent studies suggest that the reduction in cardiovascular risk is a result of global lifestyle changes and that any reduction in alcohol consumption is beneficial [39]. In the present study, among nonsmokers, both alcohol categories were not associated with increased cardiovascular risk. In contrast, among the smokers, the multiplicative adverse effect of alcohol was found for both heavy and moderate use with hazard ratios of 3.4 and 2.7, respectively. These data are in keeping with those by Shin et al., who found that the adverse effect of alcohol combined with smoking also occurred for moderate alcohol consumption [38]. In a cohort study by Xu et al., nonsmokers with moderate alcohol consumption showed a reduced risk of cardiovascular events; in contrast, no beneficial effect from alcohol was observed in smokers with moderate alcohol use [40].

Tobacco and alcohol use have reciprocal influences on potentiating cravings and interact with each other leading to more frequent use and higher consumption levels [41]. A recent US study has shown that high-risk lifestyle factors tend to cluster in the population and that the joint risk is much higher than the sum of the individual risks [42], highlighting the importance of paying attention to their unhealthy co-effects. The present study confirms that unhealthy lifestyle factors tend to cluster together, as smokers were more frequent alcohol drinkers and had more sedentary habits.

The mechanisms underlying the interactive cardiovascular effects of smoking and alcohol remain elusive. In a previous study, we observed an interactive effect of these two factors on 24 h catecholamine output, suggesting that increased sympatho-adrenergic activity may be a contributing factor to the synergistic cardiovascular effect of tobacco and alcohol use [32]. In addition, it has been shown that both alcohol consumption and smoking trigger the production of carbon monoxide and phenolic free radicals, which have proven pro-oxidant and pro-inflammatory effects, thereby increasing the likelihood of adverse clinical outcomes [43]. Through chronic inflammation and endothelial damage, both tobacco and alcohol consumption can cause a direct or indirect impairment of vascular elasticity and promote atherosclerosis [44,45].

5. Limitations

We acknowledge that the present study has several limitations. First, in our study, the status of lifestyle factors was self-reported by the participants and thus subject to misclassification. However, health behaviors were checked frequently during the follow-up, showing that lifestyle habits were constant and well-reported [32,33]. Second, the evaluation criteria of lifestyle factors in the HARVEST differ from those of other reports, which might cause differences between the studies. This limitation pertains particularly to the definition of heavy and moderate drinkers, which is inconsistent among different studies. Third, we enrolled only Caucasians and were unable to perform subgroup analyses by race or ethnicity. In addition, we could not estimate differences between men and women because of the smaller sample size and the low number of events among the women. Therefore, the present results may not be applicable to women or people of other racial backgrounds.

6. Conclusions

The present findings indicate that there is an important synergistic effect between tobacco and alcohol consumption on cardiovascular and renal outcomes in young hypertensive subjects. The multiplicative risk associated with smoking and alcohol drinking also occurred for moderate alcohol consumption, emphasizing the importance of controlling the concurrence of unhealthy lifestyle factors. Strategies for improving lifestyle behaviors are well recognized and should be applied and reinforced, particularly in young patients with hypertension. Indeed, increases in heart disease and cardiovascular mortality has been reported in recent years in younger adults, which reflect recent unfavorable trends in cardiovascular risk determinants and events [29,46]. Tobacco product use remains high among youth in Western countries [47], calling for the implementation of population-based tobacco control strategies in this segment of the population. However, only a minority of smokers state they want to quit at some point in time [48]. Thus, smokers should be aware that quitting alcohol consumption would reduce the detrimental effects of tobacco use.

Supplementary Materials: The following supporting information can be downloaded at: https://www.mdpi.com/article/10.3390/jcm12082792/s1, Figure S1: Adjusted survival curves from the Cox multivariable model for the HARVEST participants stratified according to smoking (yes/no) and moderate alcohol use (yes/no). Major adverse cardiovascular and renal events were considered as the outcome variable; Figure S2: Adjusted survival curves from the Cox multivariable model for the HARVEST participants stratified according to smoking (yes/no) and heavy alcohol use (yes/no). Major adverse cardiovascular and renal events were considered as the outcome variable. References [49–52] are cited in the supplementary materials.

Author Contributions: Conceptualization, P.P.; data curation, F.S., O.V., C.F., A.E., F.B., M.C. and M.R.; formal analysis, P.P. and M.R.; funding acquisition, L.M.; investigation, F.S., O.V., C.F., A.E., F.B., M.C. and M.R.; visualization, L.M.; writing—original draft, P.P. All authors have contributed to the work. All authors have read and agreed to the published version of the manuscript.

Funding: All studies based on HARVEST data are funded by the Associazione "18 maggio 1370", San Daniele del Friuli, Italy.

Institutional Review Board Statement: The study was approved by the Department of Clinical and Experimental Medicine of the University of Padova, Italy, on 1 April 1990. The study protocol followed the principles of the Declaration of Helsinki.

Informed Consent Statement: Written informed consent, including consent for the future publication of data, was given by the participants.

Data Availability Statement: The data that support the findings of this study are available on reasonable request from the HARVEST study group.

Conflicts of Interest: The authors declare no conflict of interest. All authors have read and agreed to the published version of the manuscript.

References

1. Doyle, J.T.; Dawber, T.R.; Kannel, W.B.; Heslin, A.S.; Kahn, H.A. Cigarette smoking and coronary heart disease. Combined experience of the Albany and Framingham studies. *N. Engl. J. Med.* **1962**, *266*, 796–801. [CrossRef] [PubMed]
2. Centers for Disease Control and Prevention (CDC). Smoking-attributable mortality, years of potential life lost, and productivity losses–United States, 2000–2004. *MMWR Morb. Mortal. Wkly. Rep.* **2008**, *57*, 1226–1228.
3. US Department of Health and Human Services. *The Health Consequences of Smoking: A Report of the Surgeon General*; US Department of Health and Human Services, Centers for Disease Control and Prevention, National Center for Chronic Disease Prevention and Health Promotion, Office on Smoking and Health: Atlanta, GA, USA, 2004.
4. Barua, R.S.; Ambrose, J.A. Mechanisms of coronary thrombosis in cigarette smoke exposure. *Arter. Thromb. Vasc. Biol.* **2013**, *33*, 1460–1467. [CrossRef] [PubMed]
5. Carter, B.D.; Abnet, C.C.; Feskanich, D.; Freedman, N.D.; Hartge, P.; Lewis, C.E.; Ockene, J.K.; Prentice, R.L.; Speizer, F.E.; Thun, M.J.; et al. Smoking and mortality—Beyond established causes. *N. Engl. J. Med.* **2015**, *372*, 631–640. [CrossRef] [PubMed]

6. World Health Organization. WHO Report on the Global Tobacco Epidemic 2021: Addressing New and Emerging Products. 2021. Available online: https://www.who.int/publications/i/item/9789240032095 (accessed on 15 July 2022).
7. Wannamethee, S.G.; Shaper, A.G.; Whincup, P.H.; Walker, M. Smoking cessation and the risk of stroke in middle-aged men. *JAMA* **1995**, *274*, 155–160. [CrossRef]
8. Rehm, J.; Mathers, C.; Popova, S.; Thavorncharoensap, M.; Teerawattananon, Y.; Patra, J. Global burden of disease and injury and economic cost attributable to alcohol use and alcohol-use disorders. *Lancet* **2009**, *373*, 2223–2233. [CrossRef]
9. Corrao, G.; Rubbiati, L.; Bagnardi, V.; Zambon, A.; Poikolainen, K. Alcohol and coronary heart disease: A meta-analysis. *Addiction* **2000**, *95*, 1505–1523. [CrossRef]
10. Rehm, J.; Baliunas, D.; Borges, G.L.G.; Graham, K.; Irving, H.; Kehoe, T.; Parry, C.D.; Patra, J.; Popova, S.; Poznyak, V.; et al. The relation between different dimensions of alcohol consumption and burden of disease: An overview. *Addiction* **2010**, *105*, 817–843. [CrossRef]
11. Freiberg, M.S.; Samet, J.H. Alcohol and coronary heart disease: The answer awaits a randomized controlled trial. *Circulation* **2005**, *112*, 1379–1381. [CrossRef]
12. O'Keefe, J.H.; Bybee, K.A.; Lavie, C.J. Alcohol and Cardiovascular Health: The Razor-Sharp Double-Edged Sword. *J. Am. Coll. Cardiol.* **2007**, *50*, 1009–1014. [CrossRef]
13. Shaper, A.; Wannamethee, G.; Walker, M. Alcohol and Mortality in British Men: Explaining the U-Shaped Curve. *Lancet* **1988**, *332*, 1267–1273. [CrossRef] [PubMed]
14. Jackson, R.; Broad, J.; Connor, J.; Wells, S. Alcohol and ischaemic heart disease: Probably no free lunch. *Lancet* **2005**, *366*, 1911–1912. [CrossRef] [PubMed]
15. Brien, S.E.; Ronksley, P.E.; Turner, B.J.; Mukamal, K.J.; Ghali, W.A. Effect of alcohol consumption on biological markers associated with risk of coronary heart disease: Systematic review and meta-analysis of interventional studies. *BMJ* **2011**, *342*, d636. [CrossRef] [PubMed]
16. Ronksley, P.E.; Brien, S.E.; Turner, B.J.; Mukamal, K.J.; Ghali, W.A. Association of alcohol consumption with selected cardiovascular disease outcomes: A systematic review and meta-analysis. *BMJ* **2011**, *342*, d671. [CrossRef]
17. Grant, B.F. Age at smoking onset and its association with alcohol consumption and DSM-IV alcohol abuse and dependence: Results from the national longitudinal alcohol epidemiologic survey. *J. Subst. Abus.* **1998**, *10*, 59–73. [CrossRef]
18. King, A.C.; Epstein, A.M. Alcohol Dose—Dependent Increases in Smoking Urge in Light Smokers. *Alcohol. Clin. Exp. Res.* **2005**, *29*, 547–552. [CrossRef]
19. McKee, S.A.; Falba, T.; O'Malley, S.S.; Sindelar, J.; O'Connor, P.G. Smoking Status as a Clinical Indicator for Alcohol Misuse in US Adults. *Arch. Intern. Med.* **2007**, *167*, 716–721. [CrossRef]
20. Husky, M.M.; Paliwal, P.; Mazure, C.M.; McKee, S.A. Gender Differences in Association with Substance Use Diagnoses and Smoking. *J. Addict. Med.* **2007**, *1*, 161–164. [CrossRef]
21. Rosengren, A.; Wilhelmsen, L.; Wedel, H. Separate and Combined Effects of Smoking and Alcohol Abuse in Middle-aged Men. *Acta Medica Scand.* **1988**, *223*, 111–118. [CrossRef]
22. Madani, A.H.; Dikshit, M.; Bhaduri, D.; Aghamolaei, T.; Moosavy, S.H.; Azarpaykan, A. Interaction of Alcohol Use and Specific Types of Smoking on the Development of Oral Cancer. *Int. J. High Risk Behav. Addict.* **2014**, *3*, e12120. [CrossRef]
23. Tanaka, F.; Yamamoto, K.; Suzuki, S.; Inoue, H.; Tsurumaru, M.; Kajiyama, Y.; Kato, H.; Igaki, H.; Furuta, K.; Fujita, H.; et al. Strong interaction between the effects of alcohol consumption and smoking on oesophageal squamous cell carcinoma among individuals with ADH1B and/or ALDH2 risk alleles. *Gut* **2010**, *59*, 1457–1464. [CrossRef] [PubMed]
24. Pelucchi, C.; Gallus, S.; Garavello, W.; Bosetti, C.; La Vecchia, C. Cancer Risk Associated with Alcohol and Tobacco Use: Focus on Upper Aero-digestive Tract and Liver. *Alcohol Res. Health J. Natl. Inst. Alcohol Abus. Alcohol.* **2006**, *29*, 193–198.
25. McKee, S.A.; Krishnan-Sarin, S.; Shi, J.; Mase, T.; O'Malley, S.S. Modeling the effect of alcohol on smoking lapse behavior. *Psychopharmacology* **2006**, *189*, 201–210. [CrossRef] [PubMed]
26. Oliver, J.A.; Drobes, D.J. Cognitive manifestations of drinking–smoking associations: Preliminary findings with a cross-primed Stroop task. *Drug Alcohol Depend.* **2014**, *147*, 81–88. [CrossRef] [PubMed]
27. Nagao, T.; Nogawa, K.; Sakata, K.; Morimoto, H.; Morita, K.; Watanabe, Y.; Suwazono, Y. Effects of Alcohol Consumption and Smoking on the Onset of Hypertension in a Long-Term Longitudinal Study in a Male Workers' Cohort. *Int. J. Environ. Res. Public Health* **2021**, *18*, 11781. [CrossRef]
28. Gao, N.; Liu, T.; Wang, Y.; Chen, M.; Yu, L.; Fu, C.; Xu, K. Assessing the association between smoking and hypertension: Smoking status, type of tobacco products, and interaction with alcohol consumption. *Front. Cardiovasc. Med.* **2023**, *10*, 1027988. [CrossRef]
29. Aggarwal, R.; Yeh, R.W.; Maddox, K.E.J.; Wadhera, R.K. Cardiovascular Risk Factor Prevalence, Treatment, and Control in US Adults Aged 20 to 44 Years, 2009 to March 2020. *JAMA* **2023**, *329*, 899. [CrossRef]
30. Mehta, N.K.; Abrams, L.R.; Myrskylä, M. US life expectancy stalls due to cardiovascular disease, not drug deaths. *Proc. Natl. Acad. Sci. USA* **2020**, *117*, 6998–7000. [CrossRef]
31. Ariss, R.W.; Minhas, A.M.K.; Lang, J.; Ramanathan, P.K.; Khan, S.U.; Kassi, M.; Warraich, H.J.; Kolte, D.; Alkhouli, M.; Nazir, S. Demographic and regional trends in stroke-related mortality in young adults in the United States, 1999 to 2019. *J. Am. Heart Assoc.* **2022**, *11*, e025903. [CrossRef]
32. Palatini, P.; Fania, C.; Mos, L.; Mazzer, A.; Saladini, F.; Casiglia, E. Alcohol intake more than doubles the risk of early cardiovascular events in young hypertensive smokers. *Am. J. Med.* **2017**, *130*, 967–974. [CrossRef]

33. Palatini, P.; Graniero, G.R.; Mormino, P.; Nicolosi, L.; Mos, L.; Visentin, P.; Pessina, A.C. Relation between physical training and ambulatory blood pressure in stage I hypertensive subjects. Results of the HARVEST Trial. Hypertension and Ambulatory Recording Venetia Study. *Circulation* **1994**, *90*, 2870–2876. [CrossRef] [PubMed]
34. Palatini, P.; Canali, C.; Graniero, G.R.; Rossi, G.; De Toni, R.; Santonastaso, M.; Follo, M.D.; Zanata, G.; Ferrarese, E.; Mormino, P.; et al. Relationship of plasma renin activity with caffeine intake and physical training in mild hypertensive men. *Eur. J. Epidemiol.* **1996**, *12*, 485–491. [CrossRef] [PubMed]
35. Palatini, P.; Mormino, P.; Dorigatti, F.; Santonastaso, M.; Mos, L.; De Toni, R.; Winnicki, M.; Follo, M.D.; Biasion, T.; Garavelli, G.; et al. Glomerular hyperfiltration predicts the development of microalbuminuria in stage 1 hypertension: The Harvest. *Kidney Int.* **2006**, *70*, 578–584. [CrossRef] [PubMed]
36. GBD 2015 Tobacco Collaborators. Smoking prevalence and attributable disease burden in 195 countries and territories, 1990–2015: A systematic analysis from the Global Burden of Disease Study 2015. *Lancet* **2017**, *389*, 1885–1906. [CrossRef] [PubMed]
37. Sanchez, E. Life's Simple 7: Vital But Not Easy. *J. Am. Heart Assoc.* **2018**, *7*, e009324. [CrossRef]
38. Shin, J.; Paik, H.Y.; Joung, H.; Shin, S. Smoking and alcohol consumption influence the risk of cardiovascular diseases in Korean adults with elevated blood pressure. *Nutr. Metab. Cardiovasc. Dis.* **2022**, *32*, 2187–2194. [CrossRef]
39. Chudzińska, M.; Wołowiec, Ł.; Banach, J.; Rogowicz, D.; Grześk, G. Alcohol and Cardiovascular Diseases—Do the Consumption Pattern and Dose Make the Difference? *J. Cardiovasc. Dev. Dis.* **2022**, *9*, 317. [CrossRef]
40. Xu, W.-H.; Zhang, X.-L.; Gao, Y.-T.; Xiang, Y.-B.; Gao, L.-F.; Zheng, W.; Shu, X.-O. Joint effect of cigarette smoking and alcohol consumption on mortality. *Prev. Med.* **2007**, *45*, 313–319. [CrossRef]
41. Verplaetse, T.L.; McKee, S.A. An overview of alcohol and tobacco/nicotine interactions in the human laboratory. *Am. J. Drug Alcohol Abus.* **2016**, *43*, 186–196. [CrossRef]
42. Li, Y.; Fan, X.; Wei, L.; Yang, K.; Jiao, M. The impact of high-risk lifestyle factors on all-cause mortality in the US non-communicable disease population. *BMC Public Health* **2023**, *23*, 422. [CrossRef]
43. Venza, I.; Visalli, M.; Oteri, R.; Teti, D.; Venza, M. Combined effects of cigarette smoking and alcohol consumption on antioxidant/oxidant balance in age-related macular degeneration. *Aging Clin. Exp. Res.* **2012**, *24*, 530–536. [PubMed]
44. Virdis, A.; Giannarelli, C.; Fritsch Neves, M.; Taddei, S.; Ghiadoni, L. Cigarette Smoking and Hypertension. *Curr. Pharm. Des.* **2010**, *16*, 2518–2525. [CrossRef] [PubMed]
45. Chatterjee, S.; Bartlett, S.E. Neuronal nicotinic acetylcholine receptors as pharmacotherapeutic targets for the treatment of alcohol use disorders. *CNS Neurol. Disord. Drug Targets* **2010**, *9*, 60–76. [CrossRef] [PubMed]
46. Chen, Y.; Freedman, N.D.; Albert, P.S.; Huxley, R.R.; Shiels, M.S.; Withrow, D.R.; Spillane, S.; Powell-Wiley, T.M.; De González, A.B. Association of Cardiovascular Disease With Premature Mortality in the United States. *JAMA Cardiol.* **2019**, *4*, 1230–1238. [CrossRef] [PubMed]
47. Bridget, M.; Kuehn, M.S.J. Tobacco use remains high in middle and high schools. *JAMA* **2022**, *328*, 2389–2390.
48. Babb, S.; Malarcher, A.; Schauer, G.; Asman, K.; Jamal, A. Quitting smoking among adults—United States, 2000–2015. *MMWR Morb. Mortal. Wkly. Rep.* **2017**, *65*, 1457–1464. [CrossRef]
49. Swales, J.D.; Ramsey, L.E.; Coope, J.R. Treating mild hypertension. Report of the British Hypertension Society working party. *BMJ* **1989**, *298*, 694–698.
50. Sever, P.; Beevers, G.; Bulpitt, C.; Lever, A.; Ramsay, L.; Reid, J.; Swales, J. Management guidelines in essential hypertension: Report of the second working party of the British Hypertension Society. *BMJ* **1993**, *306*, 983–987. [CrossRef]
51. Chalmers, J.; MacMahon, S.; Mancia, G.; Whitworth, J.; Beilin, L.; Hansson, L.; Neal, B.; Rodgers, A.; Mhurchu, C.N.; Clark, T. 1999 World Health Organization-International Society of Hypertension Guidelines for the Management of Hypertension. Guidelines Sub-Committee. *Blood Press Suppl.* **1999**, *1*, 9–43.
52. European Society of Hypertension-European Society of Cardiology Guidelines Committee. 2003 European Society of Hypertension-European Society of Cardiology guidelines for the management of arterial hypertension. *J. Hypertens.* **2003**, *21*, 1011–1053. [CrossRef]

Disclaimer/Publisher's Note: The statements, opinions and data contained in all publications are solely those of the individual author(s) and contributor(s) and not of MDPI and/or the editor(s). MDPI and/or the editor(s) disclaim responsibility for any injury to people or property resulting from any ideas, methods, instructions or products referred to in the content.

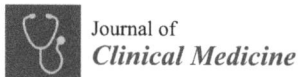 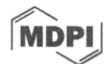

Systematic Review

Ideal Cardiovascular Health and Risk of Cardiovascular Events or Mortality: A Systematic Review and Meta-Analysis of Prospective Studies

Milan Radovanovic [1,2,*], Janko Jankovic [3,4], Stefan Mandic-Rajcevic [3,4], Igor Dumic [1,2], Richard D. Hanna [1,5] and Charles W. Nordstrom [1,2]

1. Mayo Clinic College of Medicine and Science, Rochester, MN 55905, USA
2. Department of Hospital Medicine, Mayo Clinic Health System, Eau Claire, WI 54703, USA
3. Institute of Social Medicine, Faculty of Medicine, University of Belgrade, 11000 Belgrade, Serbia
4. Centre-School of Public Health and Health Management, Faculty of Medicine, University of Belgrade, 11000 Belgrade, Serbia
5. Department of Cardiology, Mayo Clinic Health System, Eau Claire, WI 54703, USA
* Correspondence: radovanovic.milan@mayo.edu

Abstract: Cardiovascular diseases (CVD) remain the leading cause of morbidity and mortality worldwide, hence significant efforts have been made to establish behavior and risk factors associated with CVD. The American Heart Association proposed a 7-metric tool to promote ideal cardiovascular health (CVH). Recent data demonstrated that a higher number of ideal CVH metrics was associated with a lower risk of CVD, stroke, and mortality. Our study aimed to perform a systematic review and meta-analysis of prospective studies investigating the association of ideal CVH metrics and CVD, stroke, and cardiovascular mortality (CVM) in the general population. Medline and Scopus databases were searched from January 2010 to June 2022 for prospective studies reporting CVH metrics and outcomes on composite-CVD, coronary heart disease, myocardial infarction, stroke, and CVM. Each CVH metrics group was compared to another. Twenty-two studies totaling 3,240,660 adults (57.8% men) were analyzed. The follow-up duration was 12.0 ± 7.2 years. Our analysis confirmed that a higher number of ideal CVH metrics led to lower risk for CVD and CVM (statistically significant for composite-CVD, stroke, and CVM; $p < 0.05$). Conclusion: Even modest improvements in CVH are associated with CV-morbidity and mortality benefits, providing a strong public health message about the importance of a healthier lifestyle.

Keywords: cardiovascular health; Life's Simple 7; cardiovascular diseases and mortality

1. Introduction

Cardiovascular diseases (CVD) are major, global, non-communicable chronic diseases that are still the leading cause of morbidity and mortality within the United States (US) and worldwide despite declining age-standardized CVD-death rates over the second half of the 20th century [1,2]. The burden of CVD in terms of diminished quality of life, life-years lost, and direct and indirect medical costs remains substantial [2]. Nearly 50% of adults in the US have some form of CVD, and that number increases to nearly 60% among African Americans [3]. With life expectancy increasing over the past century, significant efforts have been made to establish health-related behaviors and health factors associated with CVD [1]. There is compelling evidence that unhealthy behaviors (e.g., smoking or a sedentary lifestyle) lead to unhealthy risk factors that worsen CVH and increase cardiovascular morbidity and mortality. This in turn leads to increased healthcare costs and financial burdens on individual, societal, and international levels [2]. Therefore, in 2010, the Goals and Metrics Committee of the Strategic Planning Task Force of the American Heart Association (AHA) proposed a seven-item tool as a part of their "2020 Impact Goals" to

Citation: Radovanovic, M.; Jankovic, J.; Mandic-Rajcevic, S.; Dumic, I.; Hanna, R.D.; Nordstrom, C.W. Ideal Cardiovascular Health and Risk of Cardiovascular Events or Mortality: A Systematic Review and Meta-Analysis of Prospective Studies. *J. Clin. Med.* **2023**, *12*, 4417. https://doi.org/10.3390/jcm12134417

Academic Editor: Paolo Palatini

Received: 9 June 2023
Revised: 25 June 2023
Accepted: 28 June 2023
Published: 30 June 2023

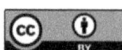

Copyright: © 2023 by the authors. Licensee MDPI, Basel, Switzerland. This article is an open access article distributed under the terms and conditions of the Creative Commons Attribution (CC BY) license (https://creativecommons.org/licenses/by/4.0/).

reduce the burden of CVD by promoting ideal CVH and primordial prevention [2,4]. The initial goal set in 2010 targeted a 20% reduction of death from CVD and stroke in the US via a 20% improvement of CVH in the American population [2]. This seven-item tool, also known as "Life's Simple 7" (LS7), consists of four health-related behaviors (not smoking, healthy dietary intake, physical activity, and body mass index [BMI]), and three health factors (total cholesterol, blood pressure, and fasting plasma glucose) [2,4]. Each of the seven CVH metrics is classified further as either poor, intermediate, or ideal; in order to numerically categorize CVH, researchers have represented these metrics as numeric scores from 0 to 2 [2]. The AHA criteria for the definition of poor, intermediate, and ideal CVH metrics are presented in Supplement Table S1.

Recent data have demonstrated that the presence of a greater number of ideal CVH metrics was associated with a lower risk of CVD, stroke, and cardiovascular mortality (CVM) [5–7]. Since the inception of CVH, there have been numerous epidemiological studies on this topic (both cohort and cross-sectional); however, there have been very few systematic reviews and meta-analyses [5–8], with the latest being published in 2018 [7]. These earlier analyses had significant shortcomings in their design, methodology, and data interpretation, and were further limited by omitting some of the important studies [9].

2. The Aim of the Study

Our study aimed to perform a systematic review and meta-analysis of prospective cohort studies investigating the association of ideal CVH metrics and CVD (composite CVD, coronary heart disease [CHD], and MI), stroke, and CVM in the general population.

3. Materials and Methods

3.1. Search Strategy, Study Selection, and Quality Assessment

A comprehensive and systematic literature search of the Medline database (via the PubMed search engine) and the Scopus database was performed according to the preferred reporting items for systematic reviews and meta-analyses (PRISMA) guidelines from the inception of the CVH concept (2010) to 30 June 2022. The review was not registered. The following search keywords (a combination of MeSH and non-MeSH terms) were used: "ideal cardiovascular health", "cardiovascular health metrics", "Life's Simple 7", "cardiovascular diseases", "coronary heart disease", "stroke", "cerebrovascular disease", "mortality", and "death". Furthermore, the reference list of identified studies was manually screened to identify additional studies that can be included in our analysis.

Two authors (M.R. and I.D.) independently and blindly screened the titles, abstracts, and full manuscripts of the identified articles, excluding duplicates and articles irrelevant to the topic. Any discrepancies or uncertainties were resolved by a third author (J.J.).

Articles included in the study were eligible if they met the following criteria: written in English, peer-reviewed, observational prospective cohort studies investigating the ideal CVH metrics and reporting cardiovascular events (e.g., composite CVD, CHD, MI, or stroke) or CVM in the general adult population. Composite CVD represents a major CVD that was not specified in the studies. All eligible studies had reported adjusted relative risks (RR) or hazard ratios (HR) with confidence intervals (CI) or standard errors (SE). Authors of eligible studies with incomplete information were contacted to provide additional data; however, if this proved either impossible or ineffective, the study was rejected. Review articles, meta-analyses, commentaries and discussions, editorials, letters to editors (except when all relevant data was available), conference papers, books, or book chapters, as well as studies conducted on children, were excluded.

The Newcastle-Ottawa Scale (NOS) for cohort studies was used for methodological quality assessment. The NOS scale is a nine-star point system used to assess the quality of non-randomized studies, including cohort studies. The scale awards up to three stars in each of three categories: the selection of study groups; the comparability of the groups; and the ascertainment of the outcome of interest [10,11]. In our analysis authors M.R. and

J.J. independently assessed the quality and calculated the NOS score for each study. Only high-quality studies with a NOS score of at least 7 were included in our analysis (Table 1).

3.2. Data Collection and Group Comparison

In addition to ideal CVH metrics, we extracted authors' names, publication year, country of the study, study name, sample size, percentage of males, population age (average or range), number of cardiovascular events including CVM, and duration of follow-up. Based on the number of ideal CVH metrics, patients were categorized into 3 groups: poor CVH group (with the fewest ideal CVH metrics: between 0 and 2), intermediate CVH group (with CVH metrics between 3 and 4), and ideal CVH group (with CVH metrics between 5 and 7). In the studies where each of the seven CVH metrics was scored from 0 to 2, patients were categorized into the poor CVH group (score 0 to 4), intermediate CVH group (score between 5 and 9), and ideal CVH group (score 10 to 14). Data were presented as mean ± SD and median (interquartile range) for continuous variables or numbers (percentages) for categorical variables.

We compared the ideal CVH group (CVH metrics 5–7 or score 10–14) to the intermediate CVH group (CVH metrics 3–4 or score 5–9) and poor CVH group (CVH metrics 0–2 or score 0–4), as well as intermediate CVH group (CVH metrics 3–4 or score 5–9) to the poor CVH group (CVH metrics 0–2 or score 0–4).

3.3. Statistical Analysis

The analysis was carried out using the log risk ratio (RR) with 95% CI as the outcome measure comparing each CVH metrics group to another. The amount of heterogeneity (i.e., T^2), was estimated using the restricted maximum-likelihood estimator [12]. In addition to the estimate of T^2, the Cochrane Q-test for heterogeneity [13] and the I^2 statistic [14] were reported. In case the I^2 statistic was higher than 50%, a random-effects (RE) model was fitted to the data, otherwise, a fixed-effects (FE) model was fitted. Sensitivity analysis was performed to investigate the robustness of the findings and results, and to determine whether a particular study accounted for the heterogeneity. Studentized residuals and Cook's distances were used to examine whether studies may be outliers and/or influential in the context of the model [15]. Studies with a studentized residual larger than the $100 \times (1 - 0.05/(2 \times k))$th percentile of a standard normal distribution were considered potential outliers (i.e., using a Bonferroni correction with two-sided $\alpha = 0.05$ for k studies included in the meta-analysis). Studies with a Cook's distance larger than the median plus 6 times the interquartile range of the Cook's distances were considered influential. The presence of publication bias was assessed graphically by funnel plots. The rank correlation test [16] and the regression test (Egger) [17], using the SE of the observed outcomes as a predictor, were used to check for funnel plot asymmetry. The analysis was carried out using R Programming Language and Environment for Statistical Computing (version 4.2.2) [18] and the metafor package (version 3.8.1) [19]. Statistical significance was reported using a two-sided p-value of <0.05.

4. Results

4.1. Literature Search and Study Characteristics

The initial search of two databases (Medline and Scopus) over the span of 12 years yielded 701 records. One study that fulfilled inclusion criteria was manually identified by checking the reference lists of identified articles [20], totaling the number of analyzed records to 702. We screened the titles and abstracts of all 400 non-duplicate records and excluded 310 irrelevant articles for the topic. A total of 90 full-text articles were reviewed for eligibility, yielding 22 studies (articles) that met the eligibility criteria for our analysis. The flow chart of detailed article selection and the final studies included in the analysis was created (Figure 1). Three studies [21–23] did not have sufficient data on CVH metric groups, however, we were able to receive additional data from the authors of one study, which we included in our analysis [21].

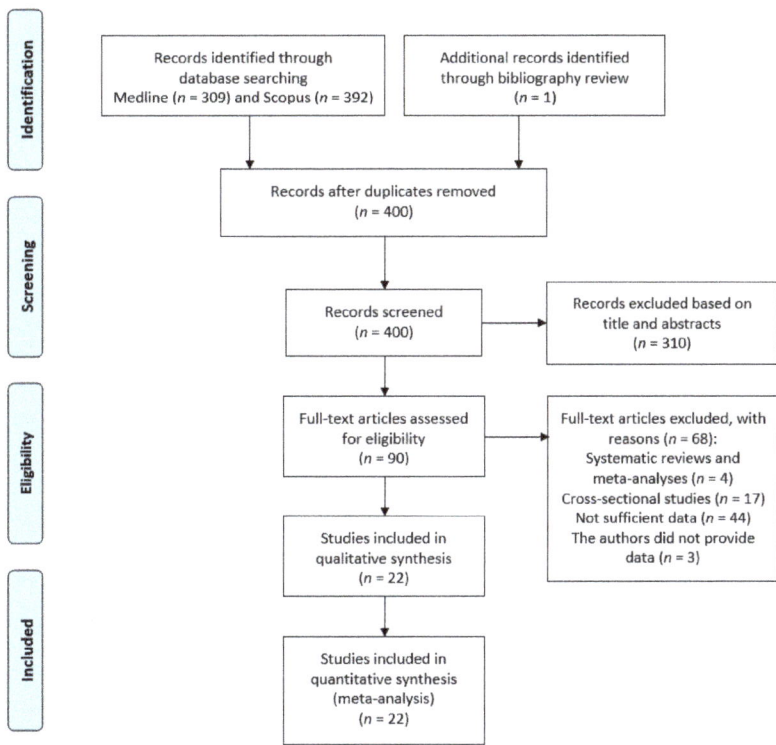

Figure 1. PRISMA flowchart detailing the search results.

All 22 selected and analyzed studies were observational prospective cohort studies, published from April 2011 [24] until June 2022 [25], that reported an association between ideal CVH metrics and the risk of CVD (composite, CHD, and MI), stroke, and CVM (Table 1). There were multiple papers published from the same large population-based studies, like Kuopio Ischemic Heart Disease (KIHD) from Finland [26–28], National Health and Nutrition Examination Survey (NHANES) from the USA [29–31], and Kailuan from China [20,32,33] (Table 1). The total number of cohort members was 3,240,660, out of which 57.8% were men. Sample sizes ranged from 2520 to 2,728,427 participants (Table 2). There were 3 published articles from the NHANES study that included only males [29–31]. Follow-up duration ranged from 3.3 to 26 years (mean 12.0 ± 7.2 years). All studies had NOS scores of 7 or 8 (Table 1).

Table 1. Characteristics of the included studies.

Reference, Year	Country	Study Name	Subjects (n)	Men (%)	Age (Range or Mean) (y)	Main Outcome	Follow-Up (y)	NOS Score
Fernandez-Lazaro et al., 2022 [25]	Spain	RIVANA	3826	44.1	52.8 ± 12.8	CVD, MI, Stroke, CVM	12.8	8
Itoh et al., 2022 [34]	Japan	JMDC database	2728427	56.2	44.9 ± 11.0	MI, stroke	3.3	8
Isiozor et al., 2021 [26]	Finland	KIHD	2520	100	42–60	Stroke	26	7
Isiozor et al., 2019 [27]	Finland	KIHD	2584	100	40–62	MI	25.2	7

Table 1. Cont.

Reference, Year	Country	Study Name	Subjects (n)	Men (%)	Age (Range or Mean) (y)	Main Outcome	Follow-Up (y)	NOS Score
Isiozor et al., 2019 [28]	Finland	KIHD	2607	100	42–60	CVM	25.8	8
Diez-Espino et al., 2019 [21]	Spain	PREDIMED	7447	42.5	67 ± 6.2	MI, stroke, CVM	4.8	8
Ahmad et al., 2019 [29]	USA	NHANES	6766	46.1	59.1 ± 13.3	CVM	14	8
Han et al., 2018 [35]	China	China-PAR	93987	40.2	51.64 ± 11.97	CVD, CHD, stroke, CVM	15	7
Gaye et al., 2017 [36]	N. Ireland, France	PRIME	9312	100	50–59	CHD, stroke	10	7
Gaye et al., 2017 [37]	France	Three-City	7371	36.7	73.82 ± 5.34	CHD, Stroke	8.6	7
Ommerborn et al., 2016 [38]	USA	Jackson Heart	3707	45.1	40–76	CVD	8.3	7
Lachman et al., 2016 [39]	UK	EPIC-Norfolk	10043	44.1	57.0 ± 9.67	CVD, CHD, stroke	10	7
Miao et al., 2015 [20]	China	Kailuan	91598	79.5	51.6 ± 12.4	CVD, MI, stroke	6.8	8
Liu et al., 2014 [32]	China	Kailuan	95429	79.7	51.46 ± 12.46	CVM	4	7
Zhang et al., 2013 [33]	China	Kailuan	91698	79.4	51.93	Stroke	4	7
Kulshreshta et al., 2013 [40]	USA	REGARDS	22915	41.9	65	Stroke	4.9	8
Kim et al., 2013 [41]	S. Korea	Seoul Male Cohort	12538	100	40–59	CVM	19	8
Yang et al., 2012 [30]	USA	NHANES	13312	49	46.8	CVM	14.5	8
Ford et al., 2012 [31]	USA	NHANES	6855	47.7	43 (median)	CVM	5.8	7
Dong et al., 2012 [42]	USA	NOMAS	2981	36.3	69 ± 10	CVD, MI, stroke, CVM	11	8
Artero et al., 2012 [43]	USA	ACLS	11993	75.7	46 ± 9.9	CVM	11.6	8
Folsom et al., 2011 [24]	USA	ARIC	12744	43.8	45–64	CVD	18.7	8

Legend: CVD—cardiovascular disease; MI—myocardial infarction; CVM—cardiovascular mortality; CHD—coronary heart disease; RIVANA—Vascular Risk in Navarra; JMDC—Japan Machine Design Center; KIHD—Kuopio Ischemic Heart Disease; PREDIMED—Prevención con Dieta Mediterránea; NHANES—National Health and Nutrition Examination Survey; PRIME—Prospective Epidemiological Study of Myocardial Infarction; EPIC—European Prospective Investigation into Cancer; REGARDS—Reasons for Geographic And Racial Differences in Stroke; NOMAS—Northern Manhattan Study; ACLS—Aerobics Center Longitudinal Study; ARIC—Atherosclerosis Risk in Communities.

Table 2. Summary of analyzed data for each outcome and CVH metrics group.

Events (n)	Subjects (n, Male %)	Poor (CVH Metrics: 0–2 or Score 0–4)		Intermediate (CVH Metrics: 3–4 or Score 5–9)		Ideal (CVH Metrics: 5–7 or Score 10–14)		Follow-Up (Average, y)
		Subjects	Events	Subjects	Events	Subjects	Events	
CVD (12069)	218786 (57.2)	18972	3370	110347	6588	89467	2111	11.8 ± 4.1
CHD (2829)	120713 (44.9)	13666	993	51972	1537	55075	299	10.9 ± 2.8
MI (7629)	2836863 (56.9)	281282	2209	1086848	3754	1468733	1666	10.6 ± 8.0
Stroke (35190)	3072125 (57.0)	342422	6539	1196199	17284	1533504	11367	9.8 ± 6.3
CVM (5500)	257741 (60.9)	62927	1945	117758	2742	77056	813	12.6 ± 6.4

Legend: CVH—cardiovascular health; CVD—cardiovascular disease; MI—myocardial infarction; CVM—cardiovascular mortality; CHD—coronary heart disease.

Table 2 represents a summary of each cardiovascular outcome and study population, with notably the highest number of events and subjects reported for stroke (the number of stroke events was 35,190, while the subject population was 3.07 million which was followed over the 9.8 ± 6.3 years).

4.2. Association between Ideal CVH Metrics and the Risk of Composite CVD

The results of our analysis demonstrated that having a higher number of ideal CVH metrics decreases the risk of developing composite CVD. When comparing the ideal to poor CVH profile, the observed RR ranged from 0.05 to 0.71, while the estimated average RR based on the RE model was 0.24 (95% CI: 0.14–0.42; $p < 0.01$; $I^2 = 97.2\%$). This demonstrates that there is a 76% lower risk of developing CVD for patients having ideal compared to poor CVH. Similarly, when comparing intermediate to poor CVH groups, the observed RR ranged from 0.41 to 0.93, and the estimated average RR based on the RE model was 0.61 (95% CI: 0.49–0.76; $p < 0.01$; $I^2 = 95.0\%$). This demonstrates that there is a 39% lower risk of developing CVD for patients having intermediate compared to poor CVH. In addition, when comparing ideal to intermediate CVH groups, the observed RR ranged from 0.11 to 0.80, and the estimated average RR based on the RE model was 0.38 (95% CI: 0.24–0.60; $p < 0.01$; $I^2 = 97.7\%$). This demonstrates that there is a 62% lower risk of developing CVD for patients having ideal compared to intermediate CVH. Forest plots showing the observed outcomes and the estimates based on the RE model are shown in Figure 2a–c. Publication bias was not detected, and funnel plots were symmetric (as shown in Supplemental Figures S1–S3 with respective $p = 0.613$, $p = 0.713$, and $p = 0.391$).

4.3. Association between Ideal CVH Metrics and the Risk of CHD

Overall, when comparing the individuals with higher numbers of ideal CVH metrics the risk for development of coronary heart disease (CHD) was lower. When comparing ideal to poor CVH groups, the observed RR ranged from 0.04 to 0.29, and the estimated average RR based on the FE model was 0.22 (95% CI: 0.18–0.26; $p = 0.05$; $I^2 = 61.5\%$). This demonstrates that there is a 78% lower risk of developing CHD for patients having ideal compared to poor CVH. Similarly, when comparing intermediate to poor CVH groups, the observed RR ranged from 0.43 to 0.59, with the estimated average RR based on the RE model was 0.51 (95% CI: 0.43–0.60; $p < 0.01$; $I^2 = 75.4\%$). This demonstrates that there is a 49% lower risk of developing CHD for patients having intermediate to poor CVH. In addition, when comparing ideal to intermediate CVH groups, the observed RR ranged from 0.08 to 0.49, with the estimated average RR based on the FE model was 0.45 (95% CI: 0.39–0.52; $p = 0.12$; $I^2 = 49.1\%$). This demonstrates that there is a 55% lower risk of developing CHD for patients having ideal compared to intermediate CVH. Forest plots showing the observed outcomes and the estimates based on the FE and RE models are shown in Figure 3a–c. Publication bias was not detected, and funnel plots were symmetric (as shown in Supplemental Figures S4–S6 with respective $p = 0.608$, $p = 0.452$, and $p = 0.330$).

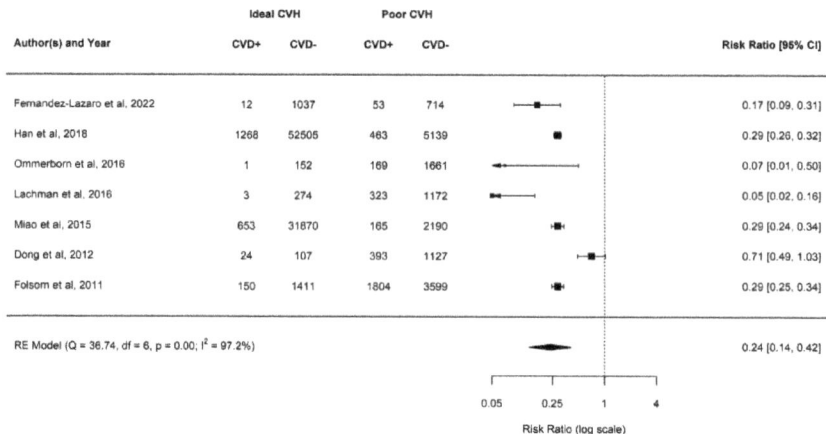

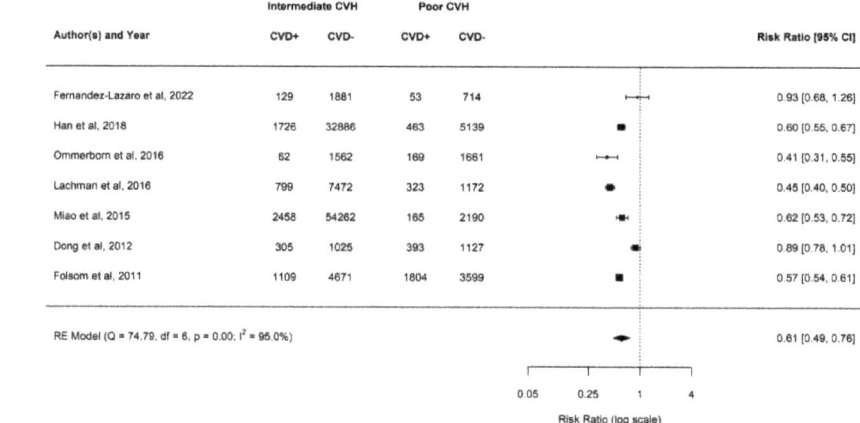

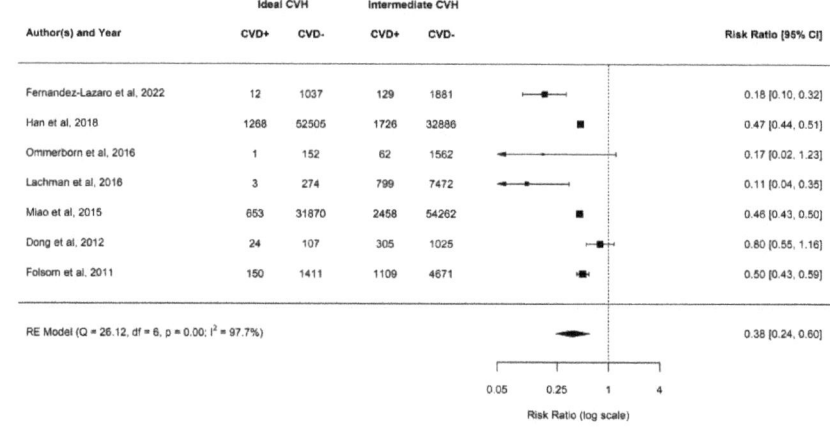

Figure 2. (**a**–**c**) Forest plots showing comparisons of CVH metrics groups for the composite CVD with RR and 95% CI [20,24,25,35,38,39,42].

4.4. Association between Ideal CVH Metrics and the Risk of MI

The results of our analysis demonstrated that having a higher number of ideal CVH metrics decreases the risk of developing MI. When comparing ideal to poor CVH groups, the observed RR ranged from 0.12 to 0.32, and the estimated average RR based on the FE model was 0.18 (95% CI: 0.17–0.20; $p = 0.12$; $I^2 = 43.2\%$). This demonstrates that there is an 82% lower risk of developing MI for patients having ideal compared to poor CVH. Similarly, when comparing intermediate to poor CVH groups, the observed RR ranged from 0.49 to 0.83, and the estimated average RR based on the RE model was 0.63 (95% CI: 0.52–0.76; $p < 0.01$; $I^2 = 74.3\%$). This demonstrates that there is a 37% lower risk of developing MI for patients having intermediate compared to poor CVH. In addition, when comparing ideal to intermediate CVH groups, the observed RR ranged from 0.17 to 0.54, and the estimated average RR based on the FE model was 0.38 (95% CI: 0.36–0.40; $p = 0.25$; $I^2 = 23.9\%$). This demonstrates that there is a 62% lower risk of developing MI for patients having ideal compared to intermediate CVH. Forest plots showing the observed outcomes and the estimates based on the FE and RE models are shown in Figure 4a–c. Publication bias was not detected for "ideal vs poor" and "ideal vs intermediate", and funnel plots were symmetric (as shown in Supplemental Figures S7 and S9 with respective $p = 0.182$, and $p = 0.837$), however, the publication bias was detected in "intermediate vs poor" with funnel plot being asymmetric (Supplemental Figure S8 with $p = 0.015$).

The study from Japan Itoh et al. [34] was identified as an influential study in the case of MI when comparing all three CVH groups by providing 96.2% of the subjects. Leave-one-out analysis indicated that the RR excluding Itoh et al. [34] would be 0.27 (95% CI: 0.20–0.36) for ideal vs poor CVH, 0.68 (95% CI: 0.58–0.79) for intermediate vs poor CVH, and 0.44 (95% CI: 0.37–0.52) for ideal vs intermediate CVH.

4.5. Association between Ideal CVH Metrics and the Risk of Stroke

Overall, when comparing the individuals with a higher number of ideal CVH metrics the risk for the development of stroke was lower. When comparing ideal to poor CVH groups, the observed RR ranged from 0.16 to 0.64, with the estimated average RR based on the RE model was 0.38 (95% CI: 0.30–0.47; $p < 0.01$; $I^2 = 85.0\%$). This demonstrates that there is a 62% lower risk of developing stroke for patients having ideal compared to poor CVH. Similarly, when comparing intermediate to poor CVH groups, the observed RR ranged from 0.53 to 0.98, and the estimated average RR based on the RE model was 0.70 (95% CI: 0.65–0.75; $p < 0.01$; $I^2 = 54.5\%$). This demonstrates that there is a 30% lower risk of developing stroke for patients having intermediate compared to poor CVH. In addition, when comparing ideal to intermediate CVH groups, the observed RR ranged from 0.16 to 0.95, and the estimated average RR based on the RE model was 0.53 (95% CI: 0.46–0.61; $p < 0.01$; $I^2 = 80.3\%$). This demonstrates that there is a 47% lower risk of developing stroke for patients having ideal compared to intermediate CVH. Forest plots showing the observed outcomes and the estimates based on the RE model are shown in Figure 5a–c. Publication bias was not detected, and funnel plots were symmetric (as shown in Supplemental Figures S10–S12 with respective $p = 0.298$, $p = 0.155$, and $p = 0.498$).

Itoh et al. [34] was identified as an influential study in the case of stroke when comparing intermediate vs poor CVH. Leave-one-out analysis indicated that the RR excluding Itoh et al. [34] would be 0.67 (95% CI: 0.63–0.72) compared to 0.70 (95% CI 0.65–0.75) when all studies are included. Although the study by Itoh et al. [34] does influence the effect size in the case of MI and stroke by providing 96.2% and 88.8% of the analyzed subjects, respectively, it does not change the direction of the effect, nor its significance.

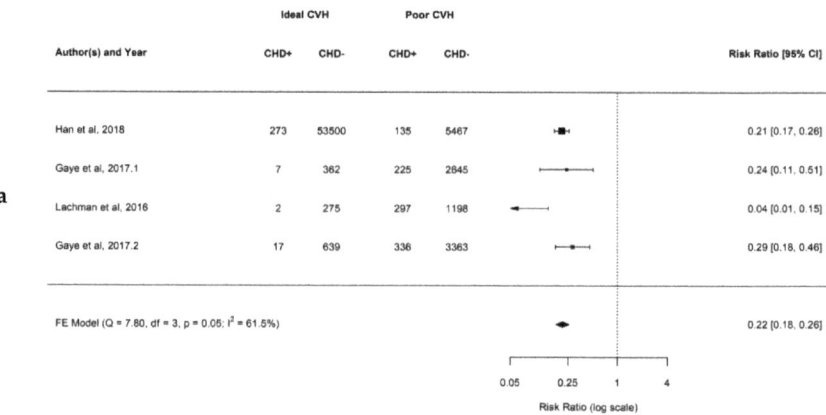
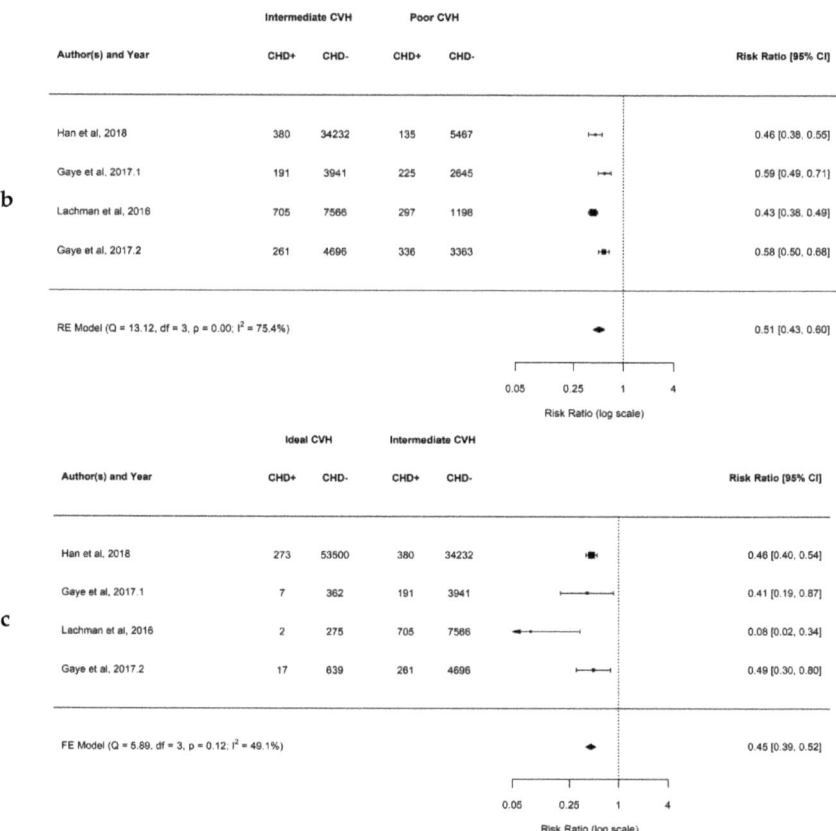

Figure 3. (a–c) Forest plots showing comparisons of CVH metrics groups for the CHD with RR and 95% CI [35–37,39].

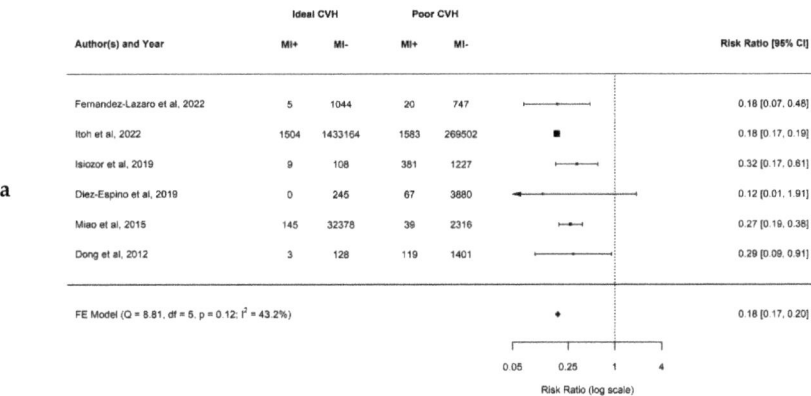

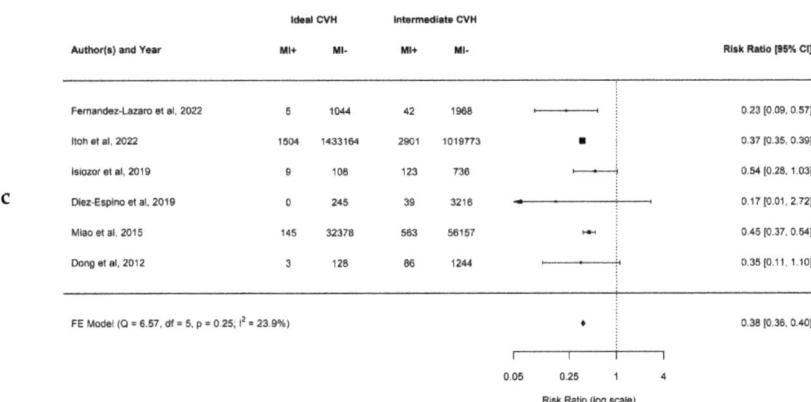

Figure 4. (**a**–**c**) Forest plots showing comparisons of CVH metrics groups for the MI with RR and 95% CI [20,21,25,27,34,42].

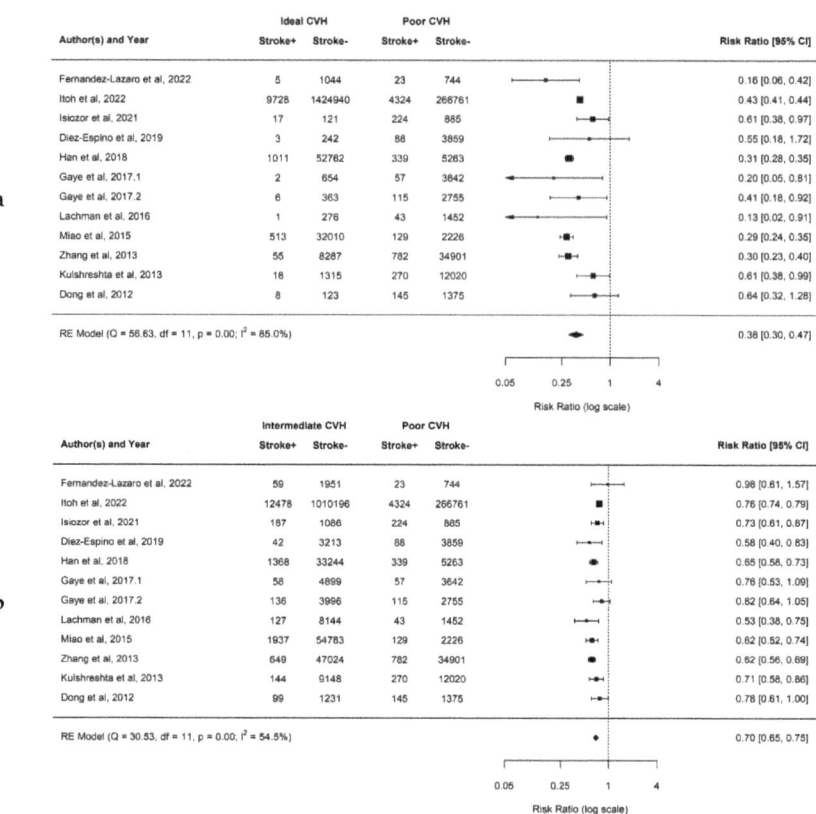

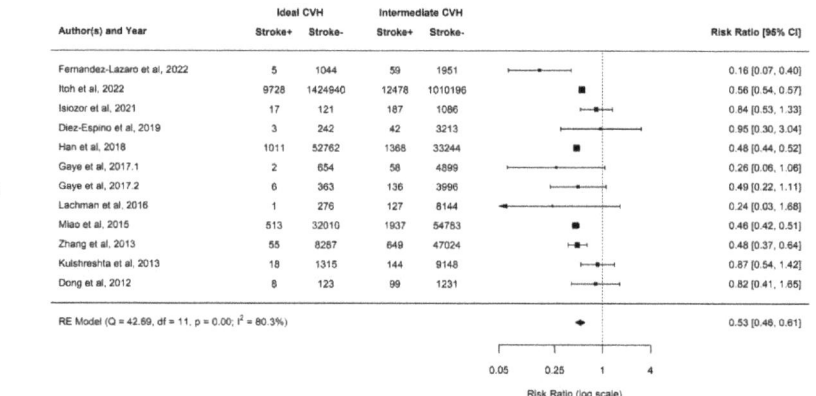

Figure 5. (**a–c**) Forest plots showing comparisons of CVH metrics groups for the Stroke with RR and 95% CI [20,21,25,26,33–37,39,40,42].

4.6. Association between Ideal CVH Metrics and the Risk of CVM

Results of our analysis demonstrated an inverse relationship showing a reduced risk of CVM with achieving a greater number of ideal CVH metrics. When comparing ideal to poor CVH groups, the observed RR ranged from 0.09 to 0.94, and the estimated average RR based on the RE model was 0.30 (95% CI: 0.21–0.42; $p < 0.01$; $I^2 = 86.3\%$). This demonstrates that there is a 70% lower risk of CVM for patients having ideal compared to poor CVH. Similarly, when comparing intermediate to poor CVH groups, the observed RR ranged from 0.41 to 1.05, while the estimated average RR based on the RE model was 0.66 (95% CI: 0.57–0.75; $p < 0.01$; $I^2 = 74.2\%$). This demonstrates that there is a 34% lower risk of CVM for patients having intermediate compared to poor CVH. In addition, when comparing ideal to intermediate CVH groups, the observed RR ranged from 0.08 to 0.94, and the estimated average RR based on the RE model was 0.49 (95% CI: 0.40–0.61; $p < 0.01$; $I^2 = 70.4\%$). This demonstrates that there is a 51% lower risk of CVM for patients having ideal compared to intermediate CVH. Forest plots showing the observed outcomes and the estimates based on the RE model are shown in Figure 6a–c. Publication bias was not detected, and funnel plots were symmetric (as shown in Supplemental Figures S13–S15 with respective $p = 0.961$, $p = 0.880$, and $p = 0.765$).

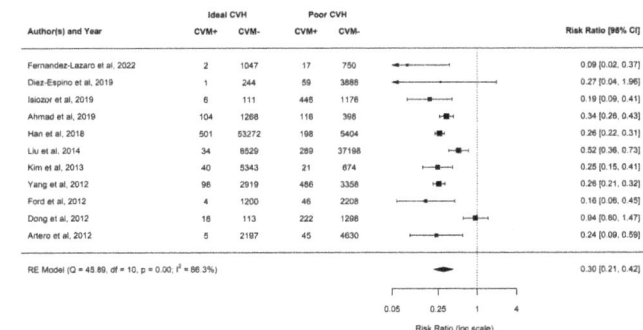

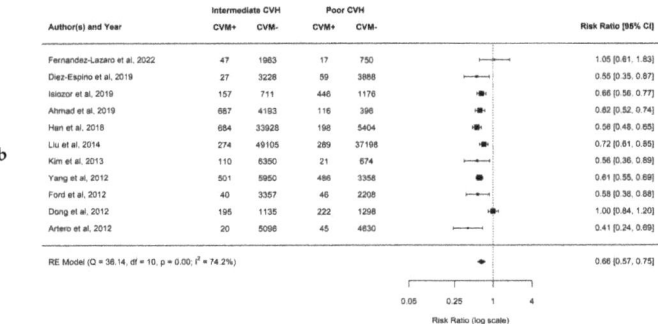

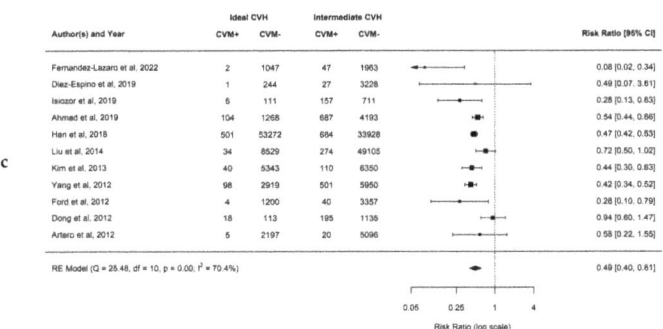

Figure 6. (a–c) Forest plots showing comparisons of CVH metrics groups for the CVM with RR and 95% CI [21,25,28–32,35,41–43].

5. Discussion

Compared to our analysis that included 22 studies, previous systematic reviews and meta-analyses on the topic of CVH [5–8] analyzed a total of 13 unique studies (ranging from 6 to 12 studies) [20,24,30–33,36,38–43], and lacked some of the important studies [9]. Except for Guo et al. [5], none of the previous meta-analyses and systematic reviews included all of the papers that fulfilled the reported inclusion criteria by the end of the performed search. The rationale for excluding eligible studies was not documented, and the selection criteria (prospective cohort studies in adults, published in the English language, and that analyzed the relationship of CVH and CVD/CVM) did not justify the exclusion of many important studies [9]. Two studies (Fang et al. [5], and Guo et al. [6]) did not examine the effect of meeting the intermediate compared to poor CVH, which is important as intermediate CVH is much more achievable in the general population than ideal CVH. Additionally, these two studies comparing ideal versus poor CVH were concerning with respect to their inconsistent and highly variable CVH group categorization as reported in "Table 1" in both papers [5,6]. Their ideal CVH group was classified as either 4–7, 5–7, or 6–7 CVH metrics; or 10–14 to 12–14 score points. Likewise, their poor CVH group was classified as either 0, 0–1, or 0–2 metrics; or 0–1, 0–2, to 0–4 score points. This variability led authors to compare dissimilar and incomparable categories of CVH. Similarly, in the paper by Aneni et al. [8], the authors compared various levels of CVH with a reference group that was un-uniform and ranged from 0, to 0–1, to 0–2 CVH metrics. This significant heterogeneity engenders substantial concerns about the validity and comparability of study results. Conversely, in our analysis, we strictly categorized data into three CVH metric groups, and if sufficient data were unavailable in the published manuscripts and supplements, we requested additional information from the study authors (from three such papers, we received additional information from only one study [21], excluding the other two studies [22,23]).

The results of our analysis confirm that achieving a higher number of ideal CVH metrics is associated with a lower risk for CVD and CVM. Our findings align with those of previous studies despite their aforementioned methodological limitations [5–8]. This was derived by comparing the 3 CVH metrics groups, having relative risk reduction with a higher number of achieved CVH metrics. In addition, Aneni et al. [8] reported an inverse linear relationship between CVH metrics and mortality, with an estimated 19% reduction in CVM for each achieved CVH metric. It was also reported in the literature that a longer duration of favorable CVH was associated with decreased cardiovascular-related morbidity and mortality [4].

The low prevalence of ideal CVH is a cause for concern. Amongst our analyzed cohort, only 12.3% qualified as ideal CVH, 39.4% fell into intermediate CVH, and 48.3% were classified as poor CVH. Similar patterns were reported in the published literature of individual studies where ideal CVH was found to be the least common (prevalence of 0.5% to 3.3% reported in the general population [44] but approaching 15% in some subgroups and specific populations [45,46]). Data from NHANES 2011–2016 reported a predominance of poor CVH in the general US population (around 59%), while merely 7.3% of adults had ideal CVH [47]. In another study, about 62% of US adults achieved 3 or fewer CVH metrics [48]. Given that even a single risk factor is associated with an increased lifetime risk of CVD, the present distribution of CVH is troubling [4,49].

Ideal CVH is difficult both to achieve and maintain. As such, it may be more realistic to improve CVH by achieving metrics that can move the population from the poor to the intermediate category. The previous systematic reviews and meta-analyses compared ideal with poor CVH. Our study, however, assessed the comparative benefits of achieving intermediate over poor CVH, which we believe to be a more attainable goal. We went one step further by assessing the risk reduction of achieving the ideal CVH in comparison to intermediate CVH, and the implications resulting from that additional improvement. The only other study that studied intermediate CVH was Ramírez-Vélez et al. [7]; however, they did not analyze ideal versus intermediate CVH, nor did they assess the effect of various CVH levels on CVM. For the composite CVD, CHD, MI, and stroke, our study reported similar results as Ramírez-Vélez et al. [7], despite our analysis of 8 additional studies (our analysis comprised a total of 22 studies; 15 after excluding studies reporting CVM, while Ramírez-Vélez et al. had 12 studies; 7 after excluding studies reporting heart failure and venous thromboembolism, which they analyzed). In both our study and that of Ramírez-Vélez et al. [7], there was a significantly lower risk when higher levels of CVH were compared to lower CVH. When comparing ideal to poor CVH, our results demonstrated that there was a lower risk of developing composite CVD, CHD, MI, and stroke of 76%, 78%, 82%, and 62%, respectively. Similarly, Ramírez-Vélez et al. [7] reported a lower risk for developing composite CVD, CHD, MI, and stroke of 77%, 79%, 76%, and 67%, respectively. When comparing intermediate to poor CVH, our results demonstrated that there was a lower risk of developing composite CVD, CHD, MI, and stroke of 39%, 49%, 37%, and 30%, respectively. Likewise, Ramírez-Vélez et al. [7] reported a lower risk for developing composite CVD, CHD, MI, and stroke of 55%, 44%, 46%, and 42% respectively. These results demonstrate that while ideal CVH confers the greatest risk reduction for CVD and stroke, achieving the more attainable goal of intermediate CVH (defined as 3–4 metrics or a score of 5–9) still offers substantial protective benefit. Due to the prevalence of poor CVH amongst the general population, Ramírez-Vélez et al. [7] point out that a realistic short-term goal should be the promotion of meeting 3 to 4 CVH metrics in order to achieve a positive outcome. The findings from our study fully support this conclusion and recommendation.

Although the beneficial effects of ideal CVH have been supported by increasing scientific evidence, the precise relationship is still not well measured. Furthermore, strong evidence of individual CVH metrics in relation to CVD, stroke, and mortality is lacking. Preliminary data on socioeconomic, gender, and racial inequalities report the unsatisfactory prevalence of ideal CVH metrics, with significant room for improvement [44]. There are many identified social determinants of health that influence an individual's psychological health and well-being, which in turn may positively or negatively affect CVH through the continuous interplay of mind-heart-body connections [45]. While a healthier lifestyle from a young age is a successful strategy for higher CVH later in life, the ability to choose and practice healthier lifestyles across the lifespan is strongly influenced by psychosocial health factors [45,50–55]. Despite CVD and CVM being improved in the US over the past decade, concerning disparities persist regarding risk factors, health behaviors, and CVM based on ethnicity, race, geography, and income [3]. Similar disparities are present globally, further efforts set by AHA ("2030 Impact Goals") and WHO are intended to improve health equity and address a broader range of factors that contribute to CVH [3].

6. Strengths and Limitations of the Study

The principal strengths of our study are its large study cohort ($n = 3,240,660$), that it has studied various CVD outcomes (including CVM) across all CVH metrics groups, and its comparison of each CVH metric group to the others. Our data interpretation, however, has several limitations that must be considered. In some cases, there was significant heterogeneity between analyzed studies, which was addressed by using the RE model. Measurements of physical activity and diet are not standardized amongst other CVH metrics, and there may have been different interpretations of ideal physical activity levels and diet. We acknowledge there is an overlap of articles published from the same studies and examined patient cohorts, however, a "leave-one-out" analysis showed no significant difference when any one study is excluded from statistical analysis. Not all eligible studies were included due to a lack of data for at least one CVH metrics group and the unavailability of authors to provide the requested information [22,23].

7. Conclusions

The results of our study clearly demonstrate that higher adherence to ideal CVH standards yields a significantly lower risk of CVD and CVM. While achieving ideal CVH metrics is associated with the lowest risk, it is imperative to recognize that achieving intermediate CVH metrics will also offer a strong protective effect. Given that the majority of the population has poor CVH, there exists tremendous potential to improve outcomes worldwide. We advocate for sending a strong public health message that even modest improvements in CVH are associated with substantial cardiovascular morbidity and mortality benefits. To that end, we should collectively promote healthier lifestyles and behaviors.

Supplementary Materials: The following supporting information can be downloaded at: https://www.mdpi.com/article/10.3390/jcm12134417/s1. Supplement Table S1. Definition of the cardiovascular health metrics and scores according to the American Heart Association. Supplement Figures S1–S3. Funnel plot publication bias for different categories of cardiovascular health and composite cardiovascular disease risk. Supplement Figures S4–S6. Funnel plot publication bias for different categories of cardiovascular health and coronary heart disease risk. Supplement Figures S7–S9. Funnel plot publication bias for different categories of cardiovascular health and myocardial infarction risk. Supplement Figures S10–S12. Funnel plot publication bias for different categories of cardiovascular health and stroke risk. Supplement Figures S13–S15. Funnel plot publication bias for different categories of cardiovascular health and cardiovascular mortality.

Author Contributions: Conceptualization, M.R. and J.J.; methodology, M.R. and J.J.; software, S.M.-R.; validation, J.J.; formal analysis, S.M.-R.; data curation, M.R., J.J. and I.D.; writing—original draft preparation, M.R. and J.J.; writing—review and editing, M.R., J.J., S.M.-R., I.D., R.D.H. and C.W.N.; supervision, J.J. All authors have read and agreed to the published version of the manuscript.

Funding: This research was supported by the Mayo Clinic Health System in Eau Claire, WI, and the Ministry of Education and Science of the Republic of Serbia (grant no. 200110).

Institutional Review Board Statement: Not applicable.

Informed Consent Statement: Not applicable.

Data Availability Statement: Not applicable.

Conflicts of Interest: The authors declare no conflict of interest.

References

1. Piepoli, M.F.; Hoes, A.W.; Agewall, S.; Albus, C.; Brotons, C.; Catapano, A.L.; Cooney, M.T.; Corrà, U.; Cosyns, B.; Deaton, C.; et al. 2016 European Guidelines on cardiovascular disease prevention in clinical practice: The Sixth Joint Task Force of the European Society of Cardiology and Other Societies on Cardiovascular Disease Prevention in Clinical Practice (constituted by representatives of 10 societies and by invited experts)Developed with the special contribution of the European Association for Cardiovascular Prevention & Rehabilitation (EACPR). *Eur. Heart J.* **2016**, *37*, 2315–2381. [PubMed]
2. Lloyd-Jones, D.M.; Hong, Y.; Labarthe, D.; Mozaffarian, D.; Appel, L.J.; Van Horn, L.; Greenlund, K.; Daniels, S.; Nichol, G.; Tomaselli, G.F.; et al. Defining and setting national goals for cardiovascular health promotion and disease reduction: The American Heart Association's strategic Impact Goal through 2020 and beyond. *Circulation* **2010**, *121*, 586–613. [CrossRef] [PubMed]
3. Angell, S.Y.; McConnell, M.V.; Anderson, C.A.M.; Bibbins-Domingo, K.; Boyle, D.S.; Capewell, S.; Ezzati, M.; de Ferranti, S.; Gaskin, D.J.; Goetzel, R.Z.; et al. The American Heart Association 2030 Impact Goal: A Presidential Advisory from the American Heart Association. *Circulation* **2020**, *141*, e120–e138. [CrossRef] [PubMed]
4. Michos, E.D.; Khan, S.S. Further understanding of ideal cardiovascular health score metrics and cardiovascular disease. *Expert Rev. Cardiovasc. Ther.* **2021**, *19*, 607–617. [CrossRef]
5. Guo, L.; Zhang, S. Association between ideal cardiovascular health metrics and risk of cardiovascular events or mortality: A meta-analysis of prospective studies. *Clin. Cardiol.* **2017**, *40*, 1339–1346. [CrossRef]
6. Fang, N.; Jiang, M.; Fan, Y. Ideal cardiovascular health metrics and risk of cardiovascular disease or mortality: A meta-analysis. *Int. J. Cardiol.* **2016**, *214*, 279–283. [CrossRef]
7. Ramírez-Vélez, R.; Saavedra, J.M.; Lobelo, F.; Celis-Morales, C.A.; Pozo-Cruz, B.D.; García-Hermoso, A. Ideal Cardiovascular Health and Incident Cardiovascular Disease Among Adults: A Systematic Review and Meta-analysis. *Mayo Clin. Proc.* **2018**, *93*, 1589–1599. [CrossRef]
8. Aneni, E.C.; Crippa, A.; Osondu, C.U.; Valero-Elizondo, J.; Younus, A.; Nasir, K.; Veledar, E. Estimates of Mortality Benefit from Ideal Cardiovascular Health Metrics: A Dose Response Meta-Analysis. *J. Am. Heart Assoc.* **2017**, *6*, e006904. [CrossRef]
9. Veledar, E.; Crippa, A.; Osondu, C.U.; Younus, A.; Nasir, K. Letter to Editor: "Ideal cardiovascular health metrics and risk of cardiovascular disease or mortality: A meta-analysis". *Int. J. Cardiol.* **2016**, *222*, 737. [CrossRef]
10. Stang, A. Critical evaluation of the Newcastle-Ottawa scale for the assessment of the quality of nonrandomized studies in meta-analyses. *Eur. J. Epidemiol.* **2010**, *25*, 603–605. [CrossRef]

11. Cook, D.A.; Reed, D.A. Appraising the quality of medical education research methods: The Medical Education Research Study Quality Instrument and the Newcastle-Ottawa Scale-Education. *Acad. Med.* **2015**, *90*, 1067–1076. [CrossRef] [PubMed]
12. Viechtbauer, W. Bias and Efficiency of Meta-Analytic Variance Estimators in the Random-Effects Model. *J. Educ. Behav. Stat.* **2005**, *30*, 261–293. [CrossRef]
13. Cochran, W.G. The combination of estimates from different experiments. *Biometrics* **1954**, *10*, 101. [CrossRef]
14. Higgins, J.P.; Thompson, S.G. Quantifying heterogeneity in a meta-analysis. *Stat. Med.* **2002**, *21*, 1539–1558. [CrossRef]
15. Viechtbauer, W.; Cheung, M.W. Outlier and influence diagnostics for meta-analysis. *Res. Synth. Methods* **2010**, *1*, 112–125. [CrossRef] [PubMed]
16. Begg, C.B.; Mazumdar, M. Operating characteristics of a rank correlation test for publication bias. *Biometrics* **1994**, *50*, 1088–1101. [CrossRef]
17. Sterne, J.A.C.; Egger, M. Regression Methods to Detect Publication and Other Bias in Meta-Analysis. In *Publication Bias in Meta-Analysis*; John Wiley & Sons, Inc.: New York, NY, USA, 2005; pp. 99–110.
18. Team, R.C. R: A Language and Environment for Statistical Computing. R Foundation for Statistical Computing. 2020. Available online: https://www.R-project.org/ (accessed on 9 June 2023).
19. Viechtbauer, W. Conducting Meta-Analyses in R with the metafor Package. *J. Stat. Softw.* **2010**, *36*, 1–48. [CrossRef]
20. Miao, C.; Bao, M.; Xing, A.; Chen, S.; Wu, Y.; Cai, J.; Chen, Y.; Yang, X. Cardiovascular Health Score and the Risk of Cardiovascular Diseases. *PLoS ONE* **2015**, *10*, e0131537. [CrossRef]
21. Díez-Espino, J.; Buil-Cosiales, P.; Babio, N.; Toledo, E.; Corella, D.; Ros, E.; Fitó, M.; Gómez-Gracia, E.; Estruch, R.; Fiol, M.; et al. Impact of Life's Simple 7 on the incidence of major cardiovascular events in high-risk Spanish adults in the PREDIMED study cohort. *Rev. Esp. Cardiol. Engl. Ed.* **2020**, *73*, 205–211. [CrossRef]
22. Dong, Y.; Hao, G.; Wang, Z.; Wang, X.; Chen, Z.; Zhang, L. Ideal Cardiovascular Health Status and Risk of Cardiovascular Disease or All-Cause Mortality in Chinese Middle-Aged Population. *Angiology* **2019**, *70*, 523–529. [CrossRef]
23. Zhou, L.; Zhao, L.; Wu, Y.; Wu, Y.; Gao, X.; Li, Y.; Mai, J.; Nie, Z.; Ou, Y.; Guo, M.; et al. Ideal cardiovascular health metrics and its association with 20-year cardiovascular morbidity and mortality in a Chinese population. *J. Epidemiol. Community Health* **2018**, *72*, 752–758. [CrossRef] [PubMed]
24. Folsom, A.R.; Yatsuya, H.; Nettleton, J.A.; Lutsey, P.L.; Cushman, M.; Rosamond, W.D.; ARIC Study Investigators. Community prevalence of ideal cardiovascular health, by the American Heart Association definition, and relationship with cardiovascular disease incidence. *J. Am. Coll. Cardiol.* **2011**, *57*, 1690–1696. [CrossRef] [PubMed]
25. Fernandez-Lazaro, C.I.; Sayon-Orea, C.; Toledo, E.; Moreno-Iribas, C.; Guembe, M.J.; RIVANA Study Investigators. Association of ideal cardiovascular health with cardiovascular events and risk advancement periods in a Mediterranean population-based cohort. *BMC Med.* **2022**, *20*, 232. [CrossRef]
26. Isiozor, N.M.; Kunutsor, S.K.; Voutilainen, A.; Kauhanen, J.; Laukkanen, J.A. Life's Simple 7 and the risk of stroke in Finnish men: A prospective cohort study. *Prev. Med.* **2021**, *153*, 106858. [CrossRef] [PubMed]
27. Isiozor, N.M.; Kunutsor, S.K.; Voutilainen, A.; Kurl, S.; Kauhanen, J.; Laukkanen, J.A. Ideal cardiovascular health and risk of acute myocardial infarction among Finnish men. *Atherosclerosis* **2019**, *289*, 126–131. [CrossRef] [PubMed]
28. Isiozor, N.M.; Kunutsor, S.K.; Voutilainen, A.; Kurl, S.; Kauhanen, J.; Laukkanen, J.A. American heart association's cardiovascular health metrics and risk of cardiovascular disease mortality among a middle-aged male Scandinavian population. *Ann. Med.* **2019**, *51*, 306–313. [CrossRef]
29. Ahmad, M.I.; Chevli, P.A.; Barot, H.; Soliman, E.Z. Interrelationships Between American Heart Association's Life's Simple 7, ECG Silent Myocardial Infarction, and Cardiovascular Mortality. *J. Am. Heart Assoc.* **2019**, *8*, e011648. [CrossRef]
30. Yang, Q.; Cogswell, M.E.; Flanders, W.D.; Hong, Y.; Zhang, Z.; Loustalot, F.; Gillespie, C.; Merritt, R.; Hu, F.B. Trends in cardiovascular health metrics and associations with all-cause and CVD mortality among US adults. *JAMA* **2012**, *307*, 1273–1283. [CrossRef]
31. Ford, E.S.; Greenlund, K.J.; Hong, Y. Ideal cardiovascular health and mortality from all causes and diseases of the circulatory system among adults in the United States. *Circulation* **2012**, *125*, 987–995. [CrossRef]
32. Liu, Y.; Chi, H.J.; Cui, L.F.; Yang, X.C.; Wu, Y.T.; Huang, Z.; Zhao, H.Y.; Gao, J.S.; Wu, S.L.; Cai, J. The ideal cardiovascular health metrics associated inversely with mortality from all causes and from cardiovascular diseases among adults in a Northern Chinese industrial city. *PLoS ONE* **2014**, *9*, e89161. [CrossRef]
33. Zhang, Q.; Zhou, Y.; Gao, X.; Wang, C.; Zhang, S.; Wang, A.; Li, N.; Bian, L.; Wu, J.; Jia, Q.; et al. Ideal cardiovascular health metrics and the risks of ischemic and intracerebral hemorrhagic stroke. *Stroke* **2013**, *44*, 2451–2456. [CrossRef] [PubMed]
34. Itoh, H.; Kaneko, H.; Okada, A.; Suzuki, Y.; Fujiu, K.; Matsuoka, S.; Michihata, N.; Jo, T.; Nakanishi, K.; Takeda, N.; et al. Age-Specific Relation of Cardiovascular Health Metrics with Incident Cardiovascular Disease. *Am. J. Cardiol.* **2022**, *177*, 34–39. [CrossRef] [PubMed]
35. Han, C.; Liu, F.; Yang, X.; Chen, J.; Li, J.; Cao, J.; Li, Y.; Shen, C.; Yu, L.; Liu, Z.; et al. Ideal cardiovascular health and incidence of atherosclerotic cardiovascular disease among Chinese adults: The China-PAR project. *Sci. China Life Sci.* **2018**, *61*, 504–514. [CrossRef] [PubMed]
36. Gaye, B.; Tafflet, M.; Arveiler, D.; Montaye, M.; Wagner, A.; Ruidavets, J.B.; Kee, F.; Evans, A.; Amouyel, P.; Ferrieres, J.; et al. Ideal Cardiovascular Health and Incident Cardiovascular Disease: Heterogeneity Across Event Subtypes and Mediating Effect of Blood Biomarkers: The PRIME Study. *J. Am. Heart Assoc.* **2017**, *6*, e006389. [CrossRef]

37. Gaye, B.; Canonico, M.; Perier, M.C.; Samieri, C.; Berr, C.; Dartigues, J.F.; Tzourio, C.; Elbaz, A.; Empana, J.P. Ideal Cardiovascular Health, Mortality, and Vascular Events in Elderly Subjects: The Three-City Study. *J. Am. Coll. Cardiol.* **2017**, *69*, 3015–3026. [CrossRef]
38. Ommerborn, M.J.; Blackshear, C.T.; Hickson, D.A.; Griswold, M.E.; Kwatra, J.; Djoussé, L.; Clark, C.R. Ideal Cardiovascular Health and Incident Cardiovascular Events: The Jackson Heart Study. *Am. J. Prev. Med.* **2016**, *51*, 502–506. [CrossRef]
39. Lachman, S.; Peters, R.J.; Lentjes, M.A.; Mulligan, A.A.; Luben, R.N.; Wareham, N.J.; Khaw, K.T.; Boekholdt, S.M. Ideal cardiovascular health and risk of cardiovascular events in the EPIC-Norfolk prospective population study. *Eur. J. Prev. Cardiol.* **2016**, *23*, 986–994. [CrossRef]
40. Kulshreshtha, A.; Vaccarino, V.; Judd, S.E.; Howard, V.J.; McClellan, W.M.; Muntner, P.; Hong, Y.; Safford, M.M.; Goyal, A.; Cushman, M. Life's Simple 7 and risk of incident stroke: The reasons for geographic and racial differences in stroke study. *Stroke* **2013**, *44*, 1909–1914. [CrossRef]
41. Kim, J.Y.; Ko, Y.J.; Rhee, C.W.; Park, B.J.; Kim, D.H.; Bae, J.M.; Shin, M.H.; Lee, M.S.; Li, Z.M.; Ahn, Y.O. Cardiovascular health metrics and all-cause and cardiovascular disease mortality among middle-aged men in Korea: The Seoul male cohort study. *J. Prev. Med. Public Health* **2013**, *46*, 319–328. [CrossRef]
42. Dong, C.; Rundek, T.; Wright, C.B.; Anwar, Z.; Elkind, M.S.; Sacco, R.L. Ideal cardiovascular health predicts lower risks of myocardial infarction, stroke, and vascular death across whites, blacks, and hispanics: The northern Manhattan study. *Circulation* **2012**, *125*, 2975–2984. [CrossRef]
43. Artero, E.G.; España-Romero, V.; Lee, D.C.; Sui, X.; Church, T.S.; Lavie, C.J.; Blair, S.N. Ideal cardiovascular health and mortality: Aerobics Center Longitudinal Study. *Mayo Clin. Proc.* **2012**, *87*, 944–952. [CrossRef]
44. Janković, J.; Mandić-Rajčević, S.; Davidović, M.; Janković, S. Demographic and socioeconomic inequalities in ideal cardiovascular health: A systematic review and meta-analysis. *PLoS ONE* **2021**, *16*, e0255959. [CrossRef] [PubMed]
45. Lloyd-Jones, D.M.; Allen, N.B.; Anderson, C.A.M.; Black, T.; Brewer, L.C.; Foraker, R.E.; Grandner, M.A.; Lavretsky, H.; Perak, A.M.; Sharma, G.; et al. Life's Essential 8: Updating and Enhancing the American Heart Association's Construct of Cardiovascular Health: A Presidential Advisory From the American Heart Association. *Circulation* **2022**, *146*, e18–e43. [CrossRef]
46. Younus, A.; Aneni, E.C.; Spatz, E.S.; Osondu, C.U.; Roberson, L.; Ogunmoroti, O.; Malik, R.; Ali, S.S.; Aziz, M.; Feldman, T.; et al. A Systematic Review of the Prevalence and Outcomes of Ideal Cardiovascular Health in US and Non-US Populations. *Mayo Clin. Proc.* **2016**, *91*, 649–670. [CrossRef]
47. Bundy, J.D.; Zhu, Z.; Ning, H.; Zhong, V.W.; Paluch, A.E.; Wilkins, J.T.; Lloyd-Jones, D.M.; Whelton, P.K.; He, J.; Allen, N.B. Estimated Impact of Achieving Optimal Cardiovascular Health Among US Adults on Cardiovascular Disease Events. *J. Am. Heart Assoc.* **2021**, *10*, e019681. [CrossRef] [PubMed]
48. Benjamin, E.J.; Muntner, P.; Alonso, A.; Bittencourt, M.S.; Callaway, C.W.; Carson, A.P.; Chamberlain, A.M.; Chang, A.R.; Cheng, S.; Das, S.R.; et al. Heart Disease and Stroke Statistics-2019 Update: A Report from the American Heart Association. *Circulation* **2019**, *139*, e56–e528. [PubMed]
49. Berry, J.D.; Dyer, A.; Cai, X.; Garside, D.B.; Ning, H.; Thomas, A.; Greenland, P.; Van Horn, L.; Tracy, R.P.; Lloyd-Jones, D.M. Lifetime risks of cardiovascular disease. *N. Engl. J. Med.* **2012**, *366*, 321–329. [CrossRef] [PubMed]
50. Pahkala, K.; Laitinen, T.T.; Niinikoski, H.; Kartiosuo, N.; Rovio, S.P.; Lagström, H.; Loo, B.M.; Salo, P.; Jokinen, E.; Magnussen, C.G.; et al. Effects of 20-year infancy-onset dietary counselling on cardiometabolic risk factors in the Special Turku Coronary Risk Factor Intervention Project (STRIP): 6-year post-intervention follow-up. *Lancet Child. Adolesc. Health* **2020**, *4*, 359–369. [CrossRef]
51. Matthews, L.A.; Matthews, L.A.; Rovio, S.P.; Jaakkola, J.M.; Niinikoski, H.; Lagström, H.; Jula, A.; Viikari, J.S.A.; Rönnemaa, T.; Simell, O.; et al. Longitudinal effect of 20-year infancy-onset dietary intervention on food consumption and nutrient intake: The randomized controlled STRIP study. *Eur. J. Clin. Nutr.* **2019**, *73*, 937–949. [CrossRef]
52. Allen, N.B.; Lloyd-Jones, D.; Hwang, S.J.; Rasmussen-Torvik, L.; Fornage, M.; Morrison, A.C.; Baldridge, A.S.; Boerwinkle, E.; Levy, D.; Cupples, L.A.; et al. Genetic loci associated with ideal cardiovascular health: A meta-analysis of genome-wide association studies. *Am. Heart J.* **2016**, *175*, 112–120. [CrossRef]
53. Liu, K.; Daviglus, M.L.; Loria, C.M.; Colangelo, L.A.; Spring, B.; Moller, A.C.; Lloyd-Jones, D.M. Healthy lifestyle through young adulthood and the presence of low cardiovascular disease risk profile in middle age: The Coronary Artery Risk Development in (Young) Adults (CARDIA) study. *Circulation* **2012**, *125*, 996–1004. [CrossRef] [PubMed]
54. Spring, B.; Moller, A.C.; Colangelo, L.A.; Siddique, J.; Roehrig, M.; Daviglus, M.L.; Polak, J.F.; Reis, J.P.; Sidney, S.; Liu, K. Healthy lifestyle change and subclinical atherosclerosis in young adults: Coronary Artery Risk Development in Young Adults (CARDIA) study. *Circulation* **2014**, *130*, 10–17. [CrossRef] [PubMed]
55. Gooding, H.C.; Shay, C.M.; Ning, H.; Gillman, M.W.; Chiuve, S.E.; Reis, J.P.; Allen, N.B.; Lloyd-Jones, D.M. Optimal Lifestyle Components in Young Adulthood Are Associated with Maintaining the Ideal Cardiovascular Health Profile into Middle Age. *J. Am. Heart Assoc.* **2015**, *4*, e002048. [CrossRef] [PubMed]

Disclaimer/Publisher's Note: The statements, opinions and data contained in all publications are solely those of the individual author(s) and contributor(s) and not of MDPI and/or the editor(s). MDPI and/or the editor(s) disclaim responsibility for any injury to people or property resulting from any ideas, methods, instructions or products referred to in the content.

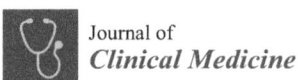

Article

Chromosome Y Haplogroup R Was Associated with the Risk of Premature Myocardial Infarction with ST-Elevation: Data from the CholeSTEMI Registry

Rebeca Lorca [1,2,3,4,5,*], Andrea Aparicio [1], María Salgado [1], Rut Álvarez-Velasco [1], Isaac Pascual [1,6], Juan Gomez [2,4,7,8], Daniel Vazquez-Coto [8], Claudia Garcia-Lago [8], Lucinda Velázquez-Cuervo [8], Elías Cuesta-Llavona [8], Pablo Avanzas [1,4,6,9,*] and Eliecer Coto [2,4,5,6,7,8]

1. Área del Corazón, Hospital Universitario Central Asturias (HUCA), 33011 Oviedo, Spain
2. Unidad de Cardiopatías Familiares, Área del Corazón y Departamento de Genética Molecular, Hospital Universitario Central Asturias, 33011 Oviedo, Spain; eliecer.coto@sespa.es (E.C.)
3. Área de Fisiología, Departamento de Biología Funcional, Universidad de Oviedo, 33003 Oviedo, Spain
4. Instituto de Investigación Sanitaria del Principado de Asturias (ISPA), 33011 Oviedo, Spain
5. Redes de Investigación Cooperativa Orientadas a Resultados en Salud (RICORs), 28029 Madrid, Spain
6. Departamento de Medicina, Universidad de Oviedo, 33003 Oviedo, Spain
7. CIBER-Enfermedades Respiratorias, 28029 Madrid, Spain
8. Genética Molecular, Hospital Universitario Central Asturias (HUCA), 33011 Oviedo, Spain
9. Centro de Investigación Biomédica en Red de Enfermedades Cardiovasculares (CIBERCV), 28029 Madrid, Spain
* Correspondence: lorcarebeca@gmail.com (R.L.); avanzas@secardiologia.es (P.A.)

Abstract: Cardiovascular disease (CVD) is the leading cause of death worldwide, with coronary artery disease (CAD) being one of its main manifestations. Both environmental and genetic factors are widely known to be related to CAD, such as smoking, diabetes mellitus, dyslipidemia, and a family history of CAD. However, there is still a lack of information about other risk factors, especially those related to genetic mutations. Sex represents a classic CAD risk factor, as men are more likely to suffer CAD, but there is lack of evidence with regard to sex-specific genetic factors. We evaluated the Y chromosome haplogroups in a cohort of young Spanish male patients who suffered from STEMI. In this cohort, haplogroup R was significantly more frequent in STEMI patients.

Keywords: coronary artery disease; genetics; cardiovascular risk factors; premature cardiovascular disease; myocardial infarction

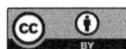

1. Introduction

Cardiovascular disease (CVD) remains the leading cause of morbidity and mortality worldwide [1,2], coronary artery disease (CAD) being a major concern. CAD is a complex disease with multiple risk factors, including genetics, lifestyle, and environmental factors [1,2]. Classic cardiovascular risk factors known to contribute to the development of CAD include smoking, high blood pressure, diabetes mellitus, high cholesterol levels or dyslipidemia (DL), a family history of CAD, obesity, a lack of physical activity, and stress [3]. Moreover, CAD has important genetic underpinnings that can be considered equivalent to environmental factors [4]. However, the role of genetic factors in CAD susceptibility, beyond familial hypercholesterolemia [5], is not yet well understood. In this regard, studying genetic susceptibility for premature CAD is of utmost importance.

Because CAD is more common among men, sex-specific factors might contribute to the risk of developing this disease. Although several loci have been identified to be associated with the genetic risk for CAD, the contribution of Y chromosome variants to CAD risk remains unclear. As a result, there has been increasing interest in the potential association between Y chromosome polymorphisms and CAD risk. Chromosome Y is male-specific and plays a determinant role in defining the biological characteristics of male sex. Chromosome Y is unique in that it is paternally inherited and passed down from father to son. Therefore, Y variants have been used to determine the patrilineal history and migration patterns of human populations [6,7]. In this regard, Y chromosome haplogroups are defined by specific sets of single-nucleotide polymorphisms (SNPs) that are passed down through the male lineage. The distribution of Y chromosome haplogroups varies significantly between populations due to differences in migration patterns, genetic drift, and natural selection, and reflects the timeline distance between human populations [6,8]. In this regard, haplogroup R (defined by SNP rs2032636, also known as M207) would have originated about 30,000 years ago in South-Asia and is present in more than half of Europeans. A subclade of R designated as R1b (SNP rs9786153 or M269) would have surged during the Upper Paleolithic (approx. 28,000 years ago) in the Caucasus region and is present in more than half of Spanish men, with higher frequencies in the Cantabrian cornice.

Some studies have suggested that Y chromosome haplogroups may also be associated with various health outcomes, including cancer or cardiovascular disease [9]. Some studies have reported an association between specific haplogroups and CAD risk [10,11]. However, other studies have failed to find such an association. In summary, the evidence linking specific haplogroups with CAD risk is still limited and controversial.

Many studies are limited by their sample sizes, differences in the definitions of CAD, presentation ages, ethnicities of the populations studied, and other potential confounding factors. Therefore, further studies are needed to elucidate the potential role of Y chromosome haplogroups in the development of CAD. Identifying genetic markers associated with CAD risk may help to develop more effective prevention and treatment strategies for this common and debilitating disease.

In this scenario, aiming to provide some insights into the genetic determinants of premature CAD in men, we aimed to evaluate the different Y chromosome haplogroups in a cohort of male patients presenting with premature myocardial infarction with ST-elevation (STEMI).

2. Materials and Methods

2.1. Study Population

Patients were recruited from the CholeSTEMI registry [5,12]. This study was approved by the local Ethical Committee (CEIMPA; registry number 2020/003) [5,12]. All participants who wished to participate in the actual investigational project had signed written consent to grant access to their genetic data for additional investigational purposes.

In this study, we review all consecutive patients referred to our center for emergency cardiac catheterization due to STEMI as reported elsewhere [5,12]. From the initial cohort of 157 male patients with premature STEMI, 35 were not studied due to lack of DNA. The main characteristics of the remaining 122 male patients with premature STEMI are shown in Table 1. All patients from this cohort were of European ancestry and from the region of Asturias (Northern Spain, total population of about 1 million). Only patients with type 1 myocardial infarction and confirmed atherothrombotic CAD by coronary angiogram, who agreed to participate in the CholeSTEMI registry, were included in this study. Patients with other kinds of myocardial infarction different to type 1 myocardial infarction (such as vasospasm, demand/supply mismatch due to hypoxemia, anemia or arryhtmia, etc.), according to ESC guidelines [13,14], were excluded from analysis.

Premature CAD for men was considered if presented before the age of 55 [15,16]. Patients without sufficient stored DNA to perform the additional Y chromosome haplogroup study were excluded from this study.

Clinical data from this cohort was already reviewed: birth date, gender, age at STEMI, and classical cardiovascular risk factors: high blood pressure, tobacco consumption, diabetes mellitus, dyslipidemia, and premature CAD.

Table 1. The 8 single nucleotide polymorphisms determined to define the Y haplogroups, genotyped with Taqman assays (Fisher scientific, Hampton, NH, USA).

NUCLEOTIDE Y Position	SNP	HAPLOGROUP	ASSAY	EUR	FREQUENCY
13407103	rs2032658 G/A	R	C___2307221_1Y	G (0.58)	0.0016
12914512	rs2032624 C/A	R1	C___2292796_20	C (0.58)	0.0016
20577481	rs9786153 T/C	R1B	C__29812961_10	C (0.53)	<0.0001
2789135	rs2534636 C/T	R1A	C__26236081_10	T (0.05)	0.0113
14436668	rs113623003 G/A	I	C_153784812_10	A (0.14)	0.0085
20587967	rs13447352 A/C	J	C__33589462_10	C (0.11)	0.1168
19617112	rs9306841 C/G	E	C__29796914_10	G (0.03)	0.0008
12915617	rs2032636 G/T	G	C___2292797_20	T (0.06)	0.0996

2.2. Control Cohort

We compare the Y chromosome haplogroup prevalence to that found in a representative control cohort of 200 individuals from the same region of the cohort of premature CAD presenting with STEMI. These male controls were aged <55 years and recruited as part of the RENASTUR project to determine the prevalence of cardiovascular risk factors in the region of Asturias [17]. For the objectives of our study, these controls were genotyped with the only purpose of determining the frequency of the main Y haplogroups in our population.

2.3. Genetic Testing

All the male patients (N = 122) and controls (N = 200) were genotyped for 8 single nucleotide polymorphisms in chromosome Y that defined the common European Y haplogroups (Table 1). The corresponding nucleotides were determined by real-time PCR with Taqman assays in an ABI7500 equipment and following the manufacturer instructions (Fisher Scientific). The allele frequencies among Europeans were obtained from the Ensembl database (www.ensembl.org).

2.4. Statistical Analysis

Statistical analysis was performed with STATA. Descriptive data for continuous variables are presented as mean ± SD and as frequencies or percentages for categorical variables. The Chi-square test was used to compare frequencies, whereas differences in continuous variables were evaluated with either Student's *t*-test or Mann–Whitney U test. A *p* value below 0.05 was considered to be significant.

3. Results

The eight single nucleotide polymorphisms determined to define the Y haplogroups are summarized in Table 1. The frequency of the allele that defined the haplogroup among Europeans is indicated in Table 1. The haplogroup labelled as "other" corresponded to the remaining haplogroups that could not be assigned based on the allele combinations at the 8 SNPs.

Prevalence of the different Y chromosome haplogroups in both control and patient's cohorts are shown in Figure 1. As expected, due to its geographical location in the Cantabrian cornice of Spain, haplogroup R was the most frequent in our population, followed by haplogroups E, H and G (Table 2). Due to it high frequency, we also evaluated R subhaplogroups, being most for them were R1 (SNP rs2032624 = M173) and R1B (Table 2).

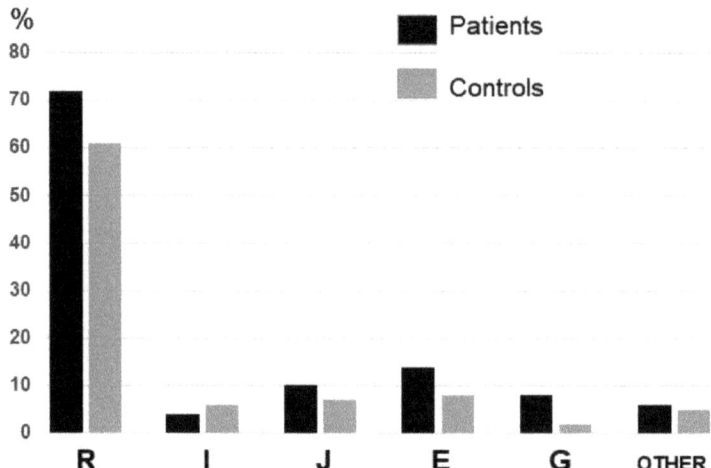

Figure 1. Prevalence of the different Y chromosome haplogroups in both control and patient's cohorts.

Table 2. Y chromosome haplogroups differences between the male control cohort and male patients with premature coronary artery disease.

Haplogroup	Control Cohort N = 200	Patients Cohort N = 122	p
R	122 (0.61)	88 (0.72)	0.04 *
R1	118 (0.59)	88 (0.72)	0.02 *
R1B	118 (0.59)	88 (0.72)	0.02 *
R1A	4 (0.02)	0	0.12
I	8 (0.04)	7 (0.06)	0.47
J	20 (0.10)	8 (0.07)	0.28
E	28 (0.14)	10 (0.08)	0.12
G	16 (0.08)	3 (0.02)	0.04 *
Other	6 (0.03)	6 (0.05)	0.38

* $p < 0.05$.

However, only 2% of the controls and none of the STEMI patients were R1A. Moreover, when we compared the frequencies of R haplogroup between patients and controls, we found that cases had a significantly increased frequency ($p = 0.04$), with an OR = 1.65 (95% CI = 1.02–2.69). In particular, we found the frequency of Y chromosome haplogroup R1B in STEMI patients to be significantly higher than in the control cohort. Thus, in our population the common Y haplogroup R seems to be a risk factor for premature STEMI in men.

In contrast, in our region, the haplogroup I was rare, representing only 4% and 6% of the control and patient cohort, respectively ($p = 0.47$). Given its low frequency, subgroups of this haplogroup were not evaluated.

Haplogroups J, E and "other" showed a frequency that was non-significantly lower in the patients than in the controls, whereas haplogroup G was significantly less frequent (Table 2). For these rare haplogroups, we believe that evaluating the effect on STEMI risk is statistically underpowered due to the reduced sample size.

General clinical characteristics of the included 122 male patients with premature STEMI are shown in Table 3. Personal history of tobacco consumption was, by far, the most frequent cardiovascular risk factor in this young population presenting with premature CAD (86%).

Table 3. Clinical characteristics of patients presenting with premature ST-elevation myocardial infarction.

	122 Male Patients with Premature STEMI
Mean age at STEMI	47.11 (±8.99)
Cardiovascular risk factors	
Previous/current smoker	95 (86.07%)
High blood pressure	34 (27.87%)
Diabetes mellitus	14 (11.48%)
Dyslipidemia	45 (36.89%)
Family history of premature CAD	30 (24.59%)

STEMI: ST-elevation myocardial infarction; CAD: coronary artery disease.

Among the population with premature STEMI, haplogroups G and I were more common in patients with a family history of premature cardiovascular disease than in those without it (Table 4). Moreover, the haplogroup "other" was significantly more frequently found in those STEMI patients who suffered diabetes mellitus when compared to those without diabetes (Table 4).

Table 4. Y chromosome haplogroup prevalence in patients with premature cardiovascular disease, depending on the presence/absence of cardiovascular risk factors.

Y Chromosome Haplogroups	No DM (108)	DM (14)	No HTN (88)	HTN (34)	No DL (77)	DL (45)	Non-Smokers (26)	Smokers (96)	No FH of PCAD (92)	FH of PCAD (30)
R	73.2%	64.3%	70.5%	76.5%	74%	68.9%	76.9%	70.8%	71.7%	73.3%
E	9.3%	-	10.2%	2.9%	7.8%	8.9%	11.5%	7.3%	9.8%	3.3%
J	5.6%	14.3%	5.7%	8.8%	6.5%	6.7%	3.9%	7.3%	6.5%	6,7%
G	2.8%	-	3.4%	-	3.9%	-	3.9%	2.1%	1.1%	6.7% *
I	6.5%	-	6.8%	2.9%	5.2%	6.7%	3.9%	6.3%	6.5% *	3.3%
Other	2.8%	21.4% *	3.4%	8.8%	2.6%	8.9%		6.3%	4.4%	6.7%

DM: diabetes mellitus; HTN: high blood pressure; DL: dyslipidemia; FH: family history; PCAD: premature coronary artery disease. * $p < 0.05$.

We did not find significant differences between the haplogroups for the mean cholesterol levels (Table 5).

Table 5. Mean cholesterol value levels in each Y chromosome haplogroup.

Mean Values (mg/dL)	R ($n = 88$)	E ($n = 10$)	J ($n = 8$)	G ($n = 3$)	I ($n = 7$)	Other ($n = 6$)
HDL cholesterol	37.6	42.7	39	34	39.57	33.33
LDL cholesterol	114.97	120.7	111.63	110	134.7	112.17
Triglycerides	173.30	157.2	152,88	140.67	191.86	242.5

4. Discussion

Premature CAD is a significant health concern that requires early diagnosis, effective management, and ongoing prevention. It is crucial to identify and manage risk factors to prevent the development of premature CAD and its associated complications. Therefore, investigating the genetics of populations with premature CAD, presenting with life threatening events like this cohort, is of utmost importance. The heritability of CAD has been estimated to be between 40% and 60%, on the basis of family and twin studies [18].

Remarkably, these heritable effects manifest more evidently in younger individuals [19]. An interesting study performed in twins reported that the probability of dying from CAD given that one's twin has already died from CAD decreased with increasing age, particularly amongst males [19].

Research studies have investigated the association between Y chromosome polymorphisms and the risk of CAD. However, the findings are not consistent and the relationship between Y haplogroups and CAD risk remains unclear. Charchar et al. studied three cohorts of British men with more than 3000 participants and found that carriers of haplogroup I had about a 50% higher age-adjusted risk of CAD than men with other Y haplogroups ($p < 0.001$; OR = 1.56, 1.24–1.97). The association between haplogroup I and increased risk of CAD was independent of traditional cardiovascular and socioeconomic risk factors [10]. These authors showed that this haplogroup was associated with the differential expression of genes related to inflammation and immunity, some of them relevant to atherosclerosis [10]. Haplogroup I has been also associated with a higher expression of chromosome Y genes linked to the immune system [11]. However, other authors failed to confirm the association between haplogroup I and CAD [20].

An analysis of men from the UK Biobank revealed that haplogroup I (Y1 subclade) was associated with an 11% increase in risk of CAD when compared with all other haplogroups combined (OR= 1.11, 95% CI = 1.04–1.189) [21]. The same authors showed that haplogroup-I1-specific variants showed enrichment for promoter and enhancer chromatin states in cells/tissues relevant to atherosclerosis, and haplogroup I1 was associated with changes in pathways involved in atherosclerosis development such as defense against pathogens, immunity, oxidative phosphorylation, mitochondrial respiration, lipids, coagulation, and extracellular matrix remodeling [21]. Due to the pivotal role of immunity and inflammation pathways in the development of atherosclerotic lesions, it is plausible that a differential immune response between the Y haplogroups could explain the reported association with CAD. These haplogroups might be associated with differences within pathways underlying almost all stages of CAD, including the initiation, growth, and rupture of atherosclerotic plaque [21–23]. A critical driver of atherosclerosis, the apolipoprotein B gene [24], was upregulated in arteries from carriers of haplogroup I1 [21]. On the contrary, CAD patients with haplogroup I1 showed the upregulation of pathways involved in platelet aggregation and arterial thrombus formation [21,25].

However, the distribution of Y chromosome haplogroups may vary from Northern to Southern European populations [8]. On the one hand, in our study, the frequency of Y haplogroup I was only slightly higher in the patients and displayed no significant difference from the controls (6% vs. 4%, $p = 0.47$, Table 2). However, it should be noted that in our population, haplogroup I was less common than in other regions where the association with CAD was reported. Moreover, the I1 subgroup is common among UK men but very rare among Spanish men (<1%). It is thus possible that the different results between populations reflect the presence of DNA variants beyond the ancestral SNP that defines the haplogroup. Thus, the sequencing of the Y-specific region is necessary to uncover the nucleotide changes that would explain the association with CAD.

On the other hand, in Southern European populations, haplogroup R1b is the most frequent (40–70%), followed by E1b1b and J2 (5–20%, respectively). In the Iberian Peninsula, the general reported prevalences are similar: 70–80% for R1B and 5–15% for E1b1b and J2, respectively [26]. In this regard, our region (Asturias) geographically belongs to the Spanish Cantabrian cornice, where haplogroup R1B is known to be the most common haplogroup. Accordingly, the frequencies from our controls were in agreement with those reported by others [26]. However, in addition, in the population of patients for whom we evaluated premature STEMI, we found significantly more patients with this particular haplogroup R1B that in the control population (Table 2).

The underlying mechanisms by which Y chromosome haplogroups influence the risk of CAD are not fully understood. However, studies have suggested that genetic variations within the Y chromosome could affect the expression of genes involved in lipid metabolism, inflammation, and thrombosis, which are key factors in the development of CAD. In this regard, Eales et al. showed that haplogroup I1 increased cardiovascular risk through the proatherosclerotic reprogramming of the transcriptome in several tissues of key relevance to CAD [21]. They observed changes in gene expression within other pathways underlying almost all stages of CAD, including the initiation, growth, and rupture of atherosclerotic plaque [21–23]. A critical driver of atherosclerosis, the apolipoprotein B gene [24], was upregulated in the arteries in carriers of haplogroup I1 [21]. On the contrary, CAD patients with haplogroup I1 showed the upregulation of pathways involved in platelet aggregation and arterial thrombus formation [21,25].

Moreover, while genetic factors play a significant role in the development of CAD, lifestyle factors such as smoking, poor diet, and lack of exercise also contribute to the risk of CAD. In this regard, some studies have shown that the association between Y chromosome haplogroups and CAD risk may vary depending on lifestyle factors. In this sense, a study by Pilbrow et al. found that men with the haplogroup I were at a higher risk of developing CAD if they smoked. In this regard, in this study of patients with premature CAD, the "rare" haplogroup was significantly more frequent among diabetic patients than non-diabetic ones. On the other hand, we found that haplogroup G was significantly more frequent in those patients with a family history of premature cardiovascular disease than in those without it.

5. Limitations

Overall, the relationship between Y chromosome haplogroups and the risk of premature CAD is complex and requires further investigation. Further studies are needed to elucidate the mechanisms underlying this association and to explore the potential clinical implications of Y chromosome haplogroups in the prevention and management of CAD. Studies with other epidemiological approaches, such as Mendelian randomization, are of interest to uncover the effect of cardio-metabolic variables in the risk for early-onset CAD. However, for this approach, a larger number of population controls and patients are required [27].

6. Conclusions

In conclusion, in our cohort of Spanish men, chromosome Y haplogroup R was significantly more frequent in premature STEMI. Y chromosome haplogroups may represent a novel avenue for understanding the genetic determinants of CAD risk in men.

Author Contributions: Conceptualization, R.L. and E.C.; Methodology, A.A., R.Á.-V., I.P., J.G., C.G.-L., L.V.-C. and E.C.; Software, R.Á.-V., J.G., D.V.-C., C.G.-L. and E.C.-L.; Validation, M.S., J.G. and E.C.; Formal analysis, A.A., R.Á.-V. and E.C.; Investigation, R.L., A.A., M.S., D.V.-C. and E.C.-L.; Resources, R.L., I.P. and E.C.; Data curation, A.A., R.Á.-V., D.V.-C., E.C.-L. and E.C.; Writing—original draft, R.L.; Writing—review & editing, R.L., I.P., P.A. and E.C.; Visualization, R.L.; Supervision, R.L., I.P., P.A. and E.C.; Project administration, P.A. and E.C.; Funding acquisition, P.A. All authors have read and agreed to the published version of the manuscript.

Funding: This research was funded by Instituto de Salud Carlos III (ISCIII) (grant number PI22/00705).

Institutional Review Board Statement: The study was conducted in accordance with the Declaration of Helsinki. Patients were recruited from the study approved by the Institutional Ethics Committee (CEIMPA; registry number 2020/003).

Informed Consent Statement: Informed consent was obtained from all subjects who underwent genetic study, for additional investigational purposes.

Conflicts of Interest: The authors declare no conflict of interest.

References

1. Arnett, D.K.; Blumenthal, R.S.; Albert, M.A.; Buroker, A.B.; Goldberger, Z.D.; Hahn, E.J.; Himmelfarb, C.D.; Khera, A.; Lloyd-Jones, D.; McEvoy, J.W.; et al. 2019 ACC/AHA Guideline on the Primary Prevention of Cardiovascular Disease: Executive Summary: A Report of the American College of Cardiology/American Heart Association Task Force on Clinical Practice Guidelines. *J. Am. Coll. Cardiol.* **2019**, *74*, 1376–1414. [CrossRef]
2. Visseren, F.L.J.; Mach, F.; Smulders, Y.M.; Carballo, D.; Koskinas, K.C.; Bäck, M.; Benetos, A.; Biffi, A.; Boavida, J.-M.; Capodanno, D.; et al. 2021 ESC Guidelines on cardiovascular disease prevention in clinical practice. *Eur. Heart J.* **2021**, *42*, 3227–3337. [CrossRef] [PubMed]
3. Yusuf, S.; Hawken, S.; Ounpuu, S.; Dans, T.; Avezum, A.; Lanas, F.; McQueen, M.; Budaj, A.; Pais, P.; Varigos, J.; et al. Effect of potentially modifiable risk factors associated with myocardial infarction in 52 countries (the INTERHEART study): Case-control study. *Lancet* **2004**, *364*, 937–952. [CrossRef]
4. McPherson, R.; Tybjaerg-Hansen, A. Genetics of Coronary Artery Disease. *Circ. Res.* **2016**, *118*, 564–578. [CrossRef] [PubMed]
5. Lorca, R.; Aparicio, A.; Cuesta-Llavona, E.; Pascual, I.; Junco, A.; Hevia, S.; Villazón, F.; Hernandez-Vaquero, D.; Rodríguez Reguero, J.J.; Moris, C.; et al. Familial Hypercholesterolemia in Premature Acute Coronary Syndrome. Insights from CholeSTEMI Registry. *J. Clin. Med.* **2020**, *9*, 3489. [CrossRef] [PubMed]
6. Jobling, M.A.; Tyler-Smith, C. The human Y chromosome: An evolutionary marker comes of age. *Nat. Rev. Genet.* **2003**, *4*, 598–612. [CrossRef]
7. Underhill, P.A.; Shen, P.; Lin, A.A.; Jin, L.; Passarino, G.; Yang, W.H.; Kauffman, E.; Bonné-Tamir, B.; Bertranpetit, J.; Francalacci, P.; et al. Y chromosome sequence variation and the history of human populations. *Nat. Genet.* **2000**, *26*, 358–361. [CrossRef]
8. Underhill, P.A.; Myres, N.M.; Rootsi, S.; Metspalu, M.; Zhivotovsky, L.A.; King, R.J.; Lin, A.A.; Chow, C.-E.T.; Semino, O.; Battaglia, V.; et al. Separating the post-Glacial coancestry of European and Asian Y chromosomes within haplogroup R1a. *Eur. J. Hum. Genet.* **2010**, *18*, 479–484. [CrossRef]
9. Wang, Z.; Parikh, H.; Jia, J.; Myers, T.; Yeager, M.; Jacobs, K.B.; Hutchinson, A.; Burdett, L.; Ghosh, A.; Thun, M.J.; et al. Y chromosome haplogroups and prostate cancer in populations of European and Ashkenazi Jewish ancestry. *Hum. Genet.* **2012**, *131*, 1173–1185. [CrossRef]
10. Charchar, F.J.; Bloomer, L.D.; Barnes, T.A.; Cowley, M.J.; Nelson, C.P.; Wang, Y.; Denniff, M.; Debiec, R.; Christofidou, P.; Nankervis, S.; et al. Inheritance of coronary artery disease in men: An analysis of the role of the Y chromosome. *Lancet* **2012**, *379*, 915–922. [CrossRef]
11. Bloomer, L.D.S.; Nelson, C.P.; Denniff, M.; Christofidou, P.; Debiec, R.; Thompson, J.; Zukowska-Szczechowska, E.; Samani, N.J.; Charchar, F.J.; Tomaszewski, M. Coronary artery disease predisposing haplogroup I of the Y chromosome, aggression and sex steroids—Genetic association analysis. *Atherosclerosis* **2014**, *233*, 160–164. [CrossRef] [PubMed]
12. Lorca, R.; Aparicio, A.; Gómez, J.; Álvarez-Velasco, R.; Pascual, I.; Avanzas, P.; González-Urbistondo, F.; Alen, A.; Vázquez-Coto, D.; González-Fernández, M.; et al. Mitochondrial Heteroplasmy as a Marker for Premature Coronary Artery Disease: Analysis of the Poly-C Tract of the Control Region Sequence. *JCM* **2023**, *12*, 2133. [CrossRef] [PubMed]
13. Thygesen, K.; Alpert, J.S.; Jaffe, A.S.; Chaitman, B.R.; Bax, J.J.; Morrow, D.A.; White, H.D.; ESC Scientific Document Group. Fourth universal definition of myocardial infarction (2018). *Eur. Heart J.* **2019**, *40*, 237–269. [CrossRef] [PubMed]
14. Collet, J.-P.; Thiele, H.; Barbato, E.; Barthélémy, O.; Bauersachs, J.; Bhatt, D.L.; Dendale, P.; Dorobantu, M.; Edvardsen, T.; Folliguet, T.; et al. 2020 ESC Guidelines for the management of acute coronary syndromes in patients presenting without persistent ST-segment elevation. *Eur. Heart J.* **2021**, *42*, 1289–1367. [CrossRef]
15. Williams, R.R.; Hunt, S.C.; Schumacher, M.C.; Hegele, R.A.; Leppert, M.F.; Ludwig, E.H.; Hopkins, P.N. Diagnosing heterozygous familial hypercholesterolemia using new practical criteria validated by molecular genetics. *Am. J. Cardiol.* **1993**, *72*, 171–176. [CrossRef] [PubMed]
16. Defesche, J.C.; Lansberg, P.J.; Umans-Eckenhausen, M.A.W.; Kastelein, J.J.P. Advanced method for the identification of patients with inherited hypercholesterolemia. *Semin. Vasc. Med.* **2004**, *4*, 59–65. [CrossRef]
17. Riobello, C.; Gómez, J.; Gil-Peña, H.; Tranche, S.; Reguero, J.R.; de la Hera, J.M.; Delgado, E.; Calvo, D.; Morís, C.; Santos, F.; et al. KCNQ1 gene variants in the risk for type 2 diabetes and impaired renal function in the Spanish Renastur cohort. *Mol. Cell. Endocrinol.* **2016**, *427*, 86–91. [CrossRef]
18. Vinkhuyzen, A.A.E.; Wray, N.R.; Yang, J.; Goddard, M.E.; Visscher, P.M. Estimation and Partition of Heritability in Human Populations Using Whole-Genome Analysis Methods. *Annu. Rev. Genet.* **2013**, *47*, 75–95. [CrossRef]
19. Zdravkovic, S.; Wienke, A.; Pedersen, N.L.; Marenberg, M.E.; Yashin, A.I.; De Faire, U. Heritability of death from coronary heart disease: A 36-year follow-up of 20,966 Swedish twins. *J. Intern. Med.* **2002**, *252*, 247–254. [CrossRef]
20. Timmers, P.R.H.J.; Wilson, J.F. Limited Effect of Y Chromosome Variation on Coronary Artery Disease and Mortality in UK Biobank-Brief Report. *Arterioscler. Thromb. Vasc. Biol.* **2022**, *42*, 1198–1206. [CrossRef]
21. Eales, J.M.; Maan, A.A.; Xu, X.; Michoel, T.; Hallast, P.; Batini, C.; Zadik, D.; Prestes, P.R.; Molina, E.; Denniff, M.; et al. Human Y Chromosome Exerts Pleiotropic Effects on Susceptibility to Atherosclerosis. *Arterioscler. Thromb. Vasc. Biol.* **2019**, *39*, 2386–2401. [CrossRef]
22. Newby, A.C. Metalloproteinases promote plaque rupture and myocardial infarction: A persuasive concept waiting for clinical translation. *Matrix Biol.* **2015**, *44–46*, 157–166. [CrossRef]

23. Ghattas, A.; Griffiths, H.R.; Devitt, A.; Lip, G.Y.H.; Shantsila, E. Monocytes in Coronary Artery Disease and Atherosclerosis. *J. Am. Coll. Cardiol.* **2013**, *62*, 1541–1551. [CrossRef] [PubMed]
24. Borén, J.; Williams, K.J. The central role of arterial retention of cholesterol-rich apolipoprotein-B-containing lipoproteins in the pathogenesis of atherosclerosis: A triumph of simplicity. *Curr. Opin. Lipidol.* **2016**, *27*, 473–483. [CrossRef] [PubMed]
25. Evans, D.J.W.; Jackman, L.E.; Chamberlain, J.; Crosdale, D.J.; Judge, H.M.; Jetha, K.; Norman, K.E.; Francis, S.E.; Storey, R.F. Platelet $P2Y_{12}$ Receptor Influences the Vessel Wall Response to Arterial Injury and Thrombosis. *Circulation* **2009**, *119*, 116–122. [CrossRef]
26. Adams, S.M.; Bosch, E.; Balaresque, P.L.; Ballereau, S.J.; Lee, A.C.; Arroyo, E.; López-Parra, A.M.; Aler, M.; Grifo, M.S.G.; Brion, M.; et al. The genetic legacy of religious diversity and intolerance: Paternal lineages of Christians, Jews, and Muslims in the Iberian Peninsula. *Am. J. Hum. Genet.* **2008**, *83*, 725–736. [CrossRef]
27. Bell, K.J.L.; Loy, C.; Cust, A.E.; Teixeira-Pinto, A. Mendelian Randomization in Cardiovascular Research: Establishing Causality When There Are Unmeasured Confounders. *Circ. Cardiovasc. Qual. Outcomes* **2021**, *14*, e005623. [CrossRef] [PubMed]

Disclaimer/Publisher's Note: The statements, opinions and data contained in all publications are solely those of the individual author(s) and contributor(s) and not of MDPI and/or the editor(s). MDPI and/or the editor(s) disclaim responsibility for any injury to people or property resulting from any ideas, methods, instructions or products referred to in the content.

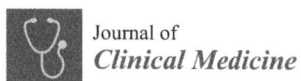

Review

Microcirculation in Hypertension: A Therapeutic Target to Prevent Cardiovascular Disease?

Damiano Rizzoni [1,*], Claudia Agabiti-Rosei [1,2], Gianluca E. M. Boari [3], Maria Lorenza Muiesan [1,2] and Carolina De Ciuceis [1,2]

1 Department of Clinical and Experimental Sciences, University of Brescia, 25121 Brescia, Italy; claudia.agabitirosei@unibs.it (C.A.-R.); marialorenza.muiesan@unibs.it (M.L.M.); carolina.deciuceis@unibs.it (C.D.C.)
2 Second Division of Medicine, Spedali Civili di Brescia, 25123 Brescia, Italy
3 Division of Medicine, Spedali Civili di Brescia, Montichiari, 25123 Brescia, Italy; gianluca@boari.net
* Correspondence: damiano.rizzoni@unibs.it

Abstract: Arterial hypertension is a common condition worldwide and an important risk factor for cardio- and cerebrovascular events, renal diseases, as well as microvascular eye diseases. Established hypertension leads to the chronic vasoconstriction of small arteries as well as to a decreased lumen diameter and the thickening of the arterial media or wall with a consequent increased media-to-lumen ratio (MLR) or wall-to-lumen ratio (WLR). This process, defined as vascular remodeling, was firstly demonstrated in small resistance arteries isolated from subcutaneous biopsies and measured by micromyography, and this is still considered the gold-standard method for the assessment of structural alterations in small resistance arteries; however, microvascular remodeling seems to represent a generalized phenomenon. An increased MLR may impair the organ flow reserve, playing a crucial role in the maintenance and, probably, also in the progressive worsening of hypertensive disease, as well as in the development of hypertension-mediated organ damage and related cardiovascular events, thus possessing a relevant prognostic relevance. New non-invasive techniques, such as scanning laser Doppler flowmetry or adaptive optics, are presently under development, focusing mainly on the evaluation of WLR in retinal arterioles; recently, also retinal microvascular WLR was demonstrated to have a prognostic impact in terms of cardio- and cerebrovascular events. A rarefaction of the capillary network has also been reported in hypertension, which may contribute to flow reduction in and impairment of oxygen delivery to different tissues. These microvascular alterations seem to represent an early step in hypertension-mediated organ damage since they might contribute to microvascular angina, stroke, and renal dysfunction. In addition, they can be markers useful in monitoring the beneficial effects of antihypertensive treatment. Additionally, conductance arteries may be affected by a remodeling process in hypertension, and an interrelationship is present in the structural changes in small and large conductance arteries. The review addresses the possible relations between structural microvascular alterations and hypertension-mediated organ damage, and their potential improvement with antihypertensive treatment.

Keywords: microcirculation; peripheral circulation; remodeling; small resistance arteries; vascular biology

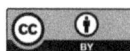

1. Introduction

Cardiovascular diseases are the main cause of death worldwide, resulting in around 18 million deaths per year (WHO, 2020) [1], and hypertension is considered as the main contributor to such a global burden [2]. Effective blood pressure (BP) control is a mandatory factor in order to improve hypertensive target organ damage and subsequent cardiovascular morbidity and mortality [2].

Functional, mechanical, and structural alterations of the microvasculature may be observed in patients with essential hypertension, even at very early stages [3–5], and contribute to the development of hypertension complications and cardiovascular prognosis [3,5]. In particular, in this setting, microvascular remodeling is a key event in triggering cardiovascular diseases [6,7].

The molecular mechanisms underlying the development of vascular remodeling are only partly understood. However, among the factors that may contribute to microvascular changes, an important role may be played by vascular inflammation with infiltration of inflammatory circulating cells and the release of inflammatory cytokines and chemokines, proliferative growth factors, as well as oxidative stress related to both a reduction in nitric oxide bioavailability and increased reaction oxygen species production [5,8,9]. These changes are promoted by mechanical, hemodynamic, or metabolic vascular insult and result in an altered vascular smooth muscle cell phenotype and the accumulation of the extracellular matrix [9]. The present review briefly summarizes the knowledge at present about microvascular remodeling and its role in hypertension-mediated organ damage and consequent cardiovascular events.

2. Microvascular Remodeling in Hypertension

Cardiovascular and metabolic diseases (in particular arterial hypertension) are very commonly associated with alterations in microcirculation [4,6,7]; morphological changes may involve small resistance arteries, arterioles, capillaries, and post-capillary venules [3,6,10]. BP is mainly influenced by vessel resistance and microcirculation is the key element of peripheral resistance regulation. As previously mentioned, microcirculation may be subdivided in small arteries, arterioles, and capillaries. Small resistance arteries are defined as arteries with a lumen diameter roughly between 350 and 100 µm. Their structure consists of an outer connective tissue adventitia, smooth muscle cell tunica media, and the endothelial layer [5,6]. Arterioles are vessels with internal diameters smaller than 100 µm, characterized by a single layer of smooth muscle cells. Small arteries and arterioles account for 45–50% of peripheral resistance and are defined as resistance arteries. These vessels have the capacity of contracting when transmural pressure increases, a feature called myogenic tone. A total of 23–30% of peripheral resistance is to be ascribed to capillaries (internal diameter less than 7 µm), whose walls are constituted only by a monolayer of endothelial cells [5,6,11–13].

It was proposed several years ago that increases in systemic vascular resistance may be a consequence of vascular smooth muscle increase and the concomitant narrowing of the arteriolar lumen [3,4,6,7,14]. Microcirculation remodeling occurs in primary hypertension [6,10]. Remodeling may be classified according to lumen and wall cross-sectional area changes [12,13]. Hence, remodeling might be inward when the internal diameter is reduced and outward when the lumen is unchanged [15,16]. On the other hand, hypertrophic remodeling occurs when the vessel wall material, i.e., media/wall cross-sectional area, increases along with media/wall thickness, whereas if the media/wall cross-sectional area does not change or is reduced, then remodeling is defined as eutrophic or hypotrophic, respectively [15,16]. Inward eutrophic remodeling is mainly observed in primary hypertension with a media thickness increase and lumen diameter decrease resulting in an unchanged media-cross sectional area [14–17]. On the contrary, hypertrophic remodeling, which may be outward or inward, has been shown in the secondary form of hypertension [17] and in cardiovascular diseases, such as diabetes mellitus [18,19], obesity [20,21], and metabolic syndrome [22], as well as in other endocrine diseases [23,24], independently, in the presence of an increase in BP increase. As result of the remodeling process, the wall-to-lumen ratio (WLR) and media-to-lumen ratio (MLR), are defined as the ratio between wall and media thickness, respectively, and lumen diameter increase.

Hypertensive patients [4,14], but also obese [25] or diabetic patients [4], present reduced basal and total capillary densities compared to the normotensive controls showing a structural anatomical rarefaction of capillaries rather than the presence of non-perfused vessels [4]. This reduction in total capillary density may consequently lead to an increase in peripheral resistances, thus negatively affecting tissue perfusion and nutrient delivery [26].

The time course of the development of hypertension in respect to the onset of microvascular alterations is not clear. An increase in the MLR of mesenteric small resistance arteries of spontaneously hypertensive rats may be present in a pre-hypertensive phase [4]. The data for humans are obviously difficult to obtain, since very few longitudinal data are presently available [4].

As previously mentioned, the hallmark of a microvascular remodeling process is an increased WLR and/or MLR. These parameters were initially measured in small resistance arteries by using wire or pressure micromyography, an in vitro ex vivo technique where a small artery is isolated from subcutaneous fat tissue and mounted on wire or glass cannulas and studied in isometric or isobaric conditions [27–29]. At present, non-invasive techniques are available [30], such as scanning laser Doppler flowmetry and adaptive optics, which allow the accurate visualization and measurement of retinal vessel morphological parameters at a high resolution providing similar information compared to the micromyographic system [31]. In particular, scanning laser Doppler flowmetry allows us to measure the external diameter of retinal arterioles in reflection images and to evaluate the internal diameter in perfusion images, according to a laser Doppler technique. A software-guided automatic comparison of the two images provides an estimation of the WLR [32,33]. With adaptive optics, the internal and external diameters of retinal arterioles are derived though an algorithm detecting the gradient of light's reflection between the lumen of the vessel and the wall; these data are then used to calculate the WLR and wall cross-sectional area [30,34] (Figure 1). Compared to scanning laser Doppler flowmetry, adaptive optics detects retinal arteriole remodeling with a lower intra-observer variability [31] and provides very high-quality images [34] (Figure 1).

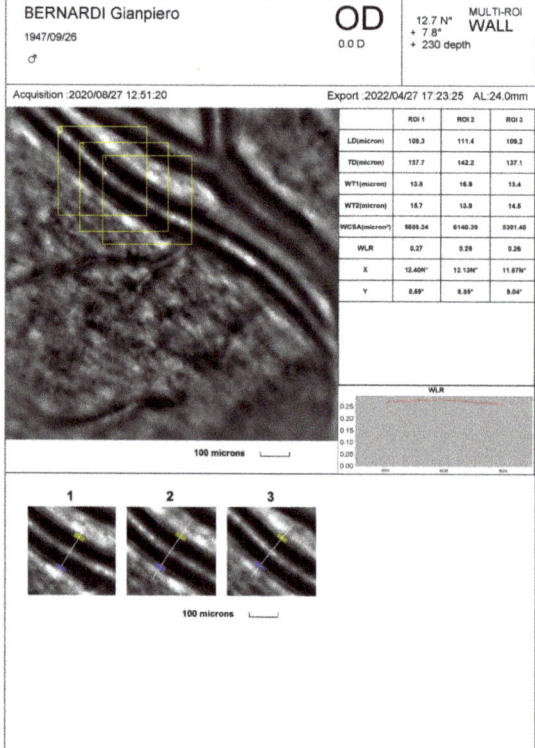

Figure 1. Evaluation of the morphology of retinal arteries by adaptive optics. Example of images obtained with adaptive optics (AO camera, Rtx-1, Imagine Eyes, Orsay, France) (**left** and **bottom**) and measurement of morphological parameters using a dedicated software (**right**). From reference [4].

The cost, advantages, disadvantages, and indications/perspectives of the different available techniques for a non-invasive investigation of microvascular structure are summarized in Table 1 [30].

Table 1. Cost, advantages, disadvantages, and indications/perspectives of the available techniques for a non-invasive investigation of microvascular structure. From reference [30].

Technique	Cost ($)	Advantages	Disadvantages	Indications/Perspectives
Forearm plethysmography	1500–2000	Relatively inexpensive	Locally invasive, needs experience	Research purposes, not for extensive clinical use
Intravital microscopy/Glycocalyx	3000–5000	Non-invasive	No prognostic data	Research purposes, not for extensive clinical use, though adoption in specific settings (i.e., critical care) is being proposed
Nailfold videocapillaroscopy	10,000–20,000	Non-invasive	No prognostic data	Research purposes in the cardiovascular setting, commonly used in rheumatology. Possible future demonstration of prognostic usefulness of such an approach might extend its clinical application to patients at elevated cardiovascular risk.
SLDF (Heidelberg Retina Flowmeter)	30,000–40,000	Some prognostic data available/possibility to assess endothelial function	No more in the market	Research purposes; potential for an extensive future clinical application in the cardiovascular field if technically developed by the producer
Adaptive optics cameras	130,000–160,000	Reliable/possibility to assess endothelial function	Cost, no prognostic data	Commonly used in ophthalmology for specific clinical purposes. Potential for an extensive future clinical application in the cardiovascular field
Dynamic Vessel Analyzer (AV ratio)	5000–6000	Some prognostic data, relatively easy to perform	Cost, some limitations in reliability	Commonly used in ophthalmology for specific purposes
OCTA	20,000–70,000	Useful vascular information on choroidal microvessels in hypertensive patients, plenty of data provided.	Imaging artefacts, high acquisition costs, role in the cardiovascular field still under evaluation	Commonly used in ophthalmology for specific purposes
Techniques for the evaluation of topological changes in the retinal vascular architecture or fractal dimensions	30,000–50,000	Some prognostic data (fractal dimensions)	Not standardized	Only research purposes
EndoPAT	2500–4000	Easy to perform, cost	Limited reliability	Only research purposes
Laser Doppler Flowmetry (skin)	1500–20,000	Easy to perform, cost	Limited reliability	Only research purposes

2.1. Pathophysiology of Microvascular Remodeling

Microvascular remodeling is the complex result of multiple factors [35]. Although the "primum movens" for the microvascular remodeling in primary hypertension is still unclear, underlying mechanisms include hemodynamic and mechanical changes, such as increased wall stress and prolonged vasoconstriction, but also hormonal factors as well as immune cell activation, inflammatory, and oxidative signaling [9]. The interaction among these factors induces alterations in the extracellular matrix (ECM), which involve integrins [36], tissue transglutaminase [37], as well as the activation of tissue metalloproteinases 2 and 9 activity with an increase in collagen deposition in the vascular wall [38]. Moreover, oxidative stress, which is, to date, defined as an imbalance between oxidants and antioxidants in favor of oxidants [39], is able to modulate ECM composition, cell growth and differentiation, and activate growth factors and pro-inflammatory genes [40].

In particular, a combination of inward vascular wall growth and apoptosis in the peripheral area of small arteries has been suggested in the development of inward eutrophic remodeling [41]. This process seems to represent a physiological protective mechanism against an increase in wall tension caused by increased BP, as wall tension is directly proportional to the lumen radius and inversely proportional to wall thickness according to Laplace's law.

On the other hand, an altered myogenic tone, which is the artery's ability to contract in response to an increased BP in order to protect distal vessels, has been hypothesized to induce hypertrophic remodeling and contribute to target organ damage [19]. In this context, reactive oxygen species (ROS), together with growth factors and mechanical injury, may switch the vascular smooth muscle cell phenotype from contractile to synthetic, thus inducing hypertrophy [42]. ROS are oxygen-derived molecules, such as superoxide (O^{2-}), nitric oxide, peroxynitrite ($OONO^-$), and hydrogen peroxide (H_2O_2), which are extremely important in the pathophysiology of hypertension and hypertension-associated target organ damage [40]. Many pro-hypertensive factors, including angiotensin II, aldosterone, endothelin 1, growth factors, immune factors, and salt, induce ROS production in endothelial cells, vascular smooth muscle cells, adventitia, and perivascular adipose tissue (PVAT), leading to vascular injury [40].

Indeed, the renin–angiotensin–aldosterone system (RAAS) and endothelin system, as well as catecholamines with sympathetic nervous system activation may play a crucial role in microvascular remodeling. Angiotensin II and endothelin exert vasoconstriction effects with diminished vasodilatation and may contribute to microvascular remodeling by regulating oxidative stress and the inflammatory mechanisms of vascular damage [7,43]. Angiotensin II elicits its deleterious effect through the angiotensin type-I receptor (AT1R) [44], a receptor that mediates pathways involved in trophic effects, hypertension, and inflammation, whereas the angiotensin 1–7/Mas receptor pathway seems to be protective [45].

Recently, PVAT dysfunction was demonstrated to be involved in microvascular alterations. PVAT seems to exert a key role in vasculature homeostasis; its activity results from the balance between the production of vasodilation and vasoconstriction substances [46]. In healthy conditions, PVAT regulates the contractile function of vessels releasing the PVAT-derived relaxing factor (ADRF), a molecule whose nature is still unknown. Adiponectin acts as a vasodilator through the activation of eNOS; it also reduces macrophage activation, vascular smooth muscle cell proliferation, oxidative stress, and increase insulin activity [46]. As the PVAT anti-contractile effect disappears when adiponectin receptors are blocked, adiponectin is considered a realistic candidate as ADRF. In particular, PVAT dysfunction occurs in systemic inflammatory states, such as obesity, where adiponectin activity and release are reduced [47]. On the other hand, under pathological conditions, such as obesity, diabetes, and hypertension, PVAT is also able to produce pro-inflammatory cytokines (IL-6, TNF-alpha, IL-8, MCP-1, TGF-Beta), prothrombotic factors (PAI-1), and vasoconstriction molecules, such as endothelin-1 and angiotensin II [48].

2.2. Role of the the Immune System in Microvascular Remodeling: Interaction with Hormonal Signals, the Sympathetic Nervous System, and PVAT

Hypertension is associated with a chronic inflammatory response due to immune cell accumulation in different hypertensive target organs, such as the kidneys, heart, brain, and blood vessels (including in the PVAT), thus exacerbating hypertension. This observation raised the hypothesis that hypertension might start as an overactivation of the central nervous system by the RAAS leading to a rise in BP with peripheral mechanical and oxidative damage [49,50]. Peripheral damage causing danger associated molecular patterns (DAMPs production) might be a trigger for immune responses as, normally, DAMPs activate the immune system and cause inflammation [50].

Animal models revealed the strong role of innate and adaptive immune cells in angiotensin II-induced hypertension [8]. In particular, adaptive immunity and, in particular, T-lymphocytes seem to play a major role [8]. Rats infused with angiotensin II elicited an increased production of T-helper (Th)-1 cytokines and a decrease in anti-inflammatory Th-2 cytokines, which may be restored by angiotensin II-receptor-1 blockers, but not by the vasodilator hydralazine, despite the similar effect on BP [51].

In order to clarify the role of the immune system in angiotensin II-mediated hypertension, many studies were conducted in immunodeficient mice. Ang II-dependent hypertension as well as vascular remodeling were demonstrated to be blunted in rats deficient in T- and B-lymphocytes [52]. T-regulatory cells (Treg), a particular subtype of T cells with the ability to suppress T-lymphocyte proliferation, seemed to also be involved in pressure regulation [53]. Indeed, rats with genetic hypertension (Dahl salt-sensitive strain) had reduced levels of Treg cytokines, less Treg cells, and more inflammatory cells in the aorta, as well as higher pressure compared with genetic normotensive rats [54]. Moreover, Treg-adoptive transfer induced a BP-lowering effect in angiotensin II rats [53]. In addition, Madhur et al. demonstrated that hypertension was associated with an increase in circulating Th17 cells and that IL-17 played an important role in Ang II-dependent hypertension [55]. Recently, it was reported that salt intake may stimulate RAAS and endothelin with consequent Th17 lymphocyte activation and a change in gut microbiome leading to intestinal wall inflammation, hence promoting microvascular damage and hypertension [56].

It has also been suggested that a splenic factor, the placental growth factor (PlGF), mediates a sympathetic stimulation of the spleen leading to costimulation and deployment in target organs of T cells promoting the onset of hypertension [57]. The spleen is innervated by sympathetic nervous system fibers that modulate immune cell responses through their neurotransmitters, thus generating a neuro-immune communication [58]. Particularly, there is a strong link between the central nervous system, RAAS, and immune system [49]. RAAS central stimulation causes an activation of peripheral T-lymphocytes and consequently vascular inflammation, further exacerbating BP [59]. This effect on T cells is centrally mediated, and it is associated with BP increase mediated by noradrenaline [60]. Noradrenaline further activates T-cell proliferation as the lymph nodes and spleen are innervated by sympathetic fibers [61].

Inflammation and oxidative stress mediated by RAAS cause PVAT dysfunction [46,47,62] and the impairment of endothelial function, thus contributing to pathophysiological hypertensive structural alterations Endothelial function is essential for microcirculation, as it regulates vascular tone, permeability, inflammation, and angiogenesis. Resistance artery endothelial function and nitric oxide (NO) availability might represent important factors involved in resistance artery remodeling, independently from cardiovascular risk factor exposure. This issue is specifically addressed elsewhere [63–65].

2.3. Prognostic Role of Microvascular Structural Alterations

The MLR of subcutaneous small resistance arteries has been suggested to represent the most prevalent and earliest form of arterial damage in essential hypertension [66] and it may be present very early on, even in the prehypertensive phase, at least in the experimental model [4].

From a physiological point of view, the reductions in the small artery and arteriole lumen are associated with an increase in flow resistance, even in condition of maximal dilatation, hence impairing the organ flow reserve [67–69]. Indeed, a relationship between the vasodilating capacity of coronary microcirculation and media-to-lumen ratio of subcutaneous small arteries was previously demonstrated [70] in patients with mild to moderate hypertension, thus suggesting that structural alterations in the subcutaneous vascular district (evaluated by wire micromyography in isolated vessels from fat biopsies obtained from the gluteal region) may be representative of similar alterations in coronary microcirculation, leading to a reduced coronary flow reserve [70,71].

Increased MLR of subcutaneous small resistance arteries has been positively related to hypertensive target organ damage, such as left ventricular hypertrophy [72,73] or carotid artery structure [73].

Importantly, the changes in small artery structure have a prognostic significance in both primary and secondary hypertension and in type-2 diabetes; indeed, an increased MLR is associated with a reduced event-free survival for cardiovascular events in high-risk patients [3,74] as well as in medium-risk ones [3,75,76]. Moreover, the presence of hypertrophic remodeling seems to be associated with an even worse prognosis compared to eutrophic remodeling [77,78]. More details about the prognostic role of the structural alterations in subcutaneous small resistance arteries evaluated by micromyography are reported in reference [3].

On the other hand, WLR evaluated by scanning laser Doppler flowmetry was proved to increase in patients with hypertension and cerebrovascular disease [32], and to directly be associated with urinary albumin excretion [79]. Likewise, an increased WLR evaluated with adaptive optics correlated with age [80,81], BP [34], and may be improved by a reduction in BP values by hypertensive treatment [46]. Most recently, the prognostic role of WLR evaluated with adaptive optics was demonstrated [80]. The event-free survival was significantly worse in 230 normotensive subjects and hypertensive patients with a baseline WLR higher than the median value of the population (0.28) according to Kaplan–Meier survival curves and multivariate analysis (Cox's proportional hazard model) [82]. The evidence was confirmed after restricting the analysis to cardiovascular events, excluding deaths and neoplastic diseases [82]. Therefore, the structural alterations of retinal arterioles evaluated by adaptive optics may predict total and cardiovascular events [82].

Most recently, it was also demonstrated that patients with coronary microvascular dysfunction, defined as the presence of a reduced myocardial flow reserve (≤ 2), evaluated by dynamic single-photon-emission computed tomography (SPECT), had higher rates of adverse outcomes that those without it [83]. However, it is not presently known whether capillary rarefaction may be related to cardiovascular events [3,4].

2.4. Possible Prevention/Regression of Microvascular Remodeling

The subsequent question to be answered is whether we should aim at correcting the structure of resistance vessels in the treatment of hypertension and whether this can affect the prognosis. Indeed, several drugs have been demonstrated to improve microvascular structure and therefore reduce the MLR, such as drugs inhibiting RAAS and dihydropyridinic calcium channel blockers, whereas diuretics and beta-blockers did not seem to have any relevant effects [5,7,84].

There is clear evidence that angiotensin-converting enzyme (ACE)-inhibitors and angiotensin-receptor blockers (ARBs) appear to be more effective than atenolol in terms of microvascular protection also in patients with diabetes mellitus [85–87]. Along this line, the direct renin inhibitor aliskiren improved microvascular structural alterations to a similar extent, compared with ramipril, in mild hypertensive patients with type-2 diabetes mellitus [88].

An improvement of microvascular remodeling was also demonstrated in the retinal vasculature. In patients with hypertension, aliskiren plus valsartan ameliorated ameliorate the WLR of retinal arterioles measured non-invasively by scanning laser Doppler flowmetry [89]. The combination of lercanidipine and enalapril was more effective in reducing the retinal arteriole WLR compared to the combination of lercanidipine and hydrochlorothiazide [90]. Using adaptive optics, the normalization of the retinal arteriole structure was observed after chronic and effective antihypertensive treatments [80]. On the contrary, a short-term reduction in BP only led to an increase in the internal diameter of retina arterioles with no changes in the wall thickness or wall cross-sectional area [80].

A complete regression of the remodeling process is difficult to obtain for patients with hypertension-mediated organ damage (i.e., left ventricular hypertrophy) or when comorbidities, such as diabetes mellitus, are present [3,4,7,84]. Usually, in such clinical situations, an improvement, but not a full normalization of the MLR of subcutaneous small resistance arteries, has been observed, despite effective BP reduction.

Several specific mechanisms may contribute to the beneficial effects of some drugs on small artery structure and outcomes compared with other pharmacological strategies. Buus NH et al. observed that, in essential hypertension, after one year of treatment with the ACE-inhibitor perindopril, the coronary flow reserve improved with the normalization of small subcutaneous arteries' structure [91]. In this study, in the parallel group treated with the beta-blocker atenolol, coronary flow was reduced and the small subcutaneous artery structure remained unchanged, despite a similar reduction in BP [91]. Therefore, it can be speculated that the beneficial effect on the hypertensive target organ damage of these drugs may be also occur to their ability to improve microvascular structure. Buus NH et al. [92] also demonstrated that MLR represents an independent predictor of cardiovascular events, beyond the extent of BP reduction, in a cohort of moderate-risk essential hypertensive patients not only including untreated patients, but also hypertensive patients during long-term effective treatment. This suggests that the assessment of the microvascular structure may also be important in treated patients, since it can allow us to identify those who may benefit from a more aggressive treatment and further risk reduction.

In addition, since vascular damage in hypertension is also caused by the inflammation, oxidative stress, and immune system activation, drugs selectively modulating these pathways can represent a potential and interesting strategy of treatment in the near future.

In patients with Conn's syndrome (primary aldosteronism due to an adenoma of the adrenals), the presence of marked or persistent vascular remodeling, as indicated by a higher MLR of subcutaneous small resistance arteries, was associated with reduced chances of BP normalization in the long-term follow-up after adrenalectomy. Thus, the severity of structural alterations in subcutaneous small resistance arteries can predict the clinical outcomes for these patients with secondary hypertension [93]. Therefore, structural alterations of small arteries can possibly be considered an important intermediate endpoint for the evaluation of the efficacy of antihypertensive treatment [4].

Antihypertensive treatment with ACE inhibitors seems to improve capillary rarefaction [90,94]; although, some methodological caveats were raised [95]. In any case, it has not yet been established whether a reversal of capillary rarefaction is associated with an improved prognosis [4].

3. Interrelationship between Microvascular and Macrovascular Remodeling

The large arteries are not only the target of high BP, but a determining factor in the pathogenesis of hypertension, particularly of isolated systolic hypertension and the increase in pulse pressure typical when aging [96,97]. The large elastic arteries allow the conduction of blood from the heart to the resistance arteries, but also for the transformation of the pulsatile flow, generated by cardiac activity, into the continuous flow observed in peripheral circulation. Part of the energy produced by the left ventricular systole is used for the stretching of arteries and it is stored in their walls. During diastole, this energy recoils the aorta and squeezes out blood into microcirculation, ensuring a continuous flow to tissues [98,99]. In essential hypertension, remodeling occurs not only in the small arteries, but also during macrocirculation [100,101]. Large conduit arteries (such as the aorta and its branches) develop arteriosclerosis of the media. This remodeling is characterized by an increase in intima-media thickness with a lumen enlargement of proximal elastic arteries, and it is a compensation mechanism used to normalize circumferential wall stress [99]. Elastic fibers in the media become thinner and frail, undergoing fragmentation with a parallel increase in collagen deposition and a consequent reduction in distensibility [96,100]. Aging and BP are the two main determinants of arterial stiffness, which is also influenced by diabetes mellitus, obesity, and metabolic syndrome. In the Framingham Heart Study, increased large-artery stiffness, measured as pulse wave velocity, and aortic root enlargement were observed to be associated with a higher risk of cardiovascular disease [5,102]. Pulse wave velocity correlates with hypertensive heart disease and microalbuminuria [103,104].

In fact, arterial stiffness has unfavorable consequences from a hemodynamic point of view. The increase in the speed of the incident and the reflected wave causes them to merge earlier, in the first part of the systole, increasing the systolic BP (with an increased afterload), reducing the diastolic BP (with a reduction in myocardial blood flow), and increasing the pulse pressure [100]. In addition, with the elastic arteries becoming more rigid than the muscular ones, a reversion in the normal center–periphery stiffness gradient occurs, which is mainly responsible for the reflection of the sphygmic wave [4,100]. Hence, the reflection site moves more distally, and the reflected wave is decreased, increasing the peripheral transmission of a large incident wave that exposes the peripheral arteries and arterioles to harmful levels of pressure plasticity, contributing to alterations of microcirculation and, in the end, of the nutrition and oxygenation of peripheral tissues (heart, brain, kidneys, and limbs), as well as the elimination of waste products [96,100].

It is still difficult to establish a temporal or linear relationship between small- and large-artery alterations in essential hypertension. The most likely relationship is actually a cross-talk between micro- and macrocirculation that may trigger a vicious cycle [96,100]. Hypertension causes the degeneration of large arteries and stiffness, with consequent higher central systolic and pulse pressures, and microvascular alterations, such as eutrophic remodeling, impaired vasodilatation, and microvascular rarefaction. Small-artery remodeling and rarefaction increase total peripheral resistance and amplify mean BP [96,100]. Indeed, in essential hypertension, the MLR of small resistance arteries and pulse wave velocity are independent determinants of central systolic BP [105]. Moreover, many indices of large-artery stiffness (e. g. pulse pressure, pulse wave velocity) are associated with indices of microvascular damage (WLR and MLR, respectively) [106,107].

Drugs that improve microvascular structure are particularly effective, also in reducing central BP, thus probably providing an additional benefit [4,62,69,74,75], most likely by slowing down the reflection of BP waves from distal reflection sites, close to microcirculation [4,96,100,103,108,109].

The pathophysiological consequences of the regression of small-artery remodeling might be: better BP control, taking advantage of reduced vascular reactivity [4,69]; an improvement of the organ flow reserve, in particular, in the heart [4,69,92]; and an effective reduction in central BP [4,96,100,103,108,109].

4. Conclusions

In hypertensive microcirculation, internal media or total wall thickness were increased in relation to the internal lumen, and this alteration contributed to the increase in peripheral resistance we observed [4]. Microvascular structural alterations might also impact the organ flow reserve [3,4,10,69,70], and this may play a role in the maintenance/progressive worsening of hypertensive disease. Therefore, an increased MLR in small resistance arteries may forecast the development of hypertension-mediated organ damage/cardiovascular events, as well as complications of the disease [77,78].

In order to allow for a wider application of the evaluation of microvascular morphology, we need non-invasive techniques to better stratify cardiovascular risk and to better evaluate the effects of antihypertensive therapy [4,30]. Techniques that allow for an evaluation of retinal artery morphology, such as scanning laser Doppler flowmetry or adaptive optics, seem to be a promising approach [30], as also stated in the 2023 ESH Guidelines for the management of arterial hypertension [110].

In conclusion, the evaluation of microvascular structure is progressively moving from bench to bedside [3,4,30,44], and can, in the near future, represent an evaluation to be performed in the majority, if not in all, hypertensive patients [3,4,30]. The most recent demonstration of the possible prognostic relevance of non-invasive measures of microvascular structure by adaptive optics represents a relevant contribution; although, this evidence has to be confirmed by other studies. In addition, we need a similar demonstration of the prognostic relevance of the changes in the indices of microvascular structure evaluated non-invasively and observed during antihypertensive treatment.

Author Contributions: D.R.: writing—original draft preparation; C.A.-R.: writing—review and editing, G.E.M.B.: writing—review and editing, M.L.M.: writing—review and editing, C.D.C.: writing—review and editing. All authors have read and agreed to the published version of the manuscript.

Funding: This research received no external funding.

Institutional Review Board Statement: Not applicable.

Informed Consent Statement: Not applicable.

Data Availability Statement: Not applicable.

Conflicts of Interest: The authors declare no conflict of interest.

References

1. World Health Organization (WHO). Cardiovascular Diseases (CVDs). Available online: https://www.who.int/news-room/fact-sheets/detail/cardiovascular-diseases-(cvds) (accessed on 14 June 2023).
2. Williams, B.; Mancia, G.; Spiering, W.; Agabiti Rosei, E.; Azizi, M.; Burnier, M.; Clement, D.L.; Coca, A.; de Simone, G.; Dominiczak, A.; et al. 2018 ESC/ESH Guidelines for the management of arterial hypertension: The Task Force for the management of arterial hypertension of the European Society of Cardiology and the European Society of Hypertension. *J. Hypertens.* **2018**, *36*, 1953–2041. [CrossRef] [PubMed]
3. Agabiti-Rosei, E.; Rizzoni, D. Microvascular structure as a prognostically relevant endpoint. *J. Hypertens.* **2017**, *35*, 914–921. [CrossRef] [PubMed]
4. Rizzoni, D.; Agabiti-Rosei, C.; De Ciuceis, C. State of the art review: Vascular remodeling in hypertension. *Am. J. Hypertens.* **2023**, *36*, 1–13. [CrossRef] [PubMed]
5. Chiarini, G.; Agabiti Rosei, C.; Lemoli, M.; Rossini, C.; Muiesan, M.L.; Rizzoni, D.; De Ciuceis, C. Organ damage in hypertension: Role of the microcirculation. *Front. Cardiovasc. Med.* 2023, submitted.
6. Mulvany, M.J.; Aalkjaer, C. Structure and function of small arteries. *Physiol. Rev.* **1990**, *70*, 921–971. [CrossRef]
7. Schiffrin, E.L. Remodeling of resistance arteries in essential hypertension and effects of antihypertensive treatment. *Am. J. Hypertens.* **2004**, *17 Pt 1*, 1192–1200. [CrossRef]
8. Rizzoni, D.; De Ciuceis, C.; Szczepaniak, P.; Paradis, P.; Schiffrin, E.L.; Guzik, T.J. Immune system and microvascular remodeling in humans. *Hypertension* **2022**, *79*, 691–705. [CrossRef]
9. Schiffrin, E.L. How structure, mechanics, and function of the vasculature contribute to BP elevation in hypertension. *Can. J. Cardiol.* **2020**, *36*, 648–658. [CrossRef]
10. Folkow, B. Physiological aspects of primary hypertension. *Physiol. Rev.* **1982**, *62*, 347–504. [CrossRef]
11. Bohlen, H.G. Localization of vascular resistance changes during hypertension. *Hypertension* **1986**, *8*, 181–183. [CrossRef]
12. Borders, J.L.; Granger, H.J. Power dissipation as a measure of peripheral resistance in vascular networks. *Hypertension* **1986**, *8*, 184–191. [CrossRef]
13. Christensen, K.L.; Mulvany, M.J. Location of resistance arteries. *J. Vasc. Res.* **2001**, *38*, 1–12. [CrossRef]
14. Rizzoni, D.; De Ciuceis, C.; Porteri, E.; Paiardi, S.; Boari, G.E.; Mortini, P.; Cornali, C.; Cenzato, M.; Rodella, L.F.; Borsani, E.; et al. Altered structure of small cerebral arteries in patients with essential hypertension. *J. Hypertens.* **2009**, *27*, 838–845. [CrossRef]
15. Heagerty, A.M.; Aalkjaer, C.; Bund, S.J.; Korsgaard, N.; Mulvany, M.J. Small artery structure in hypertension. Dual process of remodeling and growth. *Hypertension* **1993**, *21*, 391–397. [CrossRef]
16. Mulvany, M.J.; Baumbach, G.L.; Aalkjaer, C.; Heagerty, A.M.; Korsgaard, N.; Schiffrin, E.L.; Heistad, D.D. Vascular remodeling. *Hypertension* **1996**, *28*, 505–506.
17. Rizzoni, D.; Porteri, E.; Castellano, M.; Bettoni, G.; Muiesan, M.L.; Muiesan, P.; Giulini, S.M.; Agabiti Rosei, E. Vascular hypertrophy and remodeling in secondary hypertension. *Hypertension* **1996**, *28*, 785–790. [CrossRef]

18. Rizzoni, D.; Porteri, E.; Guelfi, D.; Muiesan, M.L.; Valentini, U.; Cimino, A.; Girelli, A.; Rodella, L.; Bianchi, R.; Sleiman, I.; et al. Structural alterations in subcutaneous small arteries of normotensive and hypertensive patients with non-insulin dependent diabetes mellitus. *Circulation* **2001**, *103*, 1238–1244. [CrossRef]
19. Schofield, I.; Malik, R.; Izzard, A.; Austin, C.; Heagerty, A.M. Vascular structural and functional changes in type 2 diabetes mellitus. Evidence for the role of abnormal myogenic responsiveness and dyslipidemia. *Circulation* **2002**, *106*, 3037–3043. [CrossRef]
20. Grassi, G.; Seravalle, G.; Scopelliti, F.; Dell'Oro, R.; Fattori, L.; Quarti-Trevano, F.; Brambilla, G.; Schiffrin, E.L.; Mancia, G. Structural and functional alterations of subcutaneous small resistance arteries in severe human obesity. *Obesity* **2010**, *18*, 92–98. [CrossRef]
21. De Ciuceis, C.; Porteri, E.; Rizzoni, D.; Corbellini, C.; La Boria, E.; Boari, G.E.; Pilu, A.; Mittempergher, F.; Di Betta, E.; Casella, C.; et al. Effects of weight loss on structural and functional alterations of subcutaneous small arteries in obese patients. *Hypertension* **2011**, *58*, 29–36. [CrossRef]
22. Grassi, G.; Seravalle, G.; Brambilla, G.; Facchetti, R.; Bolla, G.; Mozzi, E.; Mancia, G. Impact of the metabolic syndrome on subcutaneous microcirculation in obese patients. *J. Hypertens.* **2010**, *28*, 1708–1714. [CrossRef] [PubMed]
23. Rizzoni, D.; Porteri, E.; De Ciuceis, C.; Rodella, L.F.; Paiardi, S.; Rizzardi, N.; Platto, C.; Boari, G.E.; Pilu, A.; Tiberio, G.A.; et al. Hypertrophic remodeling of subcutaneous small resistance arteries in patients with Cushing's syndrome. *Clin. Endocrinol. Metab.* **2009**, *94*, 5010–5018. [CrossRef] [PubMed]
24. Rizzoni, D.; Porteri, E.; Giustina, A.; De Ciuceis, C.; Sleiman, I.; Boari, G.E.; Castellano, M.; Muiesan, M.L.; Bonadonna, S.; Burattin, A.; et al. Acromegalic patients show the presence of hypertrophic remodeling of subcutaneous small resistance arteries. *Hypertension* **2004**, *43*, 561–565. [CrossRef] [PubMed]
25. De Ciuceis, C.; Rossini, C.; Porteri, E.; La Boria, E.; Corbellini, C.; Mittempergher, F.; Di Betta, E.; Petroboni, B.; Sarkar, A.; Agabiti-Rosei, C.; et al. Circulating endothelial progenitor cells, microvascular density and fibrosis in obesity before and after bariatric surgery. *Blood Press.* **2013**, *22*, 165–172. [CrossRef]
26. Levy, B.I.; Schiffrin, E.L.; Mourad, J.J.; Agostini, D.; Vicaut, E.; Safar, M.E.; Struijker-Boudier, H.A. Impaired tissue perfusion: A pathology common to hypertension, obesity, and diabetes mellitus. *Circulation* **2008**, *118*, 968–976. [CrossRef]
27. Aalkjaer, C.; Heagerty, A.M.; Petersen, K.K.; Swales, J.D.; Mulvany, M.J. Evidence for increased media thickness, increased neuronal amine uptake, and depressed excitation—contraction coupling in isolated resistance vessels from essential hypertensives. *Circ. Res.* **1987**, *61*, 181–186. [CrossRef]
28. Schiffrin, E.L.; Hayoz, D. How to assess vascular remodelling in small and medium-sized muscular arteries in humans. *J. Hypertens.* **1997**, *15*, 571–584. [CrossRef]
29. Virdis, A.; Savoia, C.; Grassi, G.; Lembo, G.; Vecchione, C.; Seravalle, G.; Taddei, S.; Volpe, M.; Aganiti Rosei, E.; Rizzoni, D. Evaluation of microvascular structure in humans: A 'state-of-the-art' document of the Working Group on Macrovascular and Microvascular Alterations of the Italian Society of Arterial Hypertension. *J. Hypertens.* **2014**, *32*, 2120–2129. [CrossRef]
30. Rizzoni, D.; Mengozzi, A.; Masi, S.; Agabiti Rosei, C.; De Ciuceis, C.; Virdis, A. New noninvasive methods to evaluate microvascular structure and function. *Hypertension* **2022**, *79*, 874–886. [CrossRef]
31. De Ciuceis, C.; Agabiti Rosei, C.; Caletti, S.; Trapletti, V.; Coschignano, M.A.; Tiberio, G.A.M.; Duse, S.; Docchio, F.; Pasinetti, S.; Zambonardi, F.; et al. Comparison between invasive and noninvasive techniques of evaluation of microvascular structural alterations. *J. Hypertens.* **2018**, *36*, 1154–1163. [CrossRef]
32. Harazny, J.M.; Ritt, M.; Baleanu, D.; Ott, C.; Heckmann, J.; Schlaich, M.P.; Michelson, G.; Schmieder, R.E. Increased wall:lumen ratio of retinal arterioles in male patients with a history of a cerebrovascular event. *Hypertension* **2007**, *50*, 623–829. [CrossRef]
33. Ritt, M.; Harazny, J.M.; Ott, C.; Schlaich, M.P.; Schneider, M.P.; Michelson, G.; Schmieder, R.E. Analysis of retinal arteriolar structure in never-treated patients with essential hypertension. *J. Hypertens.* **2008**, *26*, 1427–1434. [CrossRef]
34. Koch, E.; Rosenbaum, D.; Brolly, A.; Sahel, J.A.; Chaumet-Riffaud, P.; Girerd, X.; Rossant, F.; Paques, M. Morphometric analysis of small arteries in the human retina using adaptive optics imaging: Relationship with BP and focal vascular changes. *J. Hypertens.* **2014**, *32*, 890–898. [CrossRef]
35. Heagerty, A.M.; Heerkens, E.H.; Izzard, A.S. Small artery structure and function in hypertension. *J. Cell. Mol. Med.* **2010**, *14*, 1037–1043. [CrossRef]
36. Heerkens, E.H.; Izzard, A.S.; Heagerty, A.M. Integrins, vascular remodeling, and hypertension. *Hypertension* **2007**, *49*, 1–4. [CrossRef]
37. Bakker, E.N.; Buus, C.L.; Spaan, J.A.; Perree, J.; Ganga, A.; Rolf, T.M.; Sorop, O.; Bramsen, L.H.; Mulvany, M.J.; Vanbavel, E. Small artery remodeling depends on tissue-type transglutaminase. *Circ. Res.* **2005**, *96*, 119–126. [CrossRef]
38. Rizzoni, D.; Paiardi, S.; Rodella, L.; Porteri, E.; De Ciuceis, C.; Rezzani, R.; Boari, G.E.; Zani, F.; Miclini, M.; Tiberio, G.A.; et al. Changes in extracellular matrix in subcutaneous small resistance arteries of patients with primary aldosteronism. *J. Clin. Endocrinol. Metab.* **2006**, *91*, 2638–2642. [CrossRef]
39. Lushchak, V.I. Free radicals, reactive oxygen species, oxidative stress and its classification. *Chem. Biol. Interact.* **2014**, *224*, 164–175. [CrossRef]
40. Griendling, K.K.; Camargo, L.L.; Rios, F.J.; Alves-Lopes, R.; Montezano, A.C.; Touyz, R.M. Oxidative stress and hypertension. *Circ. Res.* **2021**, *128*, 993–1020.
41. Intengan, H.D.; Schiffrin, E.L. Vascular remodeling in hypertension. *Hypertension* **2001**, *38*, 581–587. [CrossRef]

42. Touyz, R.M.; Alves-Lopes, R.; Rios, F.J.; Camargo, L.L.; Anagnostopoulou, A.; Arner, A.; Montezano, A.C. Vascular smooth muscle contraction in hypertension. *Cardiovasc. Res.* **2018**, *114*, 529–539. [CrossRef] [PubMed]
43. Mikolajczyk, T.P.; Szczepaniak, P.; Vidler, F.; Maffia, P.; Graham, G.J.; Guzik, T.J. Role of inflammatory chemokines in hypertension. *Pharmacol. Ther.* **2021**, *223*, 107799. [CrossRef] [PubMed]
44. Schiffrin, E.L.; Touyz, R.M. From bedside to bench to bedside: Role of renin-angiotensin-aldosterone system in remodeling of resistance arteries in hypertension. *Am. J. Physio. Circ. Physiol.* **2004**, *287*, H435–H446. [CrossRef] [PubMed]
45. Touyz, R.M.; Montezano, A.C. Angiotensin-(1–7) and vascular function. *Hypertension* **2018**, *71*, 68–69. [CrossRef] [PubMed]
46. Agabiti-Rosei, C.; Paini, A.; De Ciuceis, C.; Withers, S.; Greenstein, A.; Heagerty, A.M.; Rizzoni, D. Modulation of vascular reactivity by perivascular adipose tissue (PVAT). *Curr. Hypertens. Rep.* **2018**, *20*, 44. [CrossRef] [PubMed]
47. Greenstein, A.S.; Khavandi, K.; Withers, S.B.; Sonoyama, K.; Clancy, O.; Jeziorska, M.; Laing, I.; Yates, A.P.; Pemberton, P.W.; Malik, R.A.; et al. Local inflammation and hypoxia abolish the protective anticontractile properties of perivascular fat in obese patients. *Circulation* **2009**, *119*, 1661–1670. [CrossRef]
48. Meyer, M.R.; Fredette, N.C.; Barton, M.; Prossnitz, E.R. Regulation of vascular smooth muscle tone by adipose derived contracting factor. *PLoS ONE* **2013**, *8*, e79245. [CrossRef]
49. Drummond, G.R.; Vinh, A.; Guzik, T.J.; Sobey, C.G. Immune mechanisms of hypertension. *Nat. Rev. Immunol.* **2019**, *19*, 517–532. [CrossRef]
50. Harrison, D.G.; Vinh, A.; Lob, H.; Madhur, M.S. Role of the adaptive immune system in hypertension. *Curr. Opin. Pharmacol.* **2010**, *10*, 203–207. [CrossRef]
51. Shao, J.; Nangaku, M.; Miyata, T.; Inagi, R.; Yamada, K.; Kurokawa, K.; Fujita, T. Imbalance of T-cell subsets in angiotensin II-infused hypertensive rats with kidney injury. *Hypertension* **2003**, *42*, 31–38. [CrossRef]
52. Guzik, T.J.; Hoch, N.E.; Brown, K.A.; McCann, L.A.; Rahman, A.; Dikalov, S.; Goronzy, J.; Weyand, C.; Harrison, D.G. Role of the T cell in the genesis of angiotensin II induced hypertension and vascular dysfunction. *J. Exp. Med.* **2007**, *204*, 2449–2460. [CrossRef]
53. Barhoumi, T.; Kasal, D.A.; Li, M.W.; Shbat, L.; Laurant, P.; Neves, M.F.; Paradis, P.; Schiffrin, E.L. T regulatory lymphocytes prevent angiotensin II-induced hypertension and vascular injury. *Hypertension* **2011**, *57*, 469–476. [CrossRef]
54. Viel, E.C.; Lemarié, C.A.; Benkirane, K.; Paradis, P.; Schiffrin, E.L. Immune regulation and vascular inflammation in genetic hypertension. *Am. J. Physiol. Heart Circ. Physiol.* **2010**, *298*, H938–H944. [CrossRef]
55. Madhur, M.S.; Lob, H.E.; McCann, L.A.; Iwakura, Y.; Blinder, Y.; Guzik, T.J.; Harrison, D.G. Interleukin 17 promotes angiotensin II-induced hypertension and vascular dysfunction. *Hypertension* **2010**, *55*, 500–507. [CrossRef]
56. Wilck, N.; Matus, M.G.; Kearney, S.M.; Olesen, S.W.; Forslund, K.; Bartolomaeus, H.; Haase, S.; Mähler, A.; Balogh, A.; Markó, L.; et al. Salt-responsive gut commensal modulates TH17 axis and disease. *Nature* **2017**, *551*, 585–589. [CrossRef]
57. Carnevale, D.; Pallante, F.; Fardella, V.; Fardella, S.; Iacobucci, R.; Federici, M.; Cifelli, G.; De Lucia, M.; Lembo, G. The angiogenic factor PlGF mediates a neuroimmune interaction in the spleen to allow the onset of hypertension. *Immunity* **2014**, *41*, 737–752. [CrossRef]
58. Lori, A.; Perrotta, M.; Lembo, G.; Carnevale, D. The spleen: A hub connecting nervous and immune systems in cardiovascular and metabolic diseases. *Int. J. Mol. Sci.* **2017**, *18*, 1216. [CrossRef]
59. Marvar, P.J.; Thabet, S.R.; Guzik, T.J.; Lob, H.E.; McCann, L.A.; Weyand, C.; Gordon, F.J.; Harrison, D.G. Central and peripheral mechanisms of T-lymphocyte activation and vascular inflammation produced by angiotensin II-induced hypertension. *Circ. Res.* **2010**, *107*, 263–270. [CrossRef]
60. Lob, H.E.; Marvar, P.J.; Guzik, T.J.; Sharma, S.; McCann, L.A.; Weyand, C.; Gordon, F.J.; Harrison, D.G. Induction of hypertension and peripheral inflammation by reduction of extracellular superoxide dismutase in the central nervous system. *Hypertension* **2010**, *55*, 277–283. [CrossRef]
61. Case, A.J.; Zimmerman, M.C. Redox-regulated suppression of splenic T-lymphocyte activation in a model of sympathoexcitation. *Hypertension* **2015**, *65*, 916–923. [CrossRef]
62. Jones, B.H.; Standridge, M.K.; Moustaid, N. Angiotensin II increases lipogenesis in 3T3-L1 and human adipose cells. *Endocrinology* **1997**, *138*, 1512–1519. [CrossRef] [PubMed]
63. Masi, S.; Georgiopoulos, G.; Chiriacò, M.; Grassi, G.; Seravalle, G.; Savoia, C.; Volpe, M.; Taddei, S.; Rizzoni, D.; Virdis, A. The importance of endothelial dysfunction in resistance artery remodelling and cardiovascular risk. *Cardiovasc. Res.* **2020**, *116*, 429–437. [CrossRef] [PubMed]
64. Masi SRizzoni, D.; Taddei, S.; Widmer, R.J.; Montezano, A.C.; Lüscher, T.F.; Schiffrin, E.L.; Touyz, R.M.; Paneni, F.; Lerman, A.; Lanza, G.A.; et al. Assessment and pathophysiology of microvascular disease: Recent progress and clinical implications. *Eur. Heart J.* **2021**, *42*, 2590–2604. [CrossRef] [PubMed]
65. Mengozzi, A.; de Ciuceis, C.; Dell'oro, R.; Georgiopoulos, G.; Lazaridis, A.; Nosalski, R.; Pavlidis, G.; Tual-Chalot, S.; Agabiti-Rosei, C.; Anyfanti, P.; et al. The importance of microvascular inflammation in ageing and age-related diseases: A position paper from the ESH working group on small arteries, section of microvascular inflammation. *J. Hypertens.* **2023**, *ahead of print*. [CrossRef] [PubMed]
66. Park, J.B.; Schiffrin, E.L. Small artery remodeling is the most prevalent (earliest?) form of target organ damage in mild essential hypertension. *J. Hypertens.* **2001**, *19*, 921–930. [CrossRef]
67. Lever, A.F. Slow pressor mechanisms in hypertension: A role for hypertrophy of resistance vessels? *J. Hypertens.* **1986**, *4*, 515–524. [CrossRef]

68. Schiffrin, E.L. Reactivity of small blood vessel in hypertension: Relation with structural changes. *Hypertension* **1992**, *19* (Suppl. SII), II1–II9.
69. Rizzoni, D.; Agabiti-Rosei, C.; Agabiti-Rosei, E. Hemodynamic consequences of changes in microvascular structure. *Am. J. Hypertens.* **2017**, *30*, 939–946. [CrossRef]
70. Rizzoni, D.; Palombo, C.; Porteri, E.; Muiesan, M.L.; Kozàkovà, M.; La Canna, G.; Nardi, M.; Guelfi, D.; Salvetti, M.; Morizzo, C.; et al. Relationships between coronary vasodilator capacity and small artery remodeling in hypertensive patients. *J. Hypertens.* **2003**, *21*, 625–632. [CrossRef]
71. Agabiti Rosei, E.; Rizzoni, D.; Castellano, M.; Porteri, E.; Zulli, R.; Muiesan, M.L.; Bettoni, G.; Salvetti, M.; Muiesan, P.; Giulini, S.M. Media: Lumen ratio in human small resistance arteries is related to forearm minimal vascular resistance. *J. Hypertens.* **1995**, *13*, 341–347.
72. Muiesan, M.L.; Rizzoni, D.; Salvetti, M.; Porteri, E.; Monteduro, C.; Guelfi, D.; Castellano, M.; Garavelli, G.; Agabiti-Rosei, E. Structural changes in small resistance arteries and left ventricular geometry in patients with primary and secondary hypertension. *J. Hypertens.* **2002**, *20*, 1439–1444. [CrossRef]
73. Rizzoni, D.; Muiesan, M.L.; Porteri, E.; Salvetti, M.; Castellano, M.; Bettoni, G.; Tiberio, G.; Giulini, S.M.; Monteduro, C.; Garavelli, G.; et al. Relations between cardiac and vascular structure in patients with primary and secondary hypertension. *J. Am. Coll. Cardiol.* **1998**, *32*, 985–992. [CrossRef]
74. Rizzoni, D.; Porteri, E.; Boari, G.E.M.; De Ciuceis, C.; Sleiman, I.; Muiesan, M.L.; Castellano, M.; Miclini, M.; Agabiti-Rosei, E. Prognostic significance of small artery structure in hypertension. *Circulation* **2003**, *108*, 2230–2235. [CrossRef]
75. De Ciuceis, C.; Porteri, E.; Rizzoni, D.; Rizzardi, N.; Paiardi, S.; Boari, G.E.M.; Miclini, M.; Zani, F.; Muiesan, M.L.; Donato, F.; et al. Structural alterations of subcutaneous small arteries may predict major cardiovascular events in hypertensive patients. *Am. J. Hypertens.* **2007**, *20*, 846–852. [CrossRef]
76. Mathiassen, O.N.; Buus, N.H.; Sihm, I.; Thybo, N.K.; Mørn, B.; Schroeder, A.P.; Thygesen, K.; Aalkjaer, C.; Lederballe, O.; Mulvany, M.J.; et al. Small artery structure is an independent predictor of cardiovascular events in essential hypertension. *J. Hypertens.* **2007**, *25*, 1021–1026. [CrossRef]
77. Izzard, A.S.; Rizzoni, D.; Agabiti-Rosei, E.; Heagerty, A.M. Small artery structure and hypertension: Adaptive changes and target organ damage. *J. Hypertens.* **2005**, *23*, 247–250. [CrossRef]
78. Heagerty, A.M. Predicting hypertension complications from small artery structure. *J. Hypertens.* **2007**, *25*, 939–940. [CrossRef]
79. Ritt, M.; Harazny, J.M.; Ott, C.; Schneider, M.P.; Schlaich, M.P.; Michelson, G.; Schmieder, R.E. Wall-to-lumen ratio of retinal arterioles is related with urinary albumin excretion and altered vascular reactivity to infusion of the nitric oxide synthase inhibitor N-monomethyl-L-arginine. *J. Hypertens.* **2009**, *27*, 2201–2218. [CrossRef]
80. Rosenbaum, D.; Mattina, A.; Kock, E.; Rossant, F.; Gallo, A.; Kachenoura, N.; Paques, M.; Redheuil, A.; Gired, X. Effects of age, BP and antihypertensive treatment on retinal arterioles remodeling assessed by adaptive optics. *J. Hpertens.* **2016**, *34*, 1115–1122. [CrossRef]
81. Meixner, E.; Michelson, G. Measurement of retinal wall-to-lumen ratio by adaptive optics retinal camera: A clinical research. *Graefe's Arch. Clin. Exp. Ophthalmol.* **2015**, *253*, 1985–1995. [CrossRef]
82. De Ciuceis, C.; Agabiti-Rosei, C.; Malerba, P.; Rossini, C.; Chiarini, G.; Brami, V.; Famà, F.; Gaggero, A.; Nardin, M.; Lemoli, M.; et al. Prognostic significance of the wall to lumen ratio of retinal arterioles evaluated by adaptive optics in human hypertension. *Eur. J. Intern. Med.* **2023**, *41*, e63. [CrossRef]
83. Kopeva, K.; Grakova, E.; Maltseva, A.; Mochula, A.; Gusakova, A.; Smorgon, A.; Zavadovsky, K. Coronary microvascular dysfunction: Features and prognostic value. *J. Clin. Med.* **2023**, *12*, 2964. [CrossRef] [PubMed]
84. Agabiti-Rosei, E.; Heagerty, A.M.; Rizzoni, D. Effects of antihypertensive treatment on small artery remodelling. *J. Hypertens.* **2009**, *27*, 1107–1114. [CrossRef] [PubMed]
85. Savoia, C.; Touyz, R.M.; Endemann, D.H.; Pu, Q.; Ko, E.A.; De Ciuceis, C.; Schiffrin, E.L. Angiotensin receptor blocker added to previous antihypertensive agents on arteries of diabetic hypertensive patients. *Hypertension* **2006**, *48*, 271–277. [CrossRef] [PubMed]
86. Rizzoni, D.; Porteri, E.; De Ciuceis, C.; Sleiman, I.; Rodella, L.; Rezzani, R.; Paiardi, S.; Bianchi, R.; Ruggeri, G.; Boari, G.E.M.; et al. Effects of treatment with candesartan or enalapril on subcutaneous small resistance artery structure in hypertensive patients with NIDDM. *Hypertension* **2005**, *45*, 659–665. [CrossRef] [PubMed]
87. Rizzoni, D.; Agabiti Rosei, E. Small artery remodeling in diabetes mellitus. *Nutr. Metab. Cardiovasc. Dis.* **2009**, *19*, 587–592. [CrossRef]
88. De Ciuceis, C.; Savoia, C.; Arrabito, E.; Porteri, E.; Mazza, M.; Rossini, C.; Duse, S.; Semeraro, F.; Agabiti Rosei, C.; Alonzo, A.; et al. Effects of a long-term treatment with aliskiren or ramipril on structural alterations of subcutaneous small-resistance arteries of diabetic hypertensive patients. *Hypertension* **2014**, *64*, 717–724. [CrossRef]
89. Jumar, A.; Ott, C.; Kistner, I.; Friedrich, S.; Schmidt, S.; Harazny, J.M.; Schmieder, R.E. Effect of aliskiren on vascular remodelling in small retinal circulation. *J. Hypertens.* **2015**, *33*, 2491–2499. [CrossRef]
90. De Ciuceis, C.; Salvetti, M.; Rossini, C.; Muiesan, M.L.; Paini, A.; Duse, S.; La Boria, E.; Semeraro, F.; Cancarini, A.; Agabiti Rosei, C.; et al. Effect of antihypertensive treatment on microvascular structure, central BP and oxidative stress in patients with mild essential hypertension. *J. Hypertens.* **2014**, *32*, 565–574. [CrossRef]

91. Buus, N.H.; Mathiassen, O.N.; Fenger-Grøn, M.; Præstholm, M.N.; Sihm, I.; Thybo, N.K.; Schroeder, A.P.; Thygesen, K.; Aalkjær, C.; Pedersen, O.L.; et al. Small artery structure during antihypertensive therapy is an independent predictor of cardiovascular events in essential hypertension. *J. Hypertens.* **2013**, *31*, 791–797. [CrossRef]
92. Buus, N.H.; Bøttcher, M.; Jørgensen, C.G.; Christensen, K.L.; Thygesen, K.; Nielsen, T.T.; Mulvany, M.J. Myocardial perfusion during long-term angiotensin-converting enzyme inhibition or beta-blockade in patients with essential hypertension. *Hypertension* **2004**, *44*, 465–470. [CrossRef]
93. Rossi, G.P.; Bolognesi, M.; Rizzoni, D.; Seccia, T.M.; Piva, A.; Porteri, E.; Tiberio, G.A.; Giulini, S.M.; Agabiti-Rosei, E.; Pessina, A.C. Vascular remodeling and duration of hypertension predict outcome of adrenalectomy in primary aldosteronism patients. *Hypertension* **2008**, *51*, 1366–1371. [CrossRef]
94. Debbabi, H.; Uzan, L.; Mourad, J.J.; Safar, M.; Levy, B.I.; Tibirica', E. Increased skin capillary density in treated essential hypertensive patients. *Am. J. Hypertens.* **2006**, *19*, 477–483. [CrossRef]
95. Antonios, T.F. Microvascular rarefaction in hypertension--reversal or over-correction by treatment? *Am. J. Hypertens.* **2006**, *19*, 484–485. [CrossRef]
96. Laurent, S.; Agabiti-Rosei, C.; Bruno, R.M.; Rizzoni, D. Microcirculation and macrocirculation in hypertension: A dangerous cross-link? *Hypertension* **2022**, *79*, 479–490. [CrossRef]
97. Laurent, S.; Boutouyrie, P. Arterial stiffness and hypertension in the elderly. *Front. Cardiovasc. Med.* **2020**, *7*, 544302. [CrossRef]
98. Rizzoni, D.; Rizzoni, M.; Nardin, M.; Chiarini, G.; Agabiti-Rosei, C.; Aggiusti, C.; Paini, A.; Salvetti, M.; Muiesan, M.L. Vascular aging and disease of the small vessels. *High. Blood Press. Cardiovasc. Prev.* **2019**, *26*, 183–189. [CrossRef]
99. Laurent, S.; Boutouyrie, P. The structural factor of hypertension. *Circ. Res.* **2015**, *116*, 1007–1021. [CrossRef]
100. Laurent, S.; Agabiti-Rosei, E. The cross-talk between the macro- and the microcirculation. In *Early Vascular Aging (EVA): New Directions in Cardiovascular Protection*; Nilsson, P., Olsen, M.H., Laurent, S., Eds.; Elsevier: Amsterdam, The Netherlands, 2015; pp. 105–118.
101. Sasaki, R.; Yamano, S.; Yamamoto, Y.; Minami, S.; Yamamoto, J.; Nakashima, T.; Takaoka, M.; Hashimoto, T. Vascular remodeling of the carotid artery in patients with untreated essential hypertension increases with age. *Hypertens. Res.* **2002**, *25*, 373–379. [CrossRef]
102. Vasan, R.S.; Pan, S.; Xanthakis, V.; Beiser, A.; Larson, M.G.; Seshadri, S.; Mitchell, G.F. Arterial Stiffness and long-term risk of health outcomes: The Framingham Heart Study. *Hypertension* **2022**, *79*, 1045–1056. [CrossRef]
103. Laurent, S.; Briet, M.; Boutouyrie, P. Large and small artery cross-talk and recent morbidity-mortality trials in hypertension. *Hypertension* **2009**, *54*, 388–392. [CrossRef] [PubMed]
104. Mulè, G.; Cottone, S.; Vadalà, A.; Volpe, V.; Mezzatesta, G.; Mongiovì, R.; Piazza, G.; Nardi, E.; Andronico, G.; Cerasola, G. Relationship between albumin excretion rate and aortic stiffness in untreated essential hypertensive patients. *J. Intern. Med.* **2004**, *256*, 22–29. [CrossRef] [PubMed]
105. Muiesan, M.L.; Salvetti, M.; Rizzoni, D.; Paini, A.; Agabiti-Rosei, C.; Aggiusti, C.; Bertacchini, F.; Stassaldi, D.; Gavazzi, A.; Porteri, E.; et al. Pulsatile hemodynamics and microcirculation: Evidence for a close relationship in hypertensive patients. *Hypertension* **2013**, *61*, 130–136. [CrossRef] [PubMed]
106. Ott, C.; Raff, U.; Harazny, J.M.; Michelson, G.; Schmieder, R.E. Central pulse pressure is an independent determinant of vascular remodeling in the retinal circulation. *Hypertension* **2013**, *61*, 1340–1345. [CrossRef]
107. Salvetti, M.; Agabiti Rosei, C.; Paini, A.; Aggiusti, C.; Cancarini, A.; Duse, S.; Semeraro, F.; Rizzoni, D.; Agabiti Rosei, E.; Muiesan, M.L. Relationship of wall-to-lumen ratio of retinal arterioles with clinic and 24-hour BP. *Hypertension* **2014**, *63*, 1110–1115. [CrossRef]
108. Rizzoni, D.; Muiesan, M.L.; Porteri, E.; De Ciuceis, C.; Boari, G.E.; Salvetti, M.; Paini, A.; Agabiti Rosei, E. Vascular remodeling, macro- and microvessels: Therapeutic implications. *Blood Press.* **2009**, *18*, 242–246. [CrossRef]
109. Laurent, S.; Rizzoni, D. Targeting central BP through the micro-and macrocirculation cross-talk. In *Early Vascular Aging (EVA): New Directions in Cardiovascular Protection*; Nilsson, P., Olsen, M.H., Laurent, S., Eds.; Elsevier: Amsterdam, The Netherlands, 2015; pp. 297–306.
110. Mancia Chairperson, G.; Kreutz Co-Chair, R.; Brunström, M.; Burnier, M.; Grassi, G.; Januszewicz, A.; Muiesan, M.L.; Tsioufis, K.; Agabiti-Rosei, E.; Algharably, E.A.E.; et al. 2023 ESH Guidelines for the management of arterial hypertension The Task Force for the management of arterial hypertension of the European Society of Hypertension Endorsed by the European Renal Association (ERA) and the International Society of Hypertension (ISH). *J. Hypertens.* **2023**, *ahead of print*.

Disclaimer/Publisher's Note: The statements, opinions and data contained in all publications are solely those of the individual author(s) and contributor(s) and not of MDPI and/or the editor(s). MDPI and/or the editor(s) disclaim responsibility for any injury to people or property resulting from any ideas, methods, instructions or products referred to in the content.

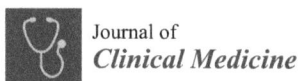 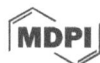

Article

Metabolic Syndrome and Its Components Have a Different Presentation and Impact as Cardiovascular Risk Factors in Psoriatic and Rheumatoid Arthritis

Fabiola Atzeni [1,*], Laura La Corte [1], Mariateresa Cirillo [1], Manuela Giallanza [1], James Galloway [2] and Javier Rodríguez-Carrio [3,4]

1. Rheumatology Unit, Department of Experimental and Internal Medicine, University of Messina, 98125 Messina, Italy
2. Centre for Rheumatic Disease, Kings College London, London WC2R 2LS, UK
3. Area of Immunology, Department of Functional Biology, Faculty of Medicine, University of Oviedo, 33006 Oviedo, Spain; rodriguezcjavier@uniovi.es
4. Instituto de Investigacíon Sanitaria del Principado de Asturias (ISPA), 33011 Oviedo, Spain
* Correspondence: atzenifabiola@hotmail.com

Abstract: Patients with chronic inflammatory arthritis have a higher cardiovascular (CV) risk than the general population. Traditional CV risk factors are clearly implicated, while the impact of metabolic syndrome (MetS) is less defined. The aim of this study was to compare MetS prevalence and impact on the CV risk in psoriatic arthritis (PsA) versus rheumatoid arthritis (RA). A retrospective analysis of real-world data of PsA and RA patients referred to a rheumatology clinic was conducted. The following data were extracted and compared: demographic data; clinical data; presence of traditional CV risk factors and MetS. Univariate and multivariate models were used to compare the impact of MetS and its components in patients with PsA versus RA. Overall, 170 patients were included (PsA: 78; RA; 92). The two groups differed significantly in mean age, disease duration, and presence of MetS, while other variables were comparable. Univariate and multivariate analysis identified distinct predictors of MetS in PsA (hypertension) and RA (dyslipidemia). The history of CV events was similar in the two groups. Predictors of CV events were MetS and most of its components in PsA, while dyslipidemia was the strongest predictor in RA. These associations were stronger in PsA than in RA. In conclusion, the impact of MetS and its components is different in PsA and RA. The association of these risk factors with CV events is stronger in PsA than in RA. This suggests the implication of different mechanisms, which may require distinct strategies for the prevention of CV events in PsA and RA.

Keywords: metabolic syndrome; arthritis; psoriatic; arthritis; rheumatoid; heart disease risk factors

Citation: Atzeni, F.; La Corte, L.; Cirillo, M.; Giallanza, M.; Galloway, J.; Rodríguez-Carrio, J. Metabolic Syndrome and Its Components Have a Different Presentation and Impact as Cardiovascular Risk Factors in Psoriatic and Rheumatoid Arthritis. *J. Clin. Med.* **2023**, *12*, 5031. https://doi.org/10.3390/jcm12155031

Academic Editor: Kikuo Isoda

Received: 4 July 2023
Revised: 28 July 2023
Accepted: 28 July 2023
Published: 31 July 2023

Copyright: © 2023 by the authors. Licensee MDPI, Basel, Switzerland. This article is an open access article distributed under the terms and conditions of the Creative Commons Attribution (CC BY) license (https://creativecommons.org/licenses/by/4.0/).

1. Introduction

Rheumatoid arthritis (RA) is associated with an increased risk of cardiovascular (CV) morbidity [1–4]. RA is now widely recognized as an independent risk factor for CV disease, similar to diabetes [5,6]. An elevated risk of CV and cerebrovascular events compared to the general population has also been reported for psoriatic arthritis (PsA) [2,7]. The increased CV risk associated with RA and other chronic inflammatory conditions is likely caused by the complex interplay of traditional CV risk factors, chronic systemic inflammation, and side effects related to the use of certain antirheumatic medications [8,9]. Although a similar figure has been proposed for PsA, to what extent these arthropathies differ is yet to be clarified.

Traditional CVD risk factors include older age, male gender, smoking, hypertension, dyslipidemia, and diabetes [10]. A specific clustering of metabolic and CV factors, known as metabolic syndrome (MetS), has also been found to substantially increase the risk of

CV events [11]. The impact of MetS on the CV risk in inflammatory arthritis is yet to be clarified.

Several studies have investigated the epidemiology of traditional CV risk factors and MetS in patients with RA and PsA [9,10,12–15]. A study based on the data from a US health insurance claim database estimated the prevalence of CV risk factors during the 12 months before diagnosis and their incidence rates during follow-up in patients with RA, PsA or psoriasis [12]. The prevalence was elevated in all diseases and ranged from 17% to 20% for hypertension, 6% to 8% for diabetes mellitus, 10% to 12% for hyperlipidemia, and 4% to 6% for obesity; incidence rates of CV risk factors were also high [12]. The largest study covering this topic, using a medical record database from United Kingdom, revealed a higher prevalence of all CV risk factors in PsA patients, whereas only diabetes and obesity were found to be increased in RA. The incidence of new diagnosis of hypertension, hyperlipidemia and diabetes mellitus was elevated in both RA and PsA [13]. However, MetS occurrence has received less attention. A recent meta-analysis compared MetS prevalence in patients with PsA versus RA and found that PsA patients were 1.6 times more likely to present with MetS than their RA counterparts [14]. Nevertheless, whether MetS clinical presentation and their components were comparable across conditions is unclear.

Overall, the epidemiologic evidence confirms the association between chronic inflammatory joint diseases and traditional CV risk factors and suggests that this association may differ among diseases [12,14,15]. These differences need to be further investigated as they may have an impact on the prevention and management of CV disease in RA and PsA. In fact, according to the 2015/2016 European Alliance of Associations for Rheumatology (EULAR) recommendations for the management of CV risk in patients with RA and other inflammatory joint disorders, current CV risk scores developed for the general population should be multiplied by 1.5 in subjects with RA [16]. However, most of the evidence came from RA studies, so CV risk management in other inflammatory joint disorders, including PsA, remains poorly established and whether different approaches may be needed is unknown.

The aim of this study was to compare the profile of traditional CV risk factors and MetS in patients with PsA and RA. The primary objective of our analysis was to evaluate the prevalence of MetS and its components in PsA versus RA real-world patients. Our secondary aim was to analyze the impact of MetS and its components on the occurrence of CV events in PsA versus RA real-world patients.

2. Materials and Methods

2.1. Study Design and Patients

This was a real-life observational study performed to primarily investigate the impact of MetS and its components in patients with PsA and RA referring to a Tertiary level rheumatology clinic in Italy between 2017 and 2022. The charts of all patients with PsA or RA referred to the clinic were reviewed between January 2021 and August 2021. Following data collection (baseline), patients were followed-up for an additional 12 months to gain insight into the course of MetS and its components. All patients with PsA fulfilled the 2006 Classification for Psoriatic Arthritis (CASPAR) criteria [17] and all patients with RA fulfilled the 2010 American College of Rheumatology (ACR)/EULAR criteria for RA [18]. MetS was defined according to the American Heart Association (AHA)/National Heart, Lung, and Blood Institute (NHLBI) by the presence of ≥ 3 of the following criteria: (1) fasting glycemia ≥ 100 mg/dL or on antihyperglycemic treatment; (2) blood pressure $\geq 130/86$ mm Hg or on antihypertension treatment; (3) triglycerides ≥ 150 mg/dl or on treatment to lower triglycerides; (4) high-density lipoprotein cholesterol (HDL-C) < 40 mg/dl in men and <50 mg/dl in women; (5) waist circumference ≥ 102 cm in men and ≥ 88 cm in women [19]. All patients gave informed consent to participate in the study, which was conducted in accordance with the Declaration of Helsinki and local regulations. The Institutional Review Board granted an exemption of ethics committee approval due to local regulations, as the participants underwent clinical and clinimetric examinations according to routine protocols used at the recruiting hospital and no further procedures were needed.

2.2. Parameters Analyzed

The following parameters were collected from patient charts: demographic and clinical characteristics (presence of autoantibodies; C-reactive protein levels; disease duration); presence of CV risk factors, including smoking, MetS, diabetes mellitus, arterial hypertension, and dyslipidemia; occurrence of CV events (ischemic heart disease, stroke, transient ischemic attack, heart failure or peripheral arterial disease). During the 12-month observation period following data extraction, the CV risk profile of the patients and the occurrence of CV events were recorded using the definitions and procedures described above. All data were anonymized before further analysis. The research process and analysis pipeline are summarized in Figure 1.

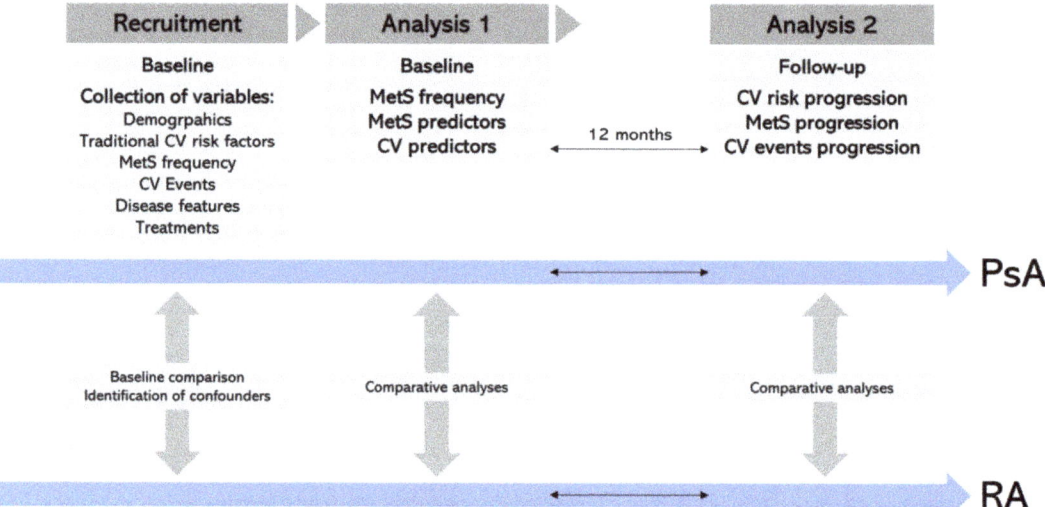

Figure 1. Research flowchart. Research flowchart showing the main steps (recruitment and analysis), stages (baseline and follow-up), and analysis pipeline of the present study. Gray, vertical arrows represent the main statistical analyses performed to compare RA and PsA groups according to the objectives of the study.

2.3. Statistical Analysis

Data were analyzed by descriptive statistics and variables were summarized here as absolute numbers and percentages or mean values ± standard deviation (SD), as appropriate. Differences between groups were evaluated using chi-square tests and binomial logistic regression analyses. Odds ratios (OR) and 95% confidence intervals (CI) were computed. Confounding factors were entered as covariables in the multivariate models. Statistical analysis was performed using the IBM SPSS Statistics software, version 27.0; IBM SPSS Statistics; Irving, TX, USA.

3. Results

3.1. Characteristics of PsA and RA Patients

Patients with PsA were significantly younger and had a significantly shorter disease duration than patients with RA (Table 1). As expected, the presence of autoantibodies (anti-citrullinated protein antibodies, ACPA, and rheumatoid factor, RF) was significantly higher in RA than in PsA patients (Table 1).

Table 1. Demographic and clinical characteristics of patients.

	PsA (n = 78)	RA (n = 92)	p-Value	p-Value (Age-Adjusted)
Demographic features				
Age, years, mean (±SD)	45.23 (16.99)	60.81 (13.19)	<0.001	
Sex, n (%)				
Female	54 (69.2)	70 (76.1)	0.316	
Male	24 (30.8)	22 (23.9)		
Clinical features				
RF, n (%)	6 (7.7)	54 (58.7)	<0.001	
ACPA, n (%)	4 (5.1)	53 (57.6)	<0.001	
CRP, mg/L, mean (±SD)	5.14 (7.91)	6.63 (9.21)	0.047	
Disease duration, months, mean (±SD)	18.86 (48.43)	176.85 (169.77)	<0.001	
Treatments				
Steroids, n (%)	12 (15.4)	37 (40.2)		
NSAIDs, n (%)	39 (50.0)	0		
Methotrexate, n (%)	13 (16.7)	44 (47.8)		
Leflunomide, n (%)	3 (3.8)	7 (7.6)		
Sulfasalazine, n (%)	5 (6.4)	4 (4.3)		
Anti-TNF, n (%)	49 (62.8)	23 (29.5)		
Anti-IL6-R, n (%)	0	8 (8.7)		
Abatacept, n (%)	0	32 (34.8)		
JAK inhibitors, n (%)	0	6 (6.5)		
Anti-CD20, n (%)	0	2 (2.2)		
Apremilast, n (%)	5 (6.4)	0		
Anti-IL17, n (%)	10 (12.8)	0		
Anti-IL12, n (%)	3 (3.8)	0		
Anti-IL23, n (%)	1 (1.3)	0		
Traditional CV risk factors				
Smoking, n (%)	22 (28.2)	26 (28.3)	0.836	0.997
MetS, n (%)	40 (51.3)	25 (27.2)	0.003	0.002
Diabetes mellitus, n (%)	26 (38.3)	33 (35.9)	0.823	0.516
Hypertension, n (%)	44 (56.4)	51 (55.4)	0.749	0.013
Dyslipidemia, n (%)	56 (71.8)	26 (28.3)	<0.001	<0.001
History of CV events				
CV events [a], n (%)	22 (28.2)	24 (26.1)	0.602	0.304

[a] Composite of ischemic heart disease, stroke, transient ischemic attack, heart failure, or peripheral arteriopathy reported in the charts of PsA and RA patients. ACPA, anti-citrullinated protein anti bodies; CRP, C-reactive protein; CV, cardiovascular; MetS, metabolic syndrome; PsA, psoriatic arthritis; RA, rheumatoid arthritis; RF, rheumatoid factor.

MetS was reported in 51.3% of PsA patients versus 27.2% of RA patients ($p = 0.002$) and dyslipidemia was reported in 71.8% of PsA patients versus 28.3% of RA patients ($p < 0.001$); these differences remained statistically significant after adjusting for the age difference (Table 1). Importantly, disease duration was not associated with MetS occurrence in RA ($p = 0.114$) nor in PsA patients ($p = 0.234$). The prevalence of the other CV risk factors considered (smoking, diabetes mellitus, hypertension) was similar in the two groups (Table 1). Moreover, the prevalence of these risk factors failed to show any association with disease duration in both conditions (Supplementary Table S1). Similar proportions of patients reported a history of CV events (28.2% of PsA patients versus 26.1% of RA patients, $p = 0.304$).

3.2. Association between the Presence of Autoantibodies and CV Risk Factors

A slight association between ACPA and smoking habit was found in RA (OR 2.55, 95% CI 0.65 to 6.89; $p = 0.060$), whereas there were no associations between the presence of ACPA and the other traditional risk factors. The autoantibody RF was associated in RA patients with diabetes mellitus (OR 0.43, 95% CI 0.18 to 1.02; $p = 0.054$). Autoantibodies were found to be unrelated to the occurrence of CV events in patients with RA (ACPA: $p = 0.691$, RF: $p = 0.600$). The small number of PsA patients with autoantibodies prevented the analysis of the association between autoantibody positivity and CV risk factors and events.

3.3. Predictors of Traditional CV Risk Factors and MetS

The occurrence of hypertension was strongly related to MetS occurrence in PsA (OR 17.88, 95% CI 5.51 to 58.00; $p < 0.001$), while it was associated with MetS (OR 11.16, 95% CI 2.99 to 41.61; $p < 0.001$), age (OR 1.09, 95% CI 1.04 to 1.14; $p < 0.001$) and dyslipidemia (OR 2.88, 95% CI 1.07 to 7.78; $p = 0.036$) in RA patients in univariate analyses. Smoking was unrelated to the other risk factors in both conditions. Dyslipidemia was slightly associated with hypertension in RA but not in PsA (Supplementary Tables S2 and S3, Supplementary Materials). Importantly, age was ruled out as a potential confounding factor in our analyses. Finally, equivalent results were observed when these associations were adjusted by treatment usage.

Univariate analyses also found a strong correlation between the occurrence of MetS and both diabetes mellitus (OR 20.71, 95% CI 4.34 to 98.78; $p < 0.001$) and hypertension (OR 17.88, 95% CI 5.51 to 57.98; $p < 0.001$) in PsA. The main predictors of MetS in RA, according to univariate analysis, were dyslipidemia (OR 18.73, 95% CI 5.77 to 60.81; $p < 0.001$) and hypertension (OR 11.16, 95% CI 2.99 to 41.61; $p < 0.001$). Multivariate analysis confirmed the differences between PsA and RA in terms of MetS predictors (Table 2): hypertension and dyslipidemia were MetS predictors in PsA, while diabetes mellitus, hypertension, and dyslipidemia were MetS predictors in RA. Notably, hypertension and dyslipidemia were the strongest MetS predictors in PsA and RA, respectively, (Table 2). Of note, age was found not to be a significant predictor in any condition, thus ruling out a major confounding effect. Similarly, adjusting for disease duration did not attenuate these associations (Table 2). Finally, adjusting for NSAIDs or anti-TNF agents did not change these results (Tables S4 and S5, Supplementary Materials). Equivalent results were observed for the rest of medications.

All these results suggest not only that not all MetS components were consistently associated with MetS presence, but also that significant differences in predictors as well as their strength of associations were observed across conditions.

3.4. Predictors of CV Events

Univariate analysis showed that MetS and some of its components (diabetes mellitus and hypertension) accounted for the history of CV events in PsA [OR (95% CI); MetS: 34.83 (4.30 to 281.99); diabetes mellitus: 7.99 (2.61 to 24.41); and hypertension: 31.00 (3.87 to 284.43); $p < 0.001$ for all associations]. In RA, MetS was also a predictor of CV events (OR 5.20, (1.84 to 14.70); $p = 0.001$), but the predictive components of MetS with statistical significance were hypertension (OR 4.27, 95% CI 1.43 to 12.77; $p = 0.007$) and dyslipidemia (OR 5.00, 95% CI 1.83 to 13.66; $p < 0.001$), while diabetes mellitus was not significantly associated with CV events. The associations were markedly stronger in PsA than in RA. Multivariate analysis confirmed these associations (Table 3): hypertension and MetS were the only predictors of CV events in PsA, while dyslipidemia was the only factor to be significantly associated with CV events in RA. Again, disease duration failed to show any association in both conditions (Table 3). Finally, equivalent findings were observed after adjusting for treatments (Table S6, Supplementary Material).

The fact that the association of traditional risk factors and MetS with CV events was stronger in PsA than in RA was corroborated by the greater coefficient of determination in PsA than in RA, indicating that in PsA approximately 70% of the variance in CV events could be explained by the variables entered in the model, compared with only 30% in RA. Adjusting for treatments did not attenuate these coefficients, thus ruling out a major effect of medications and pointing to a role of disease characteristics.

Table 2. Predictors of MetS occurrence in patients with PsA and RA. Multivariate analysis using an age-adjusted logistic regression model; the coefficient of determination R^2 of each model is indicated.

	OR (95% CI)	p-Value	OR (95% CI) [Adjusted]	p-Value [Adjusted]
PsA (R^2 = 0.543)				
Age	0.979 (0.929–1.033)	0.445	0.981 (0.933–1.033)	0.468
Sex	0.693 (0.153–3.142)	0.634	0.565 (0.121–2.634)	0.467
Smoking	2.041 (0.442–9.429)	0.361	2.626 (0.459–15.029)	0.278
Diabetes mellitus	6.465 (0.952–43.899)	0.056	6.638 (0.899–49.545)	0.065
Hypertension	11.818 (2.046–58.053)	0.002	10.457 (1.853–59.007)	0.002
Dyslipidemia	5.190 (1.118–24.092)	0.035	5.190 (1.383–49.273)	0.021
RA (R^2 = 0.669)				
Age	0.976 (0.914–1.043)	0.473	0.978 (0.915–1.046)	0.519
Sex	1.568 (0.272–9.041)	0.615	1.466 (0.250–8.583)	0.672
Smoking	0.404 (0.068–2.387)	0.317	0.395 (0.067–24487)	0.307
Diabetes mellitus	15.586 (2.418–100.453)	0.004	13.709 (2.057–91.389)	0.007
Hypertension	20.447 (2.589–161.057)	0.004	18.676 (2.359–147.859)	0.006
Dyslipidemia	43.296 (6.823–274.756)	<0.001	39.039 (6.068–251.159)	<0.001

CI, confidence interval; OR, odds ratio; RA, rheumatoid arthritis; PsA, psoriatic arthritis. OR (95% CI) [adjusted] and p-value [adjusted]: OR and p-values obtained in a multivariate analysis adjusted by disease duration.

Table 3. Predictors of cardiovascular events at baseline. Multivariate analysis using an age-adjusted logistic regression model; the coefficient of determination R^2 of each model is indicated. Baseline is defined as the time of data collection.

	p-Value	OR (95% CI)
PsA (R^2 = 0.693)		
Smoking	0.154	3.884 (0.602–25.058)
MetS	0.031	22.611 (1.323–58.655)
Diabetes mellitus	0.250	0.276 (0.031–2.468)
Hypertension	0.010	50.302 (2.583–97.661)
Sex	0.445	0.504 (0.087–2.921)
Dyslipidemia	0.241	3.225 (0.455–22.879)
CRP	0.560	0.950 (0.799–1.129)
Age	0.740	0.986 (0.910–1.069)
Disease duration	0.134	0.965 (0.921–1.011)
RA (R^2 = 0.296)		
Smoking	0.298	1.896 (0.568–6.239)
MetS	0.702	1.358 (0.282–6.531)
Diabetes mellitus	0.413	1.896 (0.568–6.329)
Hipertensión	0.129	3.004 (0.726–12.434)
Sex	0.586	0.586 (0.174–2.688)
Dyslipidemia	0.011	4.502 (1.118–16.125)
CRP	0.518	1.020 (0.961–1.081)
Age	0.669	1.012 (0.960–1.066)
Disease duration	0.329	0.997 (0.992–1.003)

CI, confidence interval; CRP, C-reactive protein; OR, odds ratio; RA, rheumatoid arthritis; PsA, psoriatic arthritis.

3.5. Outcomes after 12 Months

To evaluate the potential progression of MetS and its components in PsA and RA in the real-world setting, patients were followed up for 12 months, following recruitment in the study. Changes in the occurrence of CV risk factors and MetS over the 12-month follow-up of both PsA and RA patients were negligeable (Table 4).

Table 4. Changes in the occurrence of CV risk factors and CV events in patients with PsA and RA observed for 12 months. Baseline is defined as the time of data collection.

	Presence of CV Risk Factors, n(%)		
	Baseline	12-Month Follow-Up	*p*-Value
Patients with PsA (N = 78)			
MetS	40 (51.3)	41 (52.6)	0.207
Diabetes mellitus	26 (33.3)	26 (33.3)	
Hypertension	44 (56.4)	43 (55.1)	0.159
Patients with RA (N = 92)			
MetS	25 (27.2)	25 (27.2)	
Diabetes mellitus	33 (35.9)	33 (35.9)	
Hypertension	51 (55.4)	51 (55.4)	
	Occurrence of CV Events, n(%)		
	Baseline	12-Month Follow-Up	*p*-Value
Patients with PsA (N = 78)			
Ischemic heart disease	13 (16.7)	13 (16.7)	
Arrhythmia/Atrial fibrillation	12 (15.4)	8 (10.3)	0.023
Stroke	4 (5.1)	4 (5.1)	
Transient ischemic attack/Peripheral arterial disease	18 (23.1)	18 (23.1)	
Patients with RA (N = 92)			
Ischemic heart disease	8 (8.7)	8 (8.7)	
Arrhythmia/Atrial fibrillation	4 (4.3)	4 (4.3)	
Stroke	4 (4.3)	4 (4.3)	
Transient ischemic attack/Peripheral arterial disease	8 (8.7)	8 (8.7)	

CV, cardiovascular; MetS, metabolic syndrome; PsA, psoriatic arthritis; RA, rheumatoid arthritis.

4. Discussion

The present study confirms that several differences exist between PsA and RA in the profile of traditional CV risk factors leading to MetS occurrence and the association of these factors with the history of CV events. According to our findings, patients with PsA had a significantly higher prevalence of MetS and dyslipidemia compared to patients with RA, while the frequency of other traditional CV risk factors was comparable. Notably, the rates of CV events reported before data collection were relatively high in both groups (>25%) as expected, but similar. PsA and RA were also found to differ in terms of predictors of MetS: hypertension was the strongest predictor in PsA, while in RA the strongest predictor was dyslipidemia. Furthermore, MetS and hypertension were both shown to be significantly associated with a history of CV events in patients with PsA; in RA, only dyslipidemia was confirmed as a predictor of CV events in a multivariate model, despite exhibiting a lower frequency compared to PsA patients. Importantly, these findings remained after adjusting for age and disease duration, thereby excluding a major confounding role and pointing towards a role for disease characteristics in determining these associations. Moreover, adjusting for treatment usages did not change these associations, hence reinforcing this notion. Furthermore, equivalent differences in the profiles of associations were observed in a well characterized prospective cohort from Spain comparing RA, PsA and ankylosing spondylitis patients [20]. Taken together, these findings suggest that, although proof-of-concept, quantitative and qualitative differences regarding MetS presence could occur between RA and PsA, with potential impact on CV records across different arthropathies in real-world populations.

Several authors have investigated the role of traditional CV risk factors in chronic inflammatory conditions, with most of the efforts being devoted to RA. A study comparing the incidence of CV events in patients with RA versus the general population confirmed the higher incidence in RA [21]. After adjusting for traditional risk factors, the incidence decreased only slightly suggesting that other mechanisms are responsible for the increased rates of CV events in RA patients. Systemic inflammation, known from other studies to be involved in the development of atherosclerosis, was suggested as a possible contributor [21]. In a subsequent study, three groups of variables were tested for their effects on carotid atherosclerosis in RA, namely demographic, traditional CV risk factors, and RA manifestations [22]. The study found that demographic characteristics (age and gender) best explained the variability of atherosclerosis. The study also showed that, after adjusting for the effects of age and gender, both traditional CV risk factors and RA manifestations had a greater impact on atherosclerosis [22]. This, along with the evidence from other studies, suggested that traditional CV factors and inflammation may interact and promote atherogenesis [22,23]. An elegant study put this association into numbers, reporting that traditional CV risk factors accounted for 49% of the total risk and non-traditional risk factors (RA manifestations, inflammation, etc.) accounted for a smaller proportion (30.3%) [24]. Our results align with this evidence and may expand our knowledge about the complex interplay of CV risk factors in chronic inflammatory diseases. Traditional CV risk factors, according to the available evidence, account only for a limited fraction of the variance, which suggests the participation of other risk factors. Our findings show that MetS was independently associated with a history of CV events in multivariate models, at least in PsA, suggesting that MetS occurrence may have an additional impact, beyond that of its individual components, probably due to the existence of synergistic effects. Our findings revealed that MetS is present in a significant proportion of established PsA patients, which emphasizes the need of systematically screening and managing MetS in arthropathies. In fact, a recent meta-analysis reported a prevalence of MetS in PsA populations of 29.1%, ranging from 23.5% to 62.9% in the literature, which is in line with our cohort. Although a slightly lower prevalence was observed in a recent cohort from Spain (30.6%) [20,25], it must be noted that our cohort exhibited a higher frequency of dyslipidemia, which may explain the higher prevalence herein reported. As a consequence, MetS should be considered as a separate entity in clinical practice and routine screening of CV risk factors, but this situation may be different in different joint diseases. In this regard, it is tempting to speculate if different presentations of MetS can lead to different endotypes or pathotypes that require distinct management strategies, including screening and treatment algorithms. This may facilitate the take-decision process in the clinical setting and ensure a tailored clinical process. In fact, personalized medicine approaches have been already suggested for MetS [26–29], which may strengthen this notion.

In our analysis, the strongest predictor of CV events in patients with RA was dyslipidemia, which is known to be largely influenced by inflammation in RA [24,30]. Similar results were obtained a large, prospective Spanish cohort [25]. Importantly, this association was stronger in RA compared to PsA, despite the high prevalence in the latter, hence pointing to a relevance that may not be captured by its conventional definition/approach. It can therefore be speculated that the strong association observed may be caused, at least in part, by the lipid-inflammation crosstalk. The interaction of systemic inflammation with traditional CV risk factors is not fully understood. In RA, the evidence shows that systemic inflammation can modify traditional risk factors, especially lipid levels [3]. For example, in active RA, inflammation has been shown to modulate lipid and lipoprotein metabolism and to be associated with lower levels of lipids [3,24,30–33]. However, the decreased levels of lipids are unexpectedly associated with an increased CV risk, which is known as the "lipid paradox" [34]. A possible explanation of this paradox is that inflammation modifies low-density lipoprotein cholesterol (LDL-C) through oxidation; oxidized LDL-C is atherogenic resulting in increased CVD risk despite low serum levels [3]. However, other functions, such as enzymatic activities, pro-oxidant mechanisms, humoral response activation or pathways involving acute-phase mediators may be also implicated. In fact, the preventive effect of HDL-C on LDL-C oxidation has been shown to be impaired in RA patients compared with controls [32]. Taken together, these lines of evidence have led to a paradigm shift from the "lipid paradox" to the concept of HDL dysfunction [35]. However, HDL dysfunction phenomena in chronic inflammatory diseases still need to be thoroughly characterized [34,35]. The findings presented herein underline the central role of lipids and dyslipidemia in RA as a key factor to understand CV history, even in the presence of MetS or other traditional risk factors.

With regards to CV risk factors associated with PsA, the available evidence shows that metabolic comorbidities, obesity in particular, are involved [14,15,35]. The distinction in terms of CV risk profile from RA, despite the fact that both diseases are characterized by chronic inflammation, has been previously addressed [8,9,35,36]. It has been pointed out that, contrary to RA where systemic inflammation appears to contribute directly to the increased CV risk, in PsA traditional risk factors, including adiposity and MetS, are major contributors to the CV risk [8,35,37]. These differences were also reported in a recent study [38], although the impact of MetS was not explored. Our findings showing a significantly higher prevalence of MetS and dyslipidemia in PsA versus RA patients (despite the fact that the PsA population was significantly younger than the RA population) and the stronger association of MetS with a history of CV events in patients with PsA strongly reinforce these observations, also highlighting the differential contribution of MetS. Again, these associations were independent of disease duration, which is thought to have a different impact in RA and PsA, as evidence of a causal role is less robust in the latter [20,38,39]. Further research is needed to evaluate the impact of disease progression on MetS in the long term in inflammatory arthropathies.

During the 12-month follow-up, the prevalence of MetS and its components in both patient groups was markedly stable. This suggests that in established RA and PsA, provided that no disease flares and major treatment changes occur, the screening of CV risk factors and MetS can be performed on a yearly basis, as recommended by current EULAR guidelines [16]. Whether more frequent screening may be required in early disease or in specific patient populations (elderly, patients with comorbidities) needs to be investigated.

The fact that distinct factors are involved in the increased CV risk in different chronic inflammatory diseases raises the question as to what extent the prevention and management of CV risk should be disease specific. Compelling evidence confirms that early diagnosis and treatment may reduce the frequency of CV events and improve survival in patients with arthropathies [40]. Current practice is based on general recommendations for RA and "other forms of inflammatory joint disorders", with most of the evidence on which the recommendations are based coming from studies in patients with RA [16]. In patients with RA, it may be crucial to reduce disease activity and systemic inflammation, beside reducing traditional CV risk factors with a special focus on lipids [1,38,41]. A better understanding of this crosstalk will warrant optimal CV management. Patients with PsA, on the other hand, may benefit more from broader CV-prevention strategies that target MetS and hypertension [36]. Further research is needed to explore the feasibility and implementation in clinical practice, as well as the cost-effectiveness of disease-specific versus general recommendations for CV prevention.

Our study has several limitations including the retrospective design and the small sample size of both populations. The two populations compared were not matched in terms of mean age and disease duration; this was due to the fact that RA and PsA have a different pathogenesis and age of onset, and probably attending/organizational variables. No strict clinical features were used as inclusion/exclusion criteria in order to capture real-world populations and avoid highly selected patient samples. Therefore, this potential limitation is hard to avoid in unselected populations that are representative of patients encountered in real-life, although extensive analytical steps were performed to correct for these differences. Of note, none of these variables were observed to show a strong confounding effect. Our findings can be considered as proof-of-concept and pave the ground for future larger and prospective trials assessing the impact of MetS on inflammatory arthropathies. Furthermore, time-adjusted risk factor exposure analyses are needed to evaluate the real impact of MetS and its components.

5. Conclusions

The study shows that MetS and its components differently impact the risk of CVD in PsA and RA. The clinical presentation of MetS may differ between PsA and RA. These findings are relevant for clinical practice as a disease-specific management of CV risk may be required in distinct chronic inflammatory diseases of the joints. However, clinical validation in larger studies is needed. Further efforts are required to develop disease-specific strategies for the management of CV risk in PsA and RA.

Supplementary Materials: The following supporting information can be downloaded at https://www.mdpi.com/article/10.3390/jcm12155031/s1: Table S1: Associations between CV risk factors and disease duration; Table S2: Predictors of smoking; Table S3: Predictors of dyslipidemia; Table S4: Predictors of MetS occurrence adjusted for NSAIDs; Table S5: Predictors of MetS occurrence adjusted for anti-TNF; Table S6: Predictors of CV events at baseline.

Author Contributions: Conceptualization, F.A. and J.R.-C.; methodology, F.A. and J.R.-C.; formal analysis, F.A., J.G. and J.R.-C.; investigation, F.A., L.L.C., M.C. and M.G.; resources, F.A. and J.R.-C.; data curation, F.A., L.L.C., M.C. and M.G.; writing—original draft preparation, F.A. and J.R.-C.; writing—review and editing, F.A., L.L.C., M.C., M.G., J.G. and J.R.-C.; visualization, F.A. and J.R.-C.; supervision, F.A.; project administration, F.A.; funding acquisition, F.A. and J.R.-C. All authors have read and agreed to the published version of the manuscript.

Funding: Medical writing support was provided by Lorenza Lanini on behalf of Health Publishing & Services Srl. This support was funded by Novartis Farma Italy and Instituto de Salud Carlos III (ISCIII, Spain) with FEDER funds under the grant PI21/00054 (PI Javier Rodríguez-Carrio).

Institutional Review Board Statement: The study was conducted in accordance with the Declaration of Helsinki. The Institutional Review Board granted an exemption of ethics committee approval due to local regulations, as the participants underwent clinical and clinimetric examinations according to routine protocols used at the recruiting hospital and no further procedures were needed.

Informed Consent Statement: Informed consent was obtained from all subjects involved in the study.

Data Availability Statement: The detailed data will be available on request from the corresponding author.

Conflicts of Interest: The authors declare no conflict of interest.

References

1. Solomon, D.H.; Reed, G.W.; Kremer, J.M.; Curtis, J.R.; Farkouh, M.E.; Harrold, L.R.; Hochberg, M.C.; Tsao, P.; Greenberg, J.D. Disease activity in rheumatoid arthritis and the risk of CV events. *Arthritis Rheumatol.* **2015**, *67*, 1449–1455. [CrossRef] [PubMed]
2. Ogdie, A.; Yu, Y.; Haynes, K.; Love, T.J.; Maliha, S.; Jiang, Y.; Troxel, A.B.; Hennessy, S.; Kimmel, S.E.; Margolis, D.J.; et al. Risk of major CV events in patients with psoriatic arthritis, psoriasis and rheumatoid arthritis: A population-based cohort study. *Ann. Rheum. Dis.* **2015**, *74*, 326–332. [CrossRef] [PubMed]
3. Kerola, A.M.; Rollefstad, S.; Semb, A.G. Atherosclerotic CV Disease in Rheumatoid Arthritis: Impact of Inflammation and Antirheumatic Treatment. *Eur. Cardiol.* **2021**, *16*, e18. [CrossRef] [PubMed]
4. Dijkshoorn, B.; Raadsen, R.; Nurmohamed, M.T. CV Disease Risk in Rheumatoid Arthritis Anno 2022. *J. Clin. Med.* **2022**, *11*, 2704. [CrossRef]
5. Piepoli, M.F.; Hoes, A.W.; Agewall, S.; Albus, C.; Brotons, C.; Catapano, A.L.; Cooney, M.; Corrà, U.; Cosyns, B.; Deaton, C.; et al. 2016 European guidelines on CV disease prevention in clinical practice. The Sixth Joint Task Force of the European Society of Cardiology and Other Societies on CV Disease Prevention in Clinical Practice (constituted by representatives of 10 societies and by invited experts. Developed with the special contribution of the European Association for CV Prevention & Rehabilitation. *G. Ital. Cardiol.* **2017**, *18*, 547–612.
6. Chen, J.; Norling, L.V.; Cooper, D. Cardiac Dysfunction in Rheumatoid Arthritis: The Role of Inflammation. *Cells* **2021**, *10*, 881. [CrossRef]
7. Polachek, A.; Touma, Z.; Anderson, M.; Eder, L. Risk of CV Morbidity in Patients with Psoriatic Arthritis: A Meta-Analysis of Observational Studies. *Arthritis Care Res.* **2017**, *69*, 67–74. [CrossRef]

8. Atzeni, F.; Gerratana, E.; Francesco Masala, I.; Bongiovanni, S.; Sarzi-Puttini, P.; Rodríguez-Carrio, J. Psoriatic Arthritis and Metabolic Syndrome: Is There a Role for Disease Modifying Anti-Rheumatic Drugs? *Front. Med.* **2021**, *8*, 735150. [CrossRef]
9. Degboé, Y.; Koch, R.; Zabraniecki, L.; Jamard, B.; Couture, G.; Ruidavets, J.B.; Ferrieres, J.; Ruyssen-Witrand, A.; Constantin, A. Increased CV Risk in Psoriatic Arthritis: Results from a Case-Control Monocentric Study. *Front. Med.* **2022**, *9*, 785719. [CrossRef]
10. Symmons, D.P.; Gabriel, S.E. Epidemiology of CVD in rheumatic disease, with a focus on RA and SLE. *Nat. Rev. Rheumatol.* **2011**, *7*, 399–408. [CrossRef]
11. Qiao, Q.; Gao, W.; Zhang, L.; Nyamdorj, R.; Tuomilehto, J. Metabolic syndrome and CV disease. *Ann. Clin. Biochem.* **2007**, *44*, 232–263. [CrossRef]
12. Radner, H.; Lesperance, T.; Accortt, N.A.; Solomon, D.H. Incidence and Prevalence of CV Risk Factors Among Patients with Rheumatoid Arthritis, Psoriasis, or Psoriatic Arthritis. *Arthritis Care Res.* **2017**, *69*, 1510–1518. [CrossRef]
13. Jafri, K.; Bartels, C.M.; Shin, D.; Gelfand, J.M.; Ogdie, A. Incidence and Management of CV Risk Factors in Psoriatic Arthritis and Rheumatoid Arthritis: A Population-Based Study. *Arthritis Care Res.* **2017**, *69*, 51–57. [CrossRef] [PubMed]
14. Loganathan, A.; Kamalaraj, N.; El-Haddad, C.; Pile, K. Systematic review and meta-analysis on prevalence of metabolic syndrome in psoriatic arthritis, rheumatoid arthritis and psoriasis. *Int. J. Rheum. Dis.* **2021**, *24*, 1112–1120. [CrossRef] [PubMed]
15. Karmacharya, P.; Ogdie, A.; Eder, L. Psoriatic arthritis and the association with cardiometabolic disease: A narrative review. *Ther. Adv. Musculoskelet. Dis.* **2021**, *13*, 1759720x21998279. [CrossRef] [PubMed]
16. Agca, R.; Heslinga, S.C.; Rollefstad, S.; Heslinga, M.; McInnes, I.B.; Peters, M.J.L.; Kvien, T.K.; Dougados, M.; Radner, H.; Atzeni, F.; et al. EULAR recommendations for CV disease risk management in patients with rheumatoid arthritis and other forms of inflammatory joint disorders: 2015/2016 update. *Ann. Rheum. Dis.* **2017**, *76*, 17–28. [CrossRef] [PubMed]
17. Taylor, W.; Gladman, D.; Helliwell, P.; Marchesoni, A.; Mease, P.; Mielants, H.; CASPAR Study Group. Classification criteria for psoriatic arthritis: Development of new criteria from a large international study. *Arthritis Rheum.* **2006**, *54*, 2665–2673. [CrossRef]
18. Aletaha, D.; Neogi, T.; Silman, A.J.; Funovits, J.; Felson, D.T.; Bingham, C.O., III; Birnbaum, N.S.; Burmester, G.R.; Bykerk, V.P.; Cohen, M.D.; et al. 2010 Rheumatoid arthritis classification criteria: An American College of Rheumatology/European League Against Rheumatism collaborative initiative. *Arthritis Rheum.* **2010**, *62*, 2569–2581. [CrossRef]
19. Grundy, S.M.; Cleeman, J.I.; Daniels, S.R.; Donato, K.A.; Eckel, R.H.; Franklin, B.A.; Gordon, D.J.; Krauss, R.M.; Savage, P.J.; Smith Jr, S.C.; et al. Diagnosis and management of the metabolic syndrome: An American Heart Association/National Heart, Lung, and Blood Institute Scientific Statement. *Circulation* **2005**, *112*, 2735–2752. [CrossRef]
20. Castañeda, S.; Martín-Martínez, M.A.; González-Juanatey, C.; Llorca, J.; García-Yébenes, M.J.; Pérez-Vicente, S.; Sánchez-Costa, J.T.; Díaz-Gonzalez, F.; González-Gay, M.A.; CARMA Project Collaborative Group. Cardiovascular morbidity and associated risk factors in Spanish patients with chronic inflammatory rheumatic diseases attending rheumatology clinics: Baseline data of the CARMA Project. *Semin. Arthritis Rheum.* **2015**, *44*, 618–626. [CrossRef]
21. Del Rincón, I.; Williams, K.; Stern, M.P.; Freeman, G.L.; Escalante, A. High incidence of CV events in a rheumatoid arthritis cohort not explained by traditional cardiac risk factors. *Arthritis Rheum.* **2001**, *44*, 2737–2745. [CrossRef]
22. Del Rincón, I.; Freeman, G.L.; Haas, R.W.; O'Leary, D.H.; Escalante, A. Relative contribution of CV risk factors and rheumatoid arthritis clinical manifestations to atherosclerosis. *Arthritis Rheum.* **2005**, *52*, 3413–3423. [CrossRef] [PubMed]
23. Del Rincón, I.; Polak, J.F.; O'Leary, D.H.; Battafarano, D.F.; Erikson, J.M.; Restrepo, J.F.; Molina, E.; Escalante, A. Systemic inflammation and CV risk factors predict rapid progression of atherosclerosis in rheumatoid arthritis. *Ann. Rheum. Dis.* **2015**, *74*, 1118–1123. [CrossRef] [PubMed]
24. Crowson, C.S.; Rollefstad, S.; Ikdahl, E.; Kitas, G.D.; van Riel PL, C.M.; Gabriel, S.E.; Matteson, E.L.; Kvien, T.K.; Douglas, K.; Sandoo, A.; et al. Impact of risk factors associated with CV outcomes in patients with rheumatoid arthritis. *Ann. Rheum. Dis.* **2018**, *77*, 48–54. [CrossRef]
25. Urruticoechea-Arana, A.; Castañeda, S.; Loza, E.; Oton, T.; Benavent, D.; Martin-Martinez, M.A.; González-Gay, M.A. Prevalence of Metabolic Syndrome in Psoriatic Arthritis: Systematic Literature Review and Results from the CARMA Cohort. *J. Clin. Rheumatol.* **2022**, *28*, e388–e396. [CrossRef]
26. Stower, H. Personalizing metabolic disease therapies. *Nat. Med.* **2019**, *25*, 197. [CrossRef] [PubMed]
27. Karolina, D.S.; Tavintharan, S.; Armugam, A.; Sepramaniam, S.; Pek, S.L.T.; Wong, M.T.K.; Lim, S.C.; Sum, C.F.; Jeyaseelan, K. Circulating miRNA profiles in patients with metabolic syndrome. *J. Clin. Endocrinol. Metab.* **2012**, *97*, E2271–E2276. [CrossRef] [PubMed]
28. Lind, L.; Salihovic, S.; Sundström, J.; Elmståhl, S.; Hammar, U.; Dekkers, K.; Ärnlöv, J.; Smith, J.G.; Engström, G.; Fall, T. Metabolic Profiling of Obesity with and Without the Metabolic Syndrome: A Multisample Evaluation. *J. Clin. Endocrinol. Metab.* **2022**, *107*, 1337–1345. [CrossRef]
29. Fernandez-Berges, D.; Consuegra-Sanchez, L.; Penafiel, J.; de León, A.C.; Vila, J.; Félix-Redondo, F.J.; Segura-Fragoso, A.; Lapetra, J.; Guembe, M.J.; Vega, T.; et al. Metabolic and Inflammatory Profiles of Biomarkers in Obesity, Metabolic Syndrome, and Diabetes in a Mediterranean Population. DARIOS Inflammatory Study; Metabolic and inflammatory profiles of biomarkers in obesity, metabolic syndrome, and diabetes in a Mediterranean population. DARIOS Inflammatory study. *Rev. Esp. Cardiol.* **2014**, *67*, 624–631.
30. Choy, E.; Sattar, N. Interpreting lipid levels in the context of high-grade inflammatory states with a focus on rheumatoid arthritis: A challenge to conventional CV risk actions. *Ann. Rheum. Dis.* **2009**, *68*, 460–469. [CrossRef]

31. Robertson, J.; Peters, M.J.; McInnes, I.B.; Sattar, N. Changes in lipid levels with inflammation and therapy in RA: A maturing paradigm. *Nat. Rev. Rheumatol.* **2013**, *9*, 513–523. [CrossRef] [PubMed]
32. Dursunoğlu, D.; Evrengül, H.; Polat, B.; Tanrıverdi, H.; Çobankara, V.; Kaftan, A.; Kılıç, M. Lp(a) lipoprotein and lipids in patients with rheumatoid arthritis: Serum levels and relationship to inflammation. *Rheumatol. Int.* **2005**, *25*, 241–245. [CrossRef]
33. McMahon, M.; Grossman, J.; FitzGerald, J.; Dahlin-Lee, E.; Wallace, D.J.; Thong, B.Y.; Badsha, H.; Kalunian, K.; Charles, C.; Navab, M.; et al. Proinflammatory high-density lipoprotein as a biomarker for atherosclerosis in patients with systemic lupus erythematosus and rheumatoid arthritis. *Arthritis Rheum.* **2006**, *54*, 2541–2549. [CrossRef] [PubMed]
34. Myasoedova, E.; Crowson, C.S.; Kremers, H.M.; Roger, V.L.; Fitz-Gibbon, P.D.; Therneau, T.M.; Gabriel, S.E. Lipid paradox in rheumatoid arthritis: The impact of serum lipid measures and systemic inflammation on the risk of CV disease. *Ann. Rheum. Dis.* **2011**, *70*, 482–487. [CrossRef] [PubMed]
35. Rodriguez-Carrio, J.; Suarez, A. The HDL dysfunction gains momentum: Is it time for a new approach in rheumatic diseases? *Rheumatology* **2020**, *59*, 3121–3123. [CrossRef]
36. Ferguson, L.D.; Siebert, S.; McInnes, I.B.; Sattar, N. Cardiometabolic comorbidities in RA and PsA: Lessons learned and future directions. *Nat. Rev. Rheumatol.* **2019**, *15*, 461–474. [CrossRef] [PubMed]
37. Özkul, Ö.; Yazıcı, A.; Aktürk, A.S.; Karadağ, D.T.; Işık, Ö.O.; Tekeoğlu, S.; Cefle, A. Are there any differences among psoriasis, psoriatic arthritis and rheumatoid arthritis in terms of metabolic syndrome and CV risk factors? *Eur. J. Rheumatol.* **2019**, *6*, 174–178. [CrossRef]
38. Cooksey, R.; Brophy, S.; Kennedy, J.; Gutierrez, F.F.; Pickles, T.; Davies, R.; Piguet, V.; Choy, E. CV risk factors predicting cardiac events are different in patients with rheumatoid arthritis, psoriatic arthritis, and psoriasis. *Semin. Arthritis Rheum.* **2018**, *48*, 367–373. [CrossRef]
39. Eder, L.; Wu, Y.; Chandran, V.; Cook, R.; Gladman, D.D. Incidence and predictors for cardiovascular events in patients with psoriatic arthritis. *Ann. Rheum. Dis.* **2016**, *75*, 1680–1686. [CrossRef]
40. Castañeda, S.; González-Juanatey, C.; González-Gay, M.A. Inflammatory Arthritis and Heart Disease. *Curr. Pharm. Des.* **2018**, *24*, 262–280. [CrossRef]
41. Liao, K.P.; Solomon, D.H. Traditional CV risk factors, inflammation and CV risk in rheumatoid arthritis. *Rheumatology* **2013**, *52*, 45–52. [CrossRef] [PubMed]

Disclaimer/Publisher's Note: The statements, opinions and data contained in all publications are solely those of the individual author(s) and contributor(s) and not of MDPI and/or the editor(s). MDPI and/or the editor(s) disclaim responsibility for any injury to people or property resulting from any ideas, methods, instructions or products referred to in the content.

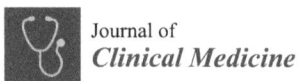

Review

Dual PPRαY Agonists for the Management of Dyslipidemia: A Systematic Review and Meta-Analysis of Randomized Clinical Trials

Antonio da Silva Menezes Junior [1,2,*,†], Vinícius Martins Rodrigues Oliveira [1,†], Izadora Caiado Oliveira [1], André Maroccolo de Sousa [1], Ana Júlia Prego Santana [1], Davi Peixoto Craveiro Carvalho [1], Ricardo Figueiredo Paro Piai [1], Fernando Henrique Matos [1], Arthur Marot de Paiva [1] and Gabriel Baêta Branquinho Reis [1]

1. Faculty of Medicine, Federal University of Goiás, Goiânia 74605020, Brazil; vinicius.martins@discente.ufg.br (V.M.R.O.); izadora.caiado@discente.ufg.br (I.C.O.); andremaroccolo@discente.ufg.br (A.M.d.S.); ana.santana@discente.ufg.br (A.J.P.S.); davi.peixoto@discente.ufg.br (D.P.C.C.); ricardopiai@discente.ufg.br (R.F.P.P.); fernando.matos@discente.ufg.br (F.H.M.); amarotdepaiva@gmail.com (A.M.d.P.); gabrielbaeta@discente.ufg.br (G.B.B.R.)
2. School of Medical and Life Sciences, Pontifical Catholic University of Goiás, Goiânia 74605050, Brazil
* Correspondence: a.menezes.junior@uol.com.br; Tel.: +55-62982711177
† These authors contributed equally to this work.

Abstract: Saroglitazar is a novel medication for dyslipidemia, but its specific effects remain unclear. Therefore, we performed a systematic review and meta-analysis to assess the efficacy and safety of saroglitazar for managing dyslipidemia. The PubMed, Scopus, and EMBASE databases were systematically searched for randomized controlled trials (RCTs) comparing 2 and 4 mg of saroglitazar with placebos for treating dyslipidemia. A random-effects model calculated the pooled mean differences for continuous outcomes with 95% confidence intervals. The study included seven RCTs involving 1975 patients. Overall, 340 (31.0%) and 513 (46.8%) participants received 2 and 4 mg of saroglitazar, respectively; 242 (22.11%) received the placebo. The mean ages ranged from 40.2 to 62.6 years, and 436 (39.8%) were women. Compared to the control group, 4 mg of saroglitazar significantly decreased the triglyceride and low-density lipoprotein (LDL) cholesterol levels but did not affect the high-density lipoprotein cholesterol level. Furthermore, the alanine aminotransferase level significantly decreased, the creatine level significantly increased, and body weight did not differ between the groups. Finally, 4 mg of saroglitazar, compared to 2 mg, significantly lowered the triglyceride level. Saroglitazar (4 mg) may be an effective treatment, but safety concerns remain.

Keywords: dual PPRαY agonist; dyslipidemia; saroglitazar

1. Introduction

Diabetic dyslipidemia is characterized by increased triglyceride levels. Specifically, atherogenic dyslipidemia is characterized by a high level of small, dense low-density lipoprotein cholesterol (LDL-C) and a low level of high-density lipoprotein cholesterol (HDL-C) [1]. Together, these are commonly called the "triad of increased triglycerides." Dyslipidemia is a frequent feature of obesity, metabolic syndrome, insulin resistance, and type 2 diabetes mellitus [2]. It is also a substantial risk factor for myocardial infarction and cardiovascular disease. In addition, small, dense LDL-C particles speed up atherosclerosis progression, leading to an increased risk of cardiovascular disease-related mortality and morbidity [3].

Effective and well-studied treatments for dyslipidemia exist, such as statins and lifestyle modifications [4,5]. Statins, fibrates, and omega-3 fatty acids can manage dyslipidemia. However, although statins reduce cardiovascular events and decrease mortality, a considerable residual cardiovascular risk persists [6]. Moreover, the recent PROMINENT study failed to show pemafibrate reducing cardiovascular outcomes, notwithstanding that the lipid profile was significantly improved [7].

PPARα/Υ is primarily expressed in the liver, lowering lipotoxicity and circulating atherogenic lipid levels [8]. Saroglitazar, (S)-a-ethoxy-4-(2-methyl-5-(4-methylthio) phenyl)] [(S)-a-ethoxy-4-(2-methyl-5-(4-methylthio) phenyl]-1H-pyrrol-1-yl]-magnesium salt of ethoxy)-benzenepropanoic acid] is a new PPAR/agonist that was produced in India by Zydus Cadila and is marketed under the name Lipaglycn. It was given the green light for use in the treatment of diabetic dyslipidemia and hypertriglyceridemia by the Drug Controller General of India (DCGI) [8]. Saroglitazar also reduces hemoglobin A1c (HbA1c) levels, in part, by lowering lipotoxicity and exerting a modest amount of PPAR-agonistic action in the body. A previous study demonstrated that adding saroglitazar to metformin treatment resulted in a greater decrease in total cholesterol and HbA1c levels compared to that with fenofibrate [9]. However, saroglitazar is controversial because of conflicting findings regarding its safety and efficacy [10]. Krishnappa et al. found no abnormal findings in all treatment groups for serum creatinine, hematocrit, respiratory rate, or body temperature [11]. However, Gawrieh et al. reported a significant increase in serum creatinine levels [12].

Consequently, saroglitazar has only been approved for use in India; other institutions, such as the United States Food and Drug Administration, have yet to approve the medication [10]. Therefore, we performed a systematic review and meta-analysis to investigate the effectiveness and safety of saroglitazar in patients at risk of dyslipidemia and type II diabetes.

2. Materials and Methods

The current systematic literature review was prospectively registered on 25 May 2023 with the International Prospective Register of Systematic Reviews (PROSPERO registration number: CRD42023426614). Results are reported following the Preferred Reporting Items for Systematic Reviews and Meta-Analyses (PRISMA) guidelines [13].

2.1. Study Eligibility Criteria

Our primary study question was: "What is the safety and effectiveness of saroglitazar for treating dyslipidemia?" Our investigation was conducted based on the following population, intervention, comparison, outcome, and time (study design) (PICOT) categories: Population (i.e., P): adult patients with diabetic hypercholesterolemia or dyslipidemia; Intervention (i.e., I): saroglitazar at 2 and 4 mg doses; Comparison (i.e., C): placebo; Outcomes (i.e., O): the effectiveness and safety of saroglitazar; and Time (i.e., T): randomized clinical trials (RCTs) lasting more than four months. Efficacy assessments comprised the effects of saroglitazar on total cholesterol, LDL-C, triglycerides, HDL-C, non-HDL-C, and fasting plasma glucose (FPG) levels. Safety assessments included serum creatinine, alanine transaminase (ALT), aspartate transaminase levels, and body weight measurements. The systematic review includes all studies that met the above-mentioned PICOT criteria. Reviews, observational and descriptive research, editorials, comments, and conference proceedings were excluded.

2.2. Data Sources and Literature Searches

The PubMed, Scopus, and Embase databases were comprehensively searched from their inception through May 2023; the first search was performed in April 2023. All Medical Subject Heading phrases and keywords linked to "saroglitazar," "hypercholesterolemia," and "diabetes" were used in the search [('saroglitazar'/exp OR saroglitazar) AND ('diabetes'/exp OR 'diabetes' OR 'hypertriglyceridemia' OR'metabolic syndrome' OR 'dyslipidemia'/exp OR 'dyslipidemia'] to collect previously published studies. The reference lists of the included studies were screened, and a snowball search was performed. The Supplementary Files present a detailed search strategy for each database.

2.3. Study Selection and Data Extraction

The titles and abstracts of the retrieved papers were evaluated, followed by the full text, using the inclusion and exclusion criteria. Extremely irrelevant studies were removed during the title and abstract search, completed by two independent reviewers (IC and VM), followed by the full-text screening. A well-defined data extraction sheet that included information regarding the study's characteristics, participants, interventions, comparator, and results was used. Two separate researchers (IC and VM) performed the study selection and data extraction, and differences were handled by consensus or discussion with a third reviewer (AM).

2.4. Risk of Bias and Quality Assessments

The Cochrane Risk of Bias Assessment Tool [14] was used to assess the methodological quality of the included studies. The studies were divided into low, high, and unclear risk of bias in each domain: randomization, allocation concealment, patient blinding, blinding of outcome measurements, incomplete outcome data, and selective reporting.

The quality of the included double-arm trials was evaluated by the National Institutes of Health Checklist [15], which consists of 12 items identifying the methodological features based on the existing study design and study-reporting guidelines. Each item carries one point, and scores of 0–4, 4–8, and 9–12 were considered poor, fair, and good-quality studies, respectively. Two independent reviewers (IC and VM) evaluated the risk of bias and quality of the included studies and resolved disagreements through consensus or a discussion with a third reviewer.

2.5. Data Synthesis

The analyses were performed using RevMan software (Review Manager [computer program], Version 5.4.1, The Cochrane Collaboration, 2004) using a meta-package. Changes in continuous outcomes were calculated for every included study arm by subtracting the value at baseline from the value after the intervention. All of the estimates of effectiveness were presented in the form of mean differences (MDs) or absolute weighted mean changes. A safety estimate, ALT, was presented in the form of standard mean differences (SMD) and 95% confidence intervals (CIs) from the baseline. Based on the Cochrane Handbook, standard deviations (SDs) were calculated from the standard error or 95% CI for a systematic review of interventions [16]. The Higgins I^2 statistics and Cochran's Q test were used to assess the potential statistical heterogeneity among trials. The meta-analysis was conducted using a fixed-effect model (using inverse variance) or a random-effect model (DerSimonian-Laird method) based on low heterogeneity (50%). If the low (<50%) and high (>50%) heterogeneity criteria resulted in a low number of studies (<10), publication bias assessments were performed using funnel plots (Figures S1 and S2).

3. Results

3.1. Study Selection and Baseline Characteristics

The electronic database search yielded 267 citations; 196 citations were screened after removing 71 duplicates. Next, 160 studies were excluded during first-pass screening after reviewing the titles and abstracts. The full texts of 36 citations were downloaded for the second-pass screening. Finally, eight articles met our inclusion criteria. Figure 1 presents the PRISMA flowchart for the study selection.

Table 1 summarizes the characteristics of the included studies. Of the 8 included studies, 7 were RCTs, and 1 was a pooled analysis of RCTs. They included 1975 patients, of whom 546 and 731 received 2 and 4 mg of saroglitazar, respectively. Furthermore, 389 and 40 patients received 30 and 45 mg of pioglitazone, respectively. Finally, 18 patients received 160 mg of fenofibrate, and 251 received a placebo.

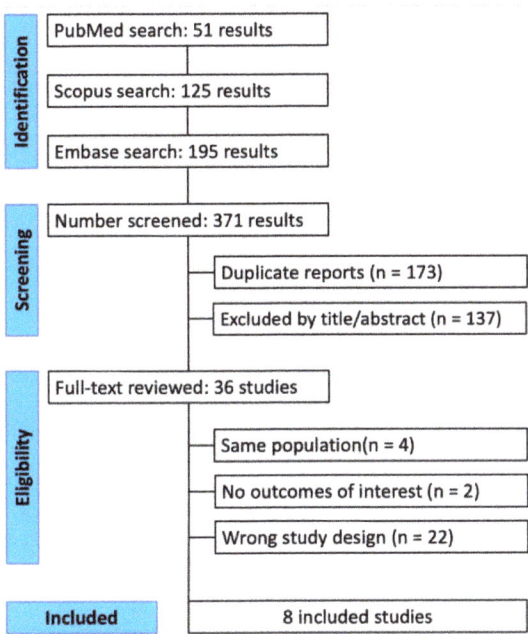

Figure 1. Preferred Reporting Items for Systematic Reviews and Meta-Analyses: Flow Diagram of the Study Screening and Selection Process.

Furthermore, five studies [12,17–20] analyzed the efficacy and safety endpoints between patients receiving saroglitazar and placebo. In 3 studies [9,11,21], the control patients received anti-lipid medications (i.e., 10 mg of atorvastatin, 160 mg of fenofibrate, 30 mg of pioglitazone, and 45 mg of pioglitazone, respectively).

Table 1. Characteristics of the included studies.

Study	Population	Country and Date	Follow-Up (Weeks)	No. of Patients
JANI et al. [17]	Patients with T2DM and hypertriglyceridemia are not on anti-dyslipidemia drugs, except for 10 mg of atorvastatin.	India, 2014	12	Saroglitazar 2 mg (n = 100) Saroglitazar 4 mg (n = 99) Placebo (n = 102)
PAI et al. [21]	Patients with T2DM with hypertriglyceridemia receiving sulphonylurea, metformin, or both for at least three months.	India, 2014	26	Saroglitazar 2 mg (n = 37) Saroglitazar 4 mg (n = 39) Pioglitazone 45 mg (n = 33)
GHOSH et al. [9]	Patients with diabetic dyslipidemia receiving 1000 mg of metformin daily.	India, 2015	12	Saroglitazar 4 mg (n = 18) Fenofibrate 160 mg (n = 18)
JAIN et al. [18]	Patients with T2DM with hypertriglyceridemia.	India, 2019	16	Saroglitazar 4 mg (n = 15) Placebo (n = 15)
KRISHNAPPA et al. [11]	Patients with T2DM with on a stable dose of metformin for at least six weeks.	India, 2020	12	Saroglitazar 2 mg (n = 380) Saroglitazar 4 mg (n = 386) Pioglitazone 30 mg (n = 389)

Table 1. *Cont.*

Study	Population	Country and Date	Follow-Up (Weeks)	No. of Patients
RASTOGI et al. [20]	Patients with T2DM and dyslipidemia on a stable dose of metformin.	India, 2020	12	Saroglitazar 4 mg ($n = 15$) Placebo ($n = 15$)
GAWRIEH et al. [12]	Patients with NAFLD not taking other lipid-lowering agents.	USA, 2021	16	Saroglitazar 2 mg ($n = 25$) Saroglitazar 4 mg ($n = 27$) Placebo ($n = 28$)
SIDDIQUI et al. [19]	Patients with NAFLD with and without statin therapy.	USA, 2023	52	Saroglitazar 4 mg ($n = 130$) Placebo ($n = 91$)

NAFLD: Nonalchoholic Fatty Liver Disease; T2DM: Type 2 diabetes mellitus.

3.2. Risk of Bias

Random sequence generation, allocation concealment, performance, and detection bias had minimal bias risks in 8/8 studies (100%). Decision bias (i.e., outcome assessment blinding) had a low risk in 6/8 studies (75%), but prejudice in reporting was identified in 4/8 (50%) studies. The "other bias" area looked at the financial sources, particularly from pharmaceutical industries, authors from pharmaceutical organizations, and conflicts of interest. Consequently, 4/8 studies (50%) had a risk of "other bias." Figure 2 summarizes the risk of biased assessments.

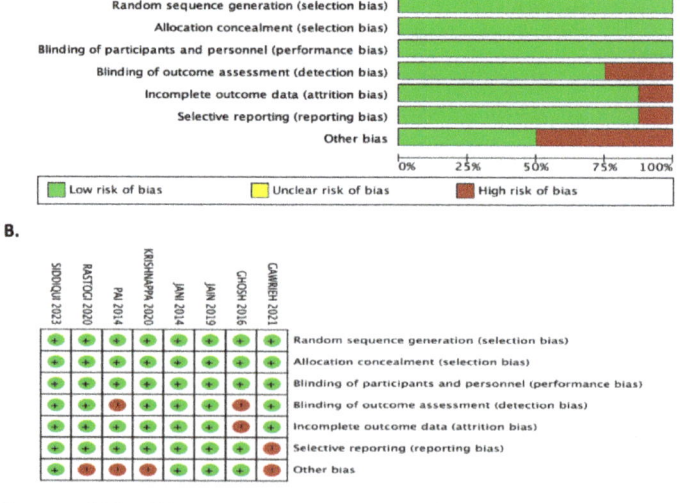

Figure 2. Risk of bias assessments (**A**) Graphical representation of the risk of bias (percentages) (**B**) Summary of the risk of bias. Risk of Bias (RoB) plot. Circles are colour coded with green indicating low RoB, yellow indicating some concerns and red indicating a high RoB. The symbols "+", "?" and "-" indicate the same RoB grades as the colours.

3.3. Pooled Analysis of All Studies

Based on a thorough endpoint analysis, our primary efficacy outcomes were the triglyceride, LDL-C, and HDL-C levels. The secondary efficacy endpoints were total cholesterol, FPG, and Hb1Ac levels. The primary safety outcomes were creatinine and ALT levels and body weight (Table 2).

Table 2. Baseline characteristics of patients in included studies.

Study	Groups	Demographic Profile		Clinical Profile		Laboratory Parameters	Lipid Parameters (mg/dL)				Safety Parameters	
		Age	Sex (F/M)	Weight (kg)	Height (cm)	HbA1c (%)	TG	TC	HDL-C	LDL-C	Cr (mg/dL)	ALT (U/L)
JANI et al. [17]	Saroglitazar 2 mg (n = 100)	50.4 ± 9.01	39/61	71.3 ± 13.56	161.9 ± 9.66	8.9 ± 1.84	273.3 ± 78.58	200.6 ± 38.11	36.6 ± 8.45	132.5 ± 30.43	NR	NR
	Saroglitazar 4 mg (n = 99)	51.2 ± 8.66	43/56	69.1 ± 10.83	160.5 ± 9.06	8.9 ± 1.77	287.3 ± 85.94	210.4 ± 37.20	39.1 ± 11.19	140.2 ± 29.36	NR	NR
	Placebo (n = 102)	49.8 ± 9.95	47/55	69.9 ± 11.53	160.9 ± 8.66	9.2 ± 1.81	286.6 ± 78.92	209.5 ± 39.31	38.5 ± 12.06	140.1 ± 33.58	NR	NR
PAI et al. [21]	Saroglitazar 2 mg (n = 41)	48.9 ± 8.98	15/26	69.8 ± 12.72	161.9 ± 9.44	8.1 ± 0.86	253.9 ± 68.44	202.4 ± 47.60	36.8 ± 12.09	134.8 ± 42.56	0.7 ± 0.21	31.5 ± 16.48
	Saroglitazar 4 mg (n = 41)	47.3 ± 9.10	16/24	73.0 ± 11.49	163.1 ± 10.17	7.9 ± 0.58	257.0 ± 52.39	197.3 ± 40.98	35.3 ± 9.64	130.8 ± 38.83	0.7 ± 0.19	29.7 ± 15.91
	Pioglitazone 45 mg (n = 40)	49.9 ± 10.98	16/24	71.0 ± 12.94	162.0 ± 10.74	8.2 ± 0.75	265.0 ± 61.66	185.8 ± 29.91	38.3 ± 10.85	116.6 ± 29.25	0.7 ± 0.2	26.3 ± 9.13
GHOSH et al. [9]	Fenofibrate 160 mg (n = 18)	58.1	20/25	NR	NR	7.1 ± 0.4	244.2 ± 20.6	NR	42.12 ± 5.19	114.1 ± 7.11	NR	NR
	Saroglitazar 4 mg (n = 18)	62.6	NR	NR	NR	6.9 ± 0.6	245.9 ± 33.9	NR	40.18 ± 5.89	114.2 ± 10.76	NR	NR
JAIN et al. [18]	Saroglitazar 4 mg (n = 15)	40.9 ± 9.6	0/15	78.7 ± 9.8	169.7 ± 5.6	NR	325.6 ± 129.3	192.4 ± 42.9	37.49 ± 9.6	116.4 ± 36.3	NR	NR
	Placebo (n = 15)	47 ± 8.8	3/12	75.6 ± 11.0	164.5 ± 11.2	NR	236.3 ± 83.1	217.6 ± 45.4	45.3 ± 8.5	146.7 ± 45.3	NR	NR
KRISHNAPPA et al. [11]	Saroglitazar 2 mg (n = 380)	51.90 ± 10.38	164/216	70.27 ± 11.84	NR	9.76 ± 1.59	163.87 ± 91.49	176.98 ± 42.67	42.39 ± 10.58	117.11 ± 36.92	NR	NR
	Saroglitazar 4 mg (n = 386)	51.34 ± 10.06	143/243	69.09 ± 11.46	NR	9.72 ± 1.58	172.52 ± 123.67	174.03 ± 39.32	41.50 ± 10.47	112.93 ± 34.89	NR	NR
	Pioglitazone 30 mg (n = 389)	51.84 ± 9.76	167/222	69.49 ± 11.59	NR	9.49 ± 1.54	166.20 ± 89.93	176.42 ± 37.83	42.64 ± 12.72	116.77 ± 32.31	NR	NR
RASTOGI et al. [20]	Saroglitazar 4 mg (n = 15)	53.1 ± 8.8	8/7	69.9 ± 12.6	159.3 ± 10.3	7.6 ± 0.9	NR	176.7 ± 41.4	37.7 ± 7.6	117.4 ± 38.4	NR	NR
	Placebo (n = 15)	54.9 ± 7.8	6/9	78.0 ± 11.7	164.1 ± 9.9	8.0 ± 1.0	NR	151.4 ± 36.4	47.4 ± 8.8	89.0 ± 36.3	NR	NR
GAWRIEH et al. [12]	Saroglitazar 1 mg (n = 25)	47.9 ± 10.4	12/13	NR	NR	6.8 ± 1.5	201.9 ± 116.6	194.0 ± 44.0	44.5 ± 7.3	124.3 ± 36.9	0.8 ± 0.2	84.8 ± 29.3
	Saroglitazar 4 mg (n = 27)	49.0 ± 11.0	12/15	NR	NR	6.1 ± 0.9	190.9 ± 98.5	204.8 ± 62.3	46.8 ± 15.8	132.7 ± 56.1	0.8 ± 0.2	83.4 ± 27.9
	Placebo (n = 28)	48.7 ± 10.5	13/15	NR	NR	6.2 ± 1.0	181.1 ± 62.2	191.7 ± 39.7	46.9 ± 12.0	121.6 ± 38.1	0.8 ± 0.2	93.4 ± 42.1
SIDDIQUI et al. [19]	Saroglitazar 4 mg (n = 130)	48.0 ± 0.9	53/77	NR	NR	6.2 ± 1.0	182.4 ± 116.1	188.8	43.3	117.5	NR	76 ± 51
	Placebo (n = 91)	47.8 ± 10.1	44/47	NR	NR	6.0 ± 0.9	171.6 ± 68.2	185.3	43.8	115.4	NR	72 ± 42

ALT: alanine transaminase; Cr: Creatine; NR: Not reported; TC: Total cholesterol; TG: Triglycerides.

3.4. Efficacy Endpoints

3.4.1. Triglycerides

A pooled analysis of six studies compared the triglyceride levels between the 4 mg saroglitazar (n = 418) and placebo (n = 372) groups [9,11,18–21]. The MD was −47.38 mg/dL (95% CI: −79.12 to −15.64 mg/dL; p = 0.03), demonstrating that 4 mg/day of saroglitazar decreased the triglyceride level compared to that in the control group in patients with dyslipidemia (Figure 3A).

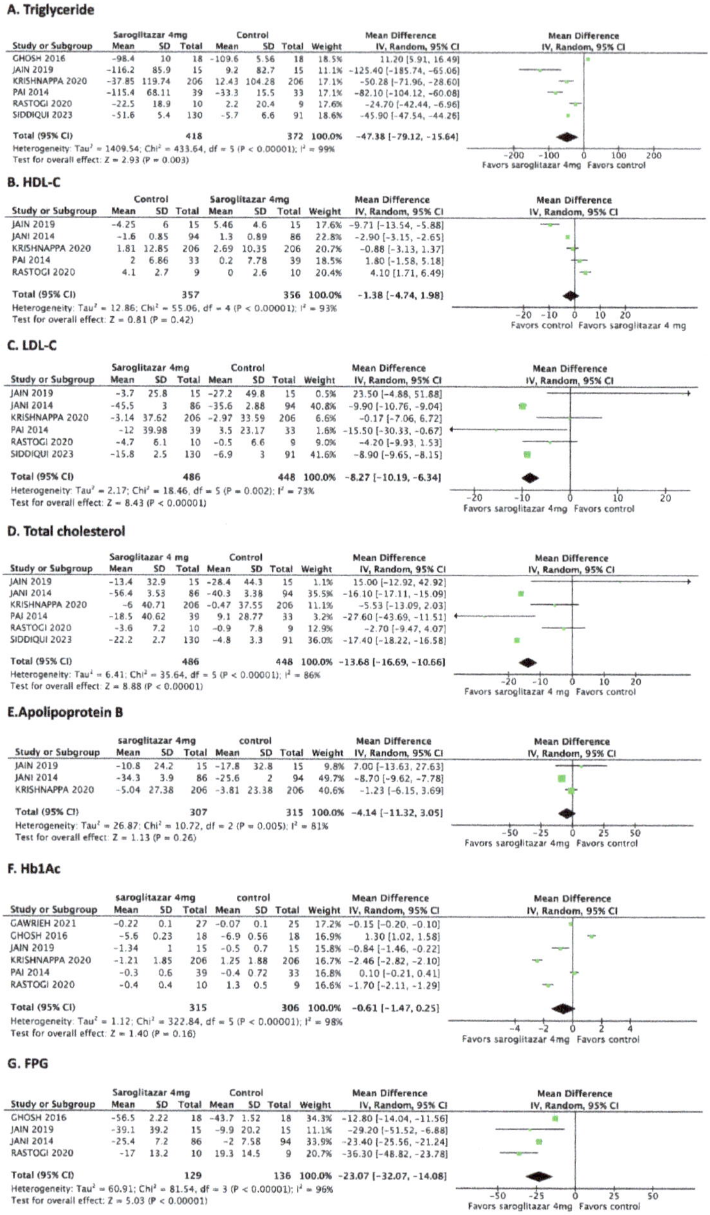

Figure 3. Forest plots comparing the efficacy endpoints between the 4 mg saroglitazar and control groups Saroglitazar (**A**) significantly reduces the triglyceride level [9,11,18–21]; (**B**) does not affect

the high-density lipoprotein cholesterol level [11,17,18,20,21]; (C) significantly reduces the low-density lipoprotein and [11,17–21] (D) total cholesterol levels [11,17–21]; (E) does not affect the apolipopotein B levels [11,17,18]; (F) does not affect the hemoglobin A1c level [9,11,12,18,20,21]; and (G) significantly decreases the fasting plasma glucose level compared to the control [9,17,18,20]. CI: confidence interval; IV: inverse variance; SD: standard deviation; The green squares represent the weighted mean difference (WMD) of each study, the horizontal line represents 95% confidence intervals (95% CI), and the black diamond represents the summary of weight mean difference.

We also compared the triglyceride level between the 2 mg (n = 256) and 4 mg (n = 270) saroglitazar groups. The MD was −32.38 mg/dL (95% CI: −53.62 to −11.14 mg/dL; p = 0.003), demonstrating that 4 mg/day of saroglitazar significantly decreased the triglyceride level compared to 2 mg/day in patients with diabetes-related dyslipidemia (Figure S3A).

3.4.2. HDL-C

A pooled analysis of five studies [11,17,18,20,21] compared the HDL-C level between the 4 mg saroglitazar (n = 357) and control (n = 356) groups. The MD was −1.38 mg/dL (95% CI: −4.74 to 1.98 mg/dL; p = 0.42). The I^2 value (93%) indicated a high level of heterogeneity among the studies (Figure 3B), suggesting that 4 mg/day of saroglitazar did not affect the HDL-C level compared to that in the control group in patients with dyslipidemia. The analysis comparing the 2 mg (n = 340) and 4 mg (n = 358) saroglitazar groups had similar results (MD: 0.03; 95% CI: −2.29 to 2.35; p = 0.98; Figure S3B).

3.4.3. LDL-C

The pooled analysis of six studies [11,17–21] compared the LDL-C level between the 4 mg saroglitazar (n = 486) and control (n = 446) groups. The MD was −8.27 mg/dL (95% CI: −10.19 to −6.34 mg/dL, p < 0.00001; I^2 = 73%; Figure 3C), demonstrating that 4 mg/day of saroglitazar significantly decreased the LDL-C level compared to that in the control group in patients with dyslipidemia.

Furthermore, a pooled analysis of 4 studies [11,12,17,21] compared the LDL-C level between the 2 mg (n = 340) and 4 mg (n = 358) saroglitazar groups; the LDL-C level did not differ between them (MD: −6.81 mg/dL; 95% CI: −14.53 to 0.90 mg/dL; p = 0.08; Figure S3C).

3.4.4. Total Cholesterol

A pooled analysis of six studies [11,17–21] compared the total cholesterol level between the 4 mg saroglitazar (n = 357) and control (n = 356) groups. The MD was −13.68 (95% CI: −16.69 to −10.66 mg/dL; p < 0.00001; I^2 = 86%; Figure 3D), demonstrating that 4 mg/day of saroglitazar significantly decreased the total cholesterol level compared to that in the control group in patients with dyslipidemia.

In contrast, the total cholesterol level did not differ between the 2 mg (n = 315) and 4 mg (n = 331) groups (MD: −3.54 mg/dL; 95% CI: −10.60 to 3.53 mg/dL; p = 0.33; Figure S4).

3.4.5. Apolipoprotein B

The pooled analysis of three studies [11,17,18] compared the apolipoprotein B level between the 4 mg saroglitazar (n = 307) and control (n = 315) groups. The MD was −4.14 (95% CI: −11.32 to 3.05; p = 0.26; Figure 3E), demonstrating that a 4 mg dose of saroglitazar did not affect the apolipoprotein B level compared to that in the control group in patients with dyslipidemia.

3.4.6. Glucose Parameters

A pooled analysis of four studies [9,17,18,20] compared the FPG level between the 4 mg saroglitazar (n = 129) and control (n = 136) groups. The FPG level was significantly lower in the 4 mg saroglitazar group than in the control group (MD: −23.07; 95% CI: −32.07

to -14.08; $p < 0.00001$; Figure 3G). However, the HbA1c level did not differ between the groups (MD: -0.61 mg/dL; 95% CI: -1.47 to 0.25; $p = 0.16$; Figure 3F).

3.5. Safety Endpoints

3.5.1. Serum Creatinine

A pooled analysis of three studies [12,17,21] compared the serum creatine levels between the 4 mg saroglitazar ($n = 150$) and control ($n = 152$) groups. The serum creatinine level significantly increased in the 4 mg saroglitazar group compared to that in the control group (MD: 0.12 mg/dL; 95% CI: 0.04 to 0.21 mg/dL; $p = 0.004$; Figure 4A). The serum creatinine level did not differ between the 2 mg ($n = 123$) and 4 mg ($n = 125$) saroglitazar groups (MD: -0.06; 95% CI: -0.15 to 0.04 mg/dL; $p = 0.26$; Figure S5A).

A. Serum creatinine

Study or Subgroup	Saroglitazar 4mg Mean	SD	Total	Control Mean	SD	Total	Weight	Mean Difference IV, Random, 95% CI
GAWRIEH 2021	0.04	0.02	25	-0.02	0.02	25	57.8%	0.06 [0.05, 0.07]
JANI 2014	0.1	0.2	86	0	0.21	94	32.8%	0.10 [0.04, 0.16]
PAI 2014	0.2	0.44	39	0	0.2	33	9.4%	0.20 [0.05, 0.35]
Total (95% CI)			**150**			**152**	**100.0%**	**0.09 [0.03, 0.14]**

Heterogeneity: Tau² = 0.00; Chi² = 4.75, df = 2 (P = 0.09); I² = 58%
Test for overall effect: Z = 3.29 (P = 0.0010)

B. ALT

Study or Subgroup	Saroglitazar 4mg Mean	SD	Total	Control Mean	SD	Total	Weight	Std. Mean Difference IV, Random, 95% CI
GAWRIEH 2021	-45.8	5.7	27	3.4	5.6	28	28.7%	-8.59 [-10.33, -6.84]
JANI 2014	-3.9	15.21	86	-0.7	12.46	102	35.8%	-0.23 [-0.52, 0.06]
PAI 2014	-0.2	0.3	39	-0.2	0.25	33	35.4%	0.00 [-0.46, 0.46]
Total (95% CI)			**152**			**163**	**100.0%**	**-2.55 [-4.62, -0.48]**

Heterogeneity: Tau² = 3.10; Chi² = 88.17, df = 2 (P < 0.00001); I² = 98%
Test for overall effect: Z = 2.41 (P = 0.02)

C. Weight

Study or Subgroup	Saroglitazar 4mg Mean	SD	Total	Control Mean	SD	Total	Weight	Mean Difference IV, Random, 95% CI
JAIN 2019	0.2	2.2	15	0.4	2.1	15	18.5%	-0.20 [-1.74, 1.34]
JANI 2014	0.3	2.83	86	-0.5	2.4	94	30.3%	0.80 [0.03, 1.57]
KRISHNAPPA 2020	-0.7	1.5	192	-0.05	1.67	206	36.9%	-0.65 [-0.96, -0.34]
PAI 2014	-0.8	5.35	37	-0.1	2.7	39	14.3%	-0.70 [-2.62, 1.22]
Total (95% CI)			**330**			**354**	**100.0%**	**-0.13 [-1.05, 0.78]**

Heterogeneity: Tau² = 0.57; Chi² = 11.87, df = 3 (P = 0.008); I² = 75%
Test for overall effect: Z = 0.29 (P = 0.77)

Figure 4. Forest plots comparing the safety endpoints between the 4 mg saroglitazar and control groups Saroglitazar (**A**) significantly increased the serum creatine level [12,17,21]; (**B**) significantly decreased the alanine transaminase level [12,17,21]; and (**C**) did not affect body weight compared to the control group [11,17,18,21]. CI: confidence interval; IV: inverse variance; SD: standard deviation. The green squares represent the weighted mean difference (WMD) of each study, the horizontal line represents 95% confidence intervals (95% CI), and the black diamond represents the summary of weight mean difference.

3.5.2. ALT

A pooled analysis of three studies [12,17,21] compared the ALT level between the 4 mg saroglitazar ($n = 152$) and control ($n = 163$) groups. The ALT level significantly decreased in the 4 mg saroglitazar group compared to that in the control group (SMD: -2.55; 95% CI: -4.62 to -0.48; $p = 0.02$; Figure 4B). However, the ALT level did not differ between the 2 mg ($n = 150$) and 4 mg ($n = 150$) saroglitazar groups (SMD: 0.91; 95% CI: -0.50 to 2.31; $p = 0.21$; $I^2 = 96\%$; Figure S5B).

3.5.3. Body Weight

A pooled analysis of four studies [11,17,18,21] compared the body weight of participants in the 4 mg saroglitazar ($n = 330$) and control ($n = 354$) groups; body weight did not differ between the groups (MD: -0.13 kg; 95% CI: -1.05 to 0.78; $p = 0.77$; $I^2 = 75\%$; Figure 4C). Body weight also did not differ between the 2 mg ($n = 331$) and 4 mg ($n = 315$) groups (MD: 0.35; 95% CI: -0.46 to 1.17; $p = 0.40$; $I^2 = 65\%$; Figure S5C).

4. Discussion

This meta-analysis provides a contemporary, comprehensive review of the efficacy and safety of saroglitazar in individuals with dyslipidemia. We found that 4 mg of saroglitazar significantly decreased the triglyceride and LDL-C levels compared to those in the controls without increasing the HDL-C level. We also found that 4 mg of saroglitazar significantly increased the serum creatinine level, significantly decreased the ALT level, and did not affect body weight compared to that in the controls.

Fibrates do not affect the HbA1c level (i.e., glycemia), whereas statins mildly increase it [19]. In this study, the FPG level was lower in the 4 mg saroglitazar group than in the anti-lipid, anti-diabetes, and placebo groups, reflecting the mild antihyperglycemic properties of saroglitazar.

Peroxisome proliferator-activated receptors are crucial in maintaining homeostasis, controlling inflammation, directing cell growth and differentiation, and limiting cell proliferation. [12] Despite its use as a lipid-lowering therapy, the PPAR-agonistic activity of fibrates is not very selective [19]. Fibrates cause serious illnesses, including myopathy, impaired renal function, and increased transaminase levels. Regarding PPAR-agonist action, thiazolidinediones reduce insulin resistance and blood glucose levels better than fibrates but can cause swelling and weight gain. [9].

In vitro and in vivo studies have investigated the pharmacodynamic action of saroglitazar in several disorders [22,23]. Our results suggest that 4 mg of saroglitazar may lower fat and glucose levels in patients with dyslipidemia, as evidenced by statistically significant reductions in total cholesterol and LDL-C levels without increasing the HDL-C level. These modifications are mostly attributable to the agonistic actions of PPAR, which are known to increase hepatic fatty acid oxidation and improve the lipid profile [19]. Increased HDL-C levels also suggest that saroglitazar might also be involved in reverse cholesterol metabolism, preventing the transfer of LDL-C. Our lipid profile results are consistent with those from studies of other glitazar-class medicines [24,25]. For instance, Dutta et al. found no change in the HbA1c or FBG levels after a comprehensive review and meta-analysis and reported that the effect of saroglitazar on glucose reduction varied based on the HbA1c level [10].

An observational study conducted by Shetty et al. [26] reported that adding saroglitazar to oral antidiabetic drugs resulted in a statistically significant improvement in glycemic (i.e., HbA1c) and lipid indices (i.e., triglycerides, total cholesterol, LDL-C, HDL-C, non-HDL, and very low-density lipoprotein cholesterol). The PPARα-agonist in this drug is responsible for the substantial triglyceride level decrease, while the PPARγ-agonist is responsible for the HbA1c level decrease [23]. Our efficacy endpoint results indicated that saroglitazar significantly decreased fasting blood glucose, postprandial plasma glucose, and HbA1c levels, which is highly expressive of its ability to reduce endothelial aggression, a key factor in the onset of the process that ultimately leads to coronary disease [1]. Goyal et al. also reported that saroglitazar significantly reduced fasting blood glucose, postprandial plasma glucose, and HbA1c levels [27]. Furthermore, they also found decreased ALT, aspartate transaminase, alkaline phosphatase, and gamma-glutamyltransferase concentrations. However, only alkaline phosphatase and gamma-glutamyltransferase levels significantly decreased among individuals with cardiometabolic illnesses treated with saroglitazar [12]. Previous research has shown that the ALT level in patients treated with saroglitazar consistently improved [20,28].

The recent PROMINENT trial demonstrated that the incidence of cardiovascular events remained comparable between patients who received fibrates and those given a placebo. Although levels of triglycerides, VLDL cholesterol, remnant cholesterol, and apolipoprotein C were lower in the fibrate group, there was no reduction in apolipoprotein B levels, and it was felt that this medication does not improve cardiovascular outcomes [7]. In light of this, we emphasize that in our analysis, saroglitazar did not significantly reduce apolipoprotein B, highlighting that in spite of the fact that there were improvements in the saroglitazar group regarding the lipid profile, this may not translate to improved cardiovascular outcomes.

Saroglitazar is not excreted via the kidneys, and thus, some adverse effects have been observed in clinical studies, including hepatotoxicity and renal toxicity [12,26]. We identified a significant association between 4 mg of saroglitazar and increased serum creatinine levels (MD: 0.12 mg/dL, $p = 0.004$). However, we cannot find evidence to explain this result. One RCT assessed the estimated glomerular filtration rate (GFR), which did not decrease. Thus, consistent with the study by Dutta et al., our meta-analysis results raise concerns regarding saroglitazar and renal safety [10]. Tesaglitazar and aleglitazar increase serum creatinine, blood urea nitrogen levels, and the GFR [29]. Thus, long-term saroglitazar users should be monitored for changes in the serum creatinine level, uremic indices, urine microalbumin, and renal architecture for at least one year. Renal hemodynamics may cause renal tubules to synthesize and secrete more creatinine [12]. However, cystatin-C, inulin clearance, and GFR markers are unaffected by fenofibrate [9]. Saroglitazar, which has a PPAR-alpha agonist action similar to fenofibrate, may have comparable effects on serum creatinine levels.

Krishnappa et al. [11] examined blood creatinine levels over 56 weeks and found no significant differences between saroglitazar and pioglitazone users. Our data suggest that saroglitazar patients require a specialized and well-powered study that examines renal parameters, including glomerular filtration rate and urine microalbumin/creatinine ratio. Finally, long-term adverse effects such as cardiovascular disease (which requires a dedicated cardiovascular outcome trial), bladder cancer (seen with some other peroxisome proliferator-activated receptor (PPAR) agonists), and liposarcomas (seen with muraglitazar) must be fully evaluated to ensure the long-term safety of saroglitazar in clinical practice [27,30–33].

With regard to future perspectives, the pleiotropic effects of saroglitazar, which affect both glucose and lipid metabolism, play an important role in its potential as a therapeutic option. Sasso et al. [34] examined type 2 diabetes subjects with albuminuria and a history of cardiovascular disease and reported that the increase in the number of risk factors at target correlates with better cardiovascular outcomes in patients with type 2 DM at high CV risk. That being so, saroglitazar could represent a potential new therapeutic option.

This study has some limitations. First, all the included studies were clinical trials, which often have a small sample size and a short follow-up time, making it difficult to determine the long-term safety and effectiveness of saroglitazar. Second, since all the included trials were performed in India, these results may not be generalizable to all individuals with dyslipidemia. Third, heterogeneity is greater than 50% in many of the outcome analyses, even though the number of studies is limited to fewer than ten (Supplementary Materials). Finally, every experiment that was considered had a shorter follow-up period with surrogate results.

5. Conclusions

This meta-analysis suggests that 4 mg of saroglitazar reduces triglyceride, LDL-C, and total cholesterol levels in patients with dyslipidemia; however, there were no significant changes in apolipoprotein B levels. Thus, it improves the lipid profile; nevertheless, it may not reduce cardiovascular outcomes. Furthermore, it significantly increased the creatinine level, which is a potential safety concern.

Supplementary Materials: The following supporting information can be downloaded at: https://www.mdpi.com/article/10.3390/jcm12175674/s1, Figure S1: Forest plots comparing the efficacy endpoints between the 2 mg and 4 mg saroglitazar groups; Figure S2: Forest plots comparing the safety endpoints between the 2 mg and 4 mg saroglitazar groups; Figure S3: Funnel plots and Egger's tests comparing the (A) triglyceride, (B) low-density lipoprotein cholesterol, (C) high-density lipoprotein cholesterol, and (D) fasting plasma glucose levels between the 2 mg and 4 mg saroglitazar groups; Figure S4: Funnel plots and Egger's tests comparing the (A) creatinine level, (B) alanine transaminase level, and (C) body weight between the 2 mg and 4 mg saroglitazar groups.

Author Contributions: Conceptualization, A.d.S.M.J., V.M.R.O. and I.C.O.; methodology, A.d.S.M.J. and V.M.R.O.; software, I.C.O., A.J.P.S. and D.P.C.C.; validation, A.M.d.S. and A.M.d.P.; formal analysis, G.B.B.R., R.F.P.P. and F.H.M.; investigation, D.P.C.C. and A.J.P.S.; data curation, A.M.d.S.; R.F.P.P. and F.H.M.; writing—original draft preparation, A.d.S.M.J., V.M.R.O. and I.C.O.; writing—review and editing, A.d.S.M.J., V.M.R.O., I.C.O. and A.M.d.S.; visualization, G.B.B.R., A.M.d.P. and F.H.M.; supervision, A.d.S.M.J.; project administration, A.d.S.M.J. and V.M.R.O.; All authors have read and agreed to the published version of the manuscript.

Funding: This research received no external funding.

Institutional Review Board Statement: Not applicable.

Informed Consent Statement: Not applicable.

Data Availability Statement: The data underlying this article will be shared on reasonable request with the corresponding author.

Acknowledgments: We gratefully acknowledge the Meta-Analysis Academy for its methodological support.

Conflicts of Interest: The authors declare no conflict of interest.

References

1. Musunuru, K. Atherogenic Dyslipidemia: Cardiovascular Risk and Dietary Intervention. *Lipids* **2010**, *45*, 907–914. [CrossRef] [PubMed]
2. Musunuru, K.; Kathiresan, S. Surprises From Genetic Analyses of Lipid Risk Factors for Atherosclerosis. *Circ. Res.* **2016**, *118*, 579–585. [CrossRef] [PubMed]
3. Vrablík, M.; Šarkanová, I.; Breciková, K.; Šedová, P.; Šatný, M.; Tichopád, A. Low LDL-C goal attainment in patients at very high cardiovascular risk due to lacking observance of the guidelines on dyslipidaemias. *PLoS ONE* **2023**, *18*, e0272883. [CrossRef]
4. Chistiakov, D.A.; Grechko, A.V.; Myasoedova, V.A.; Melnichenko, A.A.; Orekhov, A.N. Impact of the cardiovascular system-associated adipose tissue on atherosclerotic pathology. *Atherosclerosis* **2017**, *263*, 361–368. [CrossRef]
5. Gepner, Y.; Shelef, I.; Komy, O.; Cohen, N.; Schwarzfuchs, D.; Bril, N.; Rein, M.; Serfaty, D.; Kenigsbuch, S.; Zelicha, H.; et al. The beneficial effects of Mediterranean diet over low-fat diet may be mediated by decreasing hepatic fat content. *J. Hepatol.* **2019**, *71*, 379–388. [CrossRef]
6. Sampson, U.K.; Fazio, S.; Linton, M.F. Residual Cardiovascular Risk Despite Optimal LDL Cholesterol Reduction with Statins: The Evidence, Etiology, and Therapeutic Challenges. *Curr. Atheroscler. Rep.* **2012**, *14*, 1–10. [CrossRef]
7. Das Pradhan, A.; Glynn, R.J.; Fruchart, J.-C.; MacFadyen, J.G.; Zaharris, E.S.; Everett, B.M.; Campbell, S.E.; Oshima, R.; Amarenco, P.; Blom, D.J.; et al. Triglyceride Lowering with Pemafibrate to Reduce Cardiovascular Risk. *N. Engl. J. Med.* **2022**, *387*, 1923–1934. [CrossRef]
8. Durga, D.R.; Mounika, N.; Mudimala, P.; Adela, R. Efficacy and Safety of Saroglitazar in Patients with Cardiometabolic Diseases: A Systematic Review and Meta-Analysis of Randomized Controlled Trials. *Clin. Drug Investig.* **2022**, *42*, 1049–1064. [CrossRef] [PubMed]
9. Ghosh, A.; Sahana, P.K.; Das, C.; Mandal, A.; Sengupta, N. Comparison of Effectiveness and Safety of Add-on Therapy of Saroglitazar and Fenofibrate with Metformin in Indian Patients with Diabetic Dyslipidaemia. *J. Clin. Diagn. Res.* **2016**, *10*, FC01–FC04. [CrossRef]
10. Dutta, D.; Bhattacharya, S.; Surana, V.; Aggarwal, S.; Singla, R.; Khandelwal, D.; Sharma, M. Efficacy and safety of saroglitazar in managing hypertriglyceridemia in type-2 diabetes: A meta-analysis. *Diabetes Metab. Syndr. Clin. Res. Rev.* **2020**, *14*, 1759–1768. [CrossRef]
11. Krishnappa, M.; Patil, K.; Parmar, K.; Trivedi, P.; Mody, N.; Shah, C.; Faldu, K.; Maroo, S.; Desai, P.; Fatania, K.; et al. Effect of saroglitazar 2 mg and 4 mg on glycemic control, lipid profile and cardiovascular disease risk in patients with type 2 diabetes mellitus: A 56-week, randomized, double blind, phase 3 study (PRESS XII study). *Cardiovasc. Diabetol.* **2020**, *19*, 93. [CrossRef] [PubMed]
12. Gawrieh, S.; Noureddin, M.; Loo, N.; Mohseni, R.; Awasty, V.; Cusi, K.; Kowdley, K.V.; Lai, M.; Schiff, E.; Parmar, D.; et al. Saroglitazar, a PPAR-α/γ Agonist, for Treatment of NAFLD: A Randomized Controlled Double-Blind Phase 2 Trial. *Hepatology* **2021**, *74*, 1809–1824. [CrossRef] [PubMed]
13. Page, M.J.; McKenzie, J.E.; Bossuyt, P.M.; Boutron, I.; Hoffmann, T.C.; Mulrow, C.D.; Shamseer, L.; Tetzlaff, J.M.; Akl, E.A.; Brennan, S.E.; et al. The PRISMA 2020 statement: An updated guideline for reporting systematic reviews. *Int. J. Surg.* **2021**, *88*, 105906. [CrossRef]
14. Sterne, J.A.C.; Savović, J.; Page, M.J.; Elbers, R.G.; Blencowe, N.S.; Boutron, I.; Cates, C.J.; Cheng, H.Y.; Corbett, M.S.; Eldridge, S.M.; et al. RoB 2: A revised tool for assessing risk of bias in randomised trials. *BMJ* **2019**, *366*, l4898. [CrossRef]

15. National Heart LaBI. Study Quality Assessment Tool 2014. Available online: https://www.nhlbi.nih.gov/health-topics/study-quality-assessment-tools (accessed on 7 April 2023).
16. Higgins, J.P.T.; Thomas, J.; Chandler, J.; Cumpston, M.; Li, T.; Page, M.J.; Welch, V.A. (Eds.) Cochrane Handbook for Systematic Reviews of Interventions Version 6.3 (Updated February 2022). *Cochrane*. 2022. Available online: www.training.cochrane.org/handbook (accessed on 7 April 2023).
17. Jani, R.H.; Pai, V.; Jha, P.; Jariwala, G.; Mukhopadhyay, S.; Bahnsali, A.; Joshi, S. A multicenter, prospective, randomized, double-blind study to evaluate the safety and efficacy of Saroglitazar 2 and 4 mg compared with placebo in type 2 diabetes mellitus patients having hypertriglyceridemia not controlled with atorvastatin therapy (PRESS VI). *Diabetes Technol. Ther.* **2014**, *16*, 63–71. [CrossRef] [PubMed]
18. Jain, N.; Bhansali, S.; Kurpad, A.V.; Hawkins, M.; Sharma, A.; Kaur, S.; Rastogi, A.; Bhansali, A. Effect of a Dual PPAR α/γ agonist on Insulin Sensitivity in Patients of Type 2 Diabetes with Hypertriglyceridemia- Randomized double-blind placebo-controlled trial. *Sci. Rep.* **2019**, *9*, 19017. [CrossRef]
19. Siddiqui, M.S.; Parmar, D.; Sheikh, F.; Sarin, S.K.; Cisneros, L.; Gawrieh, S.; Momin, T.; Duseja, A.; Sanyal, A.J. Saroglitazar, a Dual PPAR α/γ Agonist, Improves Atherogenic Dyslipidemia in Patients With Non-Cirrhotic Nonalcoholic Fatty Liver Disease: A Pooled Analysis. *Clin. Gastroenterol. Hepatol.* **2023**, *21*, 2597–2605.e2. [CrossRef]
20. Rastogi, A.; Dunbar, R.L.; Thacker, H.P.; Bhatt, J.; Parmar, K.; Parmar, D.V. Abrogation of postprandial triglyceridemia with dual PPAR α/γ agonist in type 2 diabetes mellitus: A randomized, placebo-controlled study. *Acta Diabetol.* **2020**, *57*, 809–818. [CrossRef]
21. Pai, V.; Paneerselvam, A.; Mukhopadhyay, S.; Bahnsali, A.; Kamath, D.; Shankar, V.; Gambhire, D.; Jani, R.H.; Joshi, S.; Patel, P. A Multicenter, Prospective, Randomized, Double-blind Study to Evaluate the Safety and Efficacy of Saroglitazar 2 and 4 mg Compared to Pioglitazone 45 mg in Diabetic Dyslipidemia (PRESS V). *J. Diabetes Sci. Technol.* **2014**, *8*, 132–141. [CrossRef]
22. Kamata, S.; Ishii, I. PPARα-Ligand Binding Modes Revealed by X-ray Crystallography. *Yakugaku Zasshi* **2021**, *141*, 1267–1274. [CrossRef]
23. Nikolic, D.; Castellino, G.; Banach, M.; Toth, P.P.; Ivanova, E.; Orekhov, A.; Montalto, G.; Rizzo, M. PPAR Agonists, Athero-genic Dyslipidemia and Cardiovascular risk. *Curr. Pharm. Des.* **2017**, *23*, 894–902. [CrossRef]
24. Rotman, Y.; Sanyal, A.J. Current and Upcoming Pharmacotherapy for Non-alcoholic Fatty Liver Disease. *Gut* **2017**, *66*, 180–190. [CrossRef]
25. Staels, B.; Fruchart, J.-C. Therapeutic Roles of Peroxisome Proliferator–Activated Receptor Agonists. *Diabetes* **2005**, *54*, 2460–2470. [CrossRef] [PubMed]
26. Shetty, S.R.; Kumar, S.; Mathur, R.; Sharma, K.H.; Jaiswal, A.D. Observational study to evaluate the safety and efficacy of saroglitazar in Indian diabetic dyslipidemia patients. *Indian Heart J.* **2015**, *67*, 23–26. [CrossRef]
27. Goyal, O.; Nohria, S.; Goyal, P.; Kaur, J.; Sharma, A.; Sood, A.; Chhina, R.S. Saroglitazar in patients with non-alcoholic fatty liver disease and diabetic dyslipidemia: A prospective, observational, real world study. *Sci. Rep.* **2020**, *10*, 21117. [CrossRef] [PubMed]
28. Saboo, B.; Hasnani, D.; Saiyed, M.; Patel, F. Retrospective Observational Study Evaluating Efficacy of Saroglitazar 4mg in Type 2 Diabetic Dyslipidemic Patients at Tertiary Care Centre in India. *Atheroscler. Suppl.* **2018**, *32*, 47. [CrossRef]
29. Tenenbaum, A.; Motro, M.; Fisman, E.Z. Dual and pan-peroxisome proliferator-activated receptors (PPAR) co-agonism: The bezafibrate lessons. *Cardiovasc. Diabetol.* **2005**, *4*, 14. [CrossRef] [PubMed]
30. Jani, R.H.; Kansagra, K.; Jain, M.R.; Patel, H. Pharmacokinetics, Safety, and Tolerability of Saroglitazar (ZYH1), a Predominantly PPARα Agonist with Moderate PPARγ Agonist Activity in Healthy Human Subjects. *Clin. Drug Investig.* **2013**, *33*, 809–816. [CrossRef] [PubMed]
31. Joshi, S. One Year Post-marketing Surveillance Study of Saroglitazar in Patients with Diabetic Dyslipidemia and History of Coronary Heart Disease. *Endocr. Pract.* **2017**, *23*, 44A.
32. Chatterjee, S.; Majumder, A.; Ray, S. Observational Study of Saroglitazar on Metabolic Parameters in Indian Patients with Diabetic Dyslipidemia: 43 weeks of Clinical Experience. *Diabetes. Technol. Ther.* **2017**, *19*, A120–A121. [CrossRef]
33. Kaul, U.; Parmar, D.; Manjunath, K.; Shah, M.; Parmar, K.; Patil, K.P.; Jaiswal, A. New dual peroxisome proliferator activated receptor agonist—Saroglitazar in diabetic dyslipidemia and non-alcoholic fatty liver disease: Integrated analysis of the real world evidence. *Cardiovasc. Diabetol.* **2019**, *18*, 80. [CrossRef] [PubMed]
34. Sasso, F.C.; Simeon, V.; Galiero, R.; Caturano, A.; De Nicola, L.; Chiodini, P.; Rinaldi, L.; Salvatore, T.; Lettieri, M.; Nevola, R.; et al. The number of risk factors not at target is associated with cardiovascular risk in a type 2 diabetic population with albuminuria in primary cardiovascular prevention. Post-hoc analysis of the NID-2 trial. *Cardiovasc. Diabetol.* **2022**, *21*, 235. [CrossRef] [PubMed]

Disclaimer/Publisher's Note: The statements, opinions and data contained in all publications are solely those of the individual author(s) and contributor(s) and not of MDPI and/or the editor(s). MDPI and/or the editor(s) disclaim responsibility for any injury to people or property resulting from any ideas, methods, instructions or products referred to in the content.

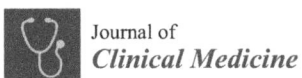

Review

Management of Residual Risk in Chronic Coronary Syndromes. Clinical Pathways for a Quality-Based Secondary Prevention

Simona Giubilato [1,*], Fabiana Lucà [2], Maurizio Giuseppe Abrignani [3], Laura Gatto [4], Carmelo Massimiliano Rao [2], Nadia Ingianni [5], Francesco Amico [1], Roberta Rossini [6], Giorgio Caretta [7], Stefano Cornara [8], Irene Di Matteo [9], Concetta Di Nora [10], Silvia Favilli [11], Anna Pilleri [12], Andrea Pozzi [13], Pier Luigi Temporelli [14], Marco Zuin [15,16], Antonio Francesco Amico [17], Carmine Riccio [18], Massimo Grimaldi [19], Furio Colivicchi [20], Fabrizio Oliva [9] and Michele Massimo Gulizia [21,22]

1. Cardiology Department, Cannizzaro Hospital, 95126 Catania, Italy; famico64@gmail.com
2. Cardiology Department, Grande Ospedale Metropolitano, AO Bianchi Melacrino Morelli, 89129 Reggio Calabria, Italy; fabiana.luca92@gmail.com (F.L.); massimo.rao@libero.it (C.M.R.)
3. Operative Unit of Cardiology, P. Borsellino Hospital, 91025 Marsala, Italy
4. Cardiology Department, San Giovanni Addolorata Hospital, 00184 Rome, Italy
5. ASP Trapani Cardiologist Marsala Castelvetrano Districts, 91022 Castelvetrano, Italy; nadiaing@hotmail.it
6. Cardiology Unit, Ospedale Santa Croce e Carle, 12100 Cuneo, Italy; roberta.rossini2@gmail.com
7. Sant'Andrea Hospital, ASL 5 Regione Liguria, 19124 La Spezia, Italy; giorgio.caretta@gmail.com
8. Arrhytmia Unit, Division of Cardiology, Ospedale San Paolo, Azienda Sanitaria Locale 2, 17100 Savona, Italy; stefano.cornara@gmail.com
9. De Gasperis Cardio Center, Niguarda Hospital, 20162 Milan, Italy; dimatteoirene@hotmail.it (I.D.M.); fabri.oliva@gmail.com (F.O.)
10. Department of Cardiothoracic Science, Azienda Sanitaria Universitaria Integrata di Udine, 33100 Udine, Italy; concetta.dinora@gmail.com
11. Department of Pediatric Cardiology, Meyer Hospital, 50139 Florence, Italy; silvia.favilli@meyer.it
12. Cardiology Unit, Brotzu Hospital, 09121 Cagliari, Italy; annapilleri@yahoo.it
13. Cardiology Unit, Papa Giovanni XXIII Hospital, 24127 Bergamo, Italy; andreawellsvabg@gmail.com
14. Division of Cardiac Rehabilitation, Istituti Clinici Scientifici Maugeri, IRCCS, 28013 Gattico-Veruno, Italy; pierluigi.temporelli@icsmaugeri.it
15. Department of Translational Medicine, University of Ferrara, 44121 Ferrara, Italy; zuinml@yahoo.it
16. Department of Cardiology, West Vicenza Hospital, 136071 Arzignano, Italy
17. CCU-Cardiology Unit, Ospedale San Giuseppe da Copertino Hospital, Copertino, 73100 Lecce, Italy
18. Cardiovascular Department, Sant'Anna e San Sebastiano Hospital, 81100 Caserta, Italy; carminericcio8@gmail.com
19. Department of Cardiology, General Regional Hospital "F. Miulli", 70021 Bari, Italy; m.grimaldi@miulli.it
20. Clinical and Rehabilitation Cardiology Unit, San Filippo Neri Hospital, 00135 Rome, Italy; furio.colivicchi@gmail.com
21. Cardiology Department, Garibaldi Nesima Hospital, 95122 Catania, Italy; michele.gulizia60@gmail.com
22. Heart Care Foundation, 50121 Florence, Italy
* Correspondence: simogiub@hotmail.com

Abstract: Chronic coronary syndrome (CCS), which encompasses a broad spectrum of clinical presentations of coronary artery disease (CAD), is the leading cause of morbidity and mortality worldwide. Recent guidelines for the management of CCS emphasize the dynamic nature of the CAD process, replacing the term "stable" with "chronic", as this disease is never truly "stable". Despite significant advances in the treatment of CAD, patients with CCS remain at an elevated risk of major cardiovascular events (MACE) due to the so-called residual cardiovascular risk. Several pathogenetic pathways (thrombotic, inflammatory, metabolic, and procedural) may distinctly contribute to the residual risk in individual patients and represent a potential target for newer preventive treatments. Identifying the level and type of residual cardiovascular risk is essential for selecting the most appropriate diagnostic tests and follow-up procedures. In addition, new management strategies and healthcare models could further support available treatments and lead to important prognostic benefits. This review aims to provide an overview of the diagnostic and therapeutic challenges in the management of patients with CCS and to promote more effective multidisciplinary care.

Keywords: chronic coronary syndromes; residual cardiovascular risk; secondary prevention; optimal medical therapy; multidisciplinary management; angina; percutaneous coronary intervention

1. Introduction

Coronary artery disease (CAD) remains a leading cause of mortality and morbidity worldwide. Recently, European [1] and American [2] guidelines have emphasized the importance of the clinical features of individuals at a higher risk of developing CAD, and the role of novel diagnostic tools in establishing a certain diagnosis. Importantly, the expression "stable" CAD has been removed and replaced with "chronic coronary syndromes (CCS)". [3]. This change in nomenclature highlights the dynamic nature of CAD, which is characterized by a "silent" progression until the onset of clinical presentations, underlining that this clinical condition is only assumed to be stable. In fact, a chronic phase may be interrupted at any time by acute events, which can further clinically destabilize the course of the disease. International consensus statements suggest a stepwise approach to the diagnostic pathway, including the assessment of a patient's history, symptoms, assessment of signs, risk factors, and comorbidities. Guidelines underscore the importance of a healthy lifestyle to prevent the onset of CAD and improve outcomes in patients with CCS. Optimal medical therapy (OMT), including antithrombotic and lipid-lowering therapy (LLT), is the first objective of CCS management for its proven prognostic efficacy. Only after intensification of pharmacological therapy should the assessment of myocardial ischemia, through both non-invasive and invasive tests, be considered to identify those patients who are likely to derive symptomatic benefit from myocardial revascularization. However, despite therapeutic advances in recent years, patients with CCS remain a population at a high risk for recurrent events [4]. Several mechanisms, including thrombotic, inflammatory, metabolic, and procedural factors, contribute to this residual risk and represent new targets for more effective and tailored secondary prevention strategies.

The aim of this review is to address the diagnostic pathways of CCS and to provide an overview of the treatment challenges in managing residual cardiovascular risk in CCS patients to promote more effective secondary prevention strategies.

2. Chronic Coronary Syndromes: Nosographic and Epidemiological Aspects

Chronic coronary syndromes (CCS) encompass a wide spectrum of different clinical entities, mainly resulting from atherosclerotic plaque buildup in the wall of the coronary arteries (obstructive CAD) but also stemming from other pathogenetic mechanisms, such as epicardial vasospasm or microvascular coronary disfunction (non-obstructive CAD). From a nosographic perspective, the ESC guidelines have further classified CCS into six separate entities (Table 1) [1], facilitating the identification and categorization of these patients.

Table 1. CCS categories according to the ESC 2019 guidelines [1].

CCS Categories	Description
1	Patients with supposed CAD and "stable" symptoms
2	Patients with new onset of heart failure or left ventricular dysfunction and suspected CAD
3	Asymptomatic and symptomatic patients <1 year after an ACS or revascularization
4	Patients >1 year after angina diagnosis or revascularization
5	Symptomatic patients with suspected vasospastic or microvascular disease
6	Asymptomatic patients in whom CAD is discovered at screening

ACS: acute coronary syndrome CAD: coronary artery disease; CCS: chronic coronary syndromes.

From an epidemiological perspective, CCS represents an important and challenging public health issue. It has been reported that in the US, the incidence of CCS is approximately twice that of myocardial infarction (MI) and is expected to affect roughly 18% of adults by 2030 [5]. In contrast, the majority of the epidemiological and clinical evidence regarding the European population with CCS comes from the ongoing ESC EURObservational Research Programme (EORP) Chronic Ischemic Cardiovascular Disease Long Term (CICD LT) registry. This registry provides up-to-date information from 20 ESC countries regarding the management and outcomes of European patients with CCS [6]. The prevalence and mortality rate of patients with CCS varies slightly between European countries reflecting the existing differences in the treatment of acute coronary syndromes (ACS) and the promotion of secondary cardiovascular (CV) preventive strategies [6]. These differences are observed in the management of both women and elderly patients, as also previously reported in larger registries of patients with stable CAD. These groups are less likely to receive guideline-directed optimal medical therapy (OMT), resulting in poorer prognosis [7–9]. Conversely, the hospitalization rate of European patients with CCS remains high, with one in five patients being hospitalized for CV reasons <1 year after CCS diagnosis [7]. Furthermore, the risk of CV events was higher among CCS patients with multiple non-cardiac comorbidities, including chronic kidney disease (CKD), chronic obstructive pulmonary disease (COPD), obesity, etc. Nevertheless, the rate of major adverse CV events (MACE) has substantially decreased in European patients with CCS, reflecting developments in their management [10]. Considering the recent introduction of a new CCS definition in clinical practice, in addition to the recent concomitant COVID-19 pandemic, which significantly limits the recruitment of patients in multicenter registries and trials, further analyses are necessary to better define the contemporary epidemiological features of CCS in different European member states, to improve the management and treatment of such patients.

3. Residual Risk in Chronic Coronary Syndromes

Both the increased application of evidence-based therapy and the newer generation of drug-eluting stents (DES) have recently led to improvements in the treatment of patients with CAD. The revolutionary advancements have been linked with a significant reduction in the rates of recurrent MACE and stent thrombosis. However, despite the undoubtedly better approach, the risk of subsequent events remains very high, especially in patients with poly-vascular disease and comorbidities [11,12]. The high rate of recurrent CV events, despite a strong secondary prevention strategy, leads to the notion of residual ischemic risk. Clinical trials in patients with CCS have demonstrated a persistent risk of MACE of 2–4% per year [13–15]. Even in the most recent studies that introduced the proprotein convertase subtilisin/kexin type 9 inhibitors (PCSK9i) in the clinical arena, the occurrence of subsequent events in the treated arms remained around 9%, despite the drastic LDL cholesterol (LDL-C) reductions [16,17]. Moreover, real-world data from registries and observational studies demonstrated even more unfavorable outcomes: The REACH (Reduction of Atherothrombosis for Continued Health) registry reported an approximate 5% risk of 1-year recurrent CV events in patients with CAD or with multiple risk factors associated with atherothrombosis [18]. A comprehensive national Swedish registry, including over 108,000 post-MI patients, found that nearly 20% experienced a recurrent MACE in the year following the index ACS event. This residual CV risk persists and increases over time: In the Swedish registry, one in five patients who persisted stable in the first year after MI had a new recurrent event in the following 3 years [19]. The GRACE (Global Registry of Acute Coronary Events) registry, which recruited 3721 post-ACS patients from the United Kingdom (UK) and Belgium for a five-year follow-up period, presented a 13% occurrence of CV mortality and a 9.3% incidence of recurrent MI [20].

CCS patients with non-obstructive CAD (Category 5 according to the ESC Classification) also exhibit an elevated risk of MACE and all-cause mortality and deserve special attention [21]. Notably, women not only have a higher incidence of non-obstructive CAD but also have a worse prognosis than men [22].

Specifically, we have gained a deeper understanding of the prognosis of patients with microvascular angina. Several studies have shown that the detection of abnormal Coronary Flow Reserve (CFR) in patients with CCS without significant obstructive CAD is strongly associated with an increased risk of MACE in the long term [23,24]. Furthermore, Murthy VL et al. have shown that among diabetic patients, those without obstructive CAD but with an abnormal CFR have a CV mortality rate similar to those with obstructive CAD during 1.4 years of follow-up [25].

A large and growing body of research has demonstrated that around 6–8% of all MI occur in the absence of coronary artery obstruction. Myocardial infarction with non-obstructive CAD (MINOCA) is a heterogenous group of diseases with various potential etiologies, including coronary artery spasm, coronary thromboembolism, plaque disruption, spontaneous coronary artery dissection, and supply–demand mismatch [26]. Patients with a history of MINOCA exhibit a comparable, or only slightly lower, rate of recurrent MACE during follow-up when compared to post-MI patients with obstructive CAD, despite their younger age and fewer comorbidities [27]. The diagnosis of MINOCA is a working diagnosis in which intracoronary imaging techniques performed during the acute phase help to better evaluate coronary arteries that appear normal on angiography. In particular, optical coherence tomography (OCT), providing high-resolution, detailed images of the coronary arteries, plays a crucial role in understanding underlying etiopathogenetic mechanisms of MINOCA, such as plaque erosion, dissection, or thromboembolism. OCT's ability to elucidate the etiology of MINOCA in more than half of patients holds significant therapeutic and prognostic implications. This allows for the customization of secondary prevention management strategies aimed at enhancing the overall prognosis of this CCS patient category [27,28]. In the future, the advancement of artificial intelligence-assisted techniques for characterizing coronary atherosclerotic plaques has the potential to improve the diagnostic power of both invasive and non-invasive approaches in suspected MINOCA cases [29].

When CCS coexists with heart failure (HF), the risk of recurrent CV events becomes even more pronounced. Previous studies have indicated that the development of HF over time in patients with stable CAD has significant prognostic implications [30,31]. More recently, findings from the CORONOR Registry have supported the notion that reduced left ventricular ejection fraction (LVEF) and a history of HF are the main causes of CV death in a modern population of patients with stable CAD who are extensively managed with guideline-directed medical therapy (GDMT) [32]. The CORONOR Registry also reported a 5.7% risk of hospitalization for HF over a 5-year period in this patient cohort. The study further highlighted that hospitalization for HF is a robust predictor of mortality with a 28% risk after 1 year and a 43% risk after 2 years [33].

There are several elements contributing to the residual risk, including traditional CV risk factors, HF, CKD, and psychological and socio-cultural factors. However, other promoters of residual risk are beginning to emerge. These are related to thrombotic, metabolic, and inflammatory pathways that can contribute to the development of recurrent events and are often not adequately addressed in common clinical practice [34]. Furthermore, in revascularized CCS patients, other factors, such as incomplete/suboptimal revascularization or complex PCI, may contribute to a residual ischemic risk. Figure 1 shows pathways of residual CV risk in CCS patients.

3.1. Prognostic Stratification

The residual CV risk has been associated with some clinical characteristics (diabetes, prior ACS, stroke, HF, poly-vascular disease, extent of CAD, completeness of revascularization) and biomarkers, such as troponins, N-terminal pro-B-type natriuretic peptide (NT-proBNP), and C-Reactive protein (CRP) [35]. Identifying patients with high residual CV risk is crucial for the secondary prevention strategies.

Risk scores are useful bedside tools for a rapid prognostic definition. The Dual Antiplatelet Therapy (DAPT) score was developed from the DAPT Study to predict ischemic and bleeding risk in patients who underwent percutaneous coronary intervention (PCI). Patients with a DAPT score ≥ 2 have a high ischemic risk and a low bleeding risk and were found to benefit from prolonged DAPT beyond 12 months. On the other hand, patients with a DAPT score < 2 present a high bleeding risk and a low ischemic risk and were found to benefit from a shorter duration of DAPT [36]. Following the development of the DAPT score, many studies have tried to define its validity in different study populations with disappointing results. Chicharron et al. confirmed the ability of the DAPT score to identify an ischemic risk, detecting an approximately twofold higher incidence of CV events in patients with a DAPT score ≥ 2 [37]. In contrast, Ueda et al. showed that in an extensive Swedish registry, this score did not effectively discriminate between bleeding and ischemic risk [38]. In a recent analysis, including 100,211 post-PCI patients, a DAPT score ≥ 2 was able to accurately recognize patients at high ischemic and low bleeding risk [39].

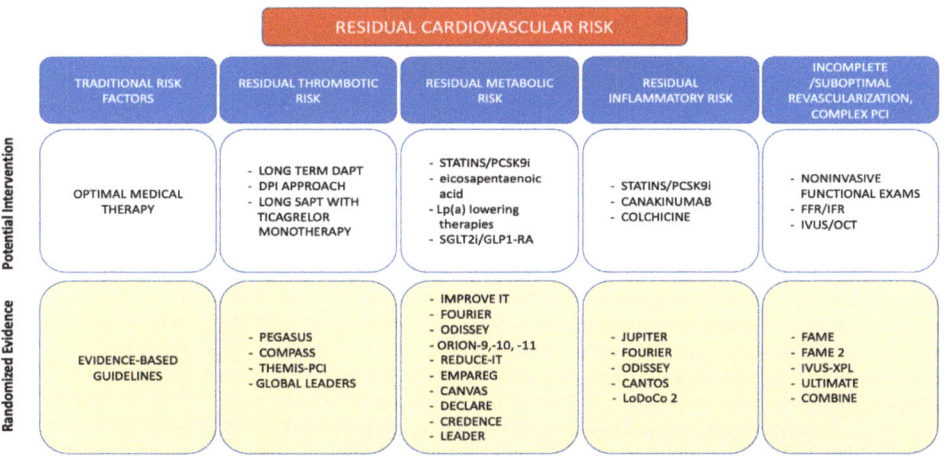

Figure 1. Pathways of residual CV risk, scientific evidence, and potential targeting interventions.

More recently, the Predicting Bleeding Complication in Patients Undergoing Stent Implantation and Subsequent Dual Antiplatelet Therapy (PRECISE-DAPT) score, specifically designed for the prediction of bleeding, was introduced [40]. A recent meta-analysis involving over 50,000 patients established that a PRECISE DAPT score > 25 was linked to an increased likelihood of major bleeding and an elevated risk of MACE [41].

Although the overlap between ischemia and bleeding is clear, Lindholm et al. demonstrated that as the number of CV risk factors increases, the risk of ischemic events increases more than the risk of bleeding. Furthermore, when patients with a history of bleeding are excluded, an increased number of CV risk factors is linked with a significant rise in ischemic events, with no significant difference in the rate of bleeding [42].

A 4-year analysis of the REACH registry demonstrated that a correct prognostic stratification cannot ignore the identification of some clinical predictors of future CV events. Subjects with atherothrombosis are extremely heterogeneous and consequently have a highly variable risk of events. This risk varies from 7% in patients with only CV risk factors, excluding diabetes, to 25% in individuals with a history of ischemic events and/or polyvascular disease. Notably, patients with previous acute CV events have a higher residual risk compared to those with stable CAD, especially during the first year; in turn, individuals with stable CAD have a higher risk compared to those with CV risk factors but without atherosclerosis. Among all risk factors, diabetes has been confirmed to raise the ischemic risk, whereas, in the subjects with atherothrombosis, the presence of poly-vascular disease has been identified as the strongest independent risk factor for recurrent MACE [43].

Subsequent ischemic events may be due to the coronary artery that was originally treated or to other sites because of disease progression. In the previously mentioned Swedish registry, the risk of recurrent ACS due to an untreated or a non-culprit lesion was twice as high as the risk of recurrent ACS due to a previously stented lesion. Predictors of recurrent ACS from an untreated lesion were male sex, multivessel disease, and a longer interval between the index and the recurrent event [35].

Intracoronary imaging techniques, identifying lesions with features suggestive of plaque vulnerability, may be useful in the prognostic stratification of patients with CCS. The Providing Regional Observations to Study Predictors of Events in the Coronary Tree (PROSPECT) study enrolled 697 ACS patients who underwent three-vessel intravascular ultrasound (IVUS) imaging after PCI. During three years of follow-up, the recurrent events were equally attributable to culprit and non-culprit lesions. Common imaging-based characteristics of non-culprit lesions associated with recurrences were angiographically mild lesions with a large plaque burden, thin-cap fibroatheroma (<65 mm), and small luminal area [44]. In the Relationship between OCT Coronary Plaque Morphology and Clinical Outcome (CLIMA) Study, which involved 1003 patients who underwent OCT imaging of the untreated proximal left anterior descending (LAD) coronary artery, the simultaneous occurrence of four high-risk OCT plaque characteristics (lipid arc > 180°, minimal lumen area < 3.5 mm^2, minimum thickness of the fibrous cap < 75 μm, presence of macrophages) was linked to an increased MACE risk [45].

3.2. Therapeutic Targets

3.2.1. Lifestyle

Improving healthy behaviors and medical adherence are the cornerstone of secondary CV prevention. In fact, a healthy diet, regular physical activity, stopping smoking, and maintaining an optimal body mass index (BMI) significantly reduce the recurrence of MACE, even after adjusting for guideline-recommended secondary prevention treatments [46–48]. Table 2 shows lifestyle recommendations.

Table 2. Lifestyle ESC Guidelines recommendations for CCS patients [1,49].

	Intervention	Relative Risk Reduction %
Stopping Smoking	Use the 'Very brief advice' for smoking cessation: - ASK: establishing and recording smoking status - ADVISE: advising on the best methods of stopping - ACT: offering help	36 (mortality)
Healthy diet	High in vegetables, fruits, and grains. Saturated fats <10% of total intake. Limit alcohol to <100 g/week or 15 g/day.	31 (MACE)
Physical activity	30–60 min of moderate-intensity aerobic activity ≥5 days per week.	27 (mortality)
Weight loss	BMI ≤ 25 kg/m^2	33 (MACE)

Additionally, the ESC guidelines recommend cognitive-behavioral interventions to support CCS patients to adopt healthy behaviors, which may require a multidisciplinary team of experts (cardiologists, nurses, dieticians, general practitioners, physiotherapists, and psychologists), exercise-based cardiac rehabilitation, and the annual flu vaccination, particularly in patients older than 65 years and in those with HF [48–51].

3.2.2. Psychosocial Risk Factors

The onset and progression of CAD are closely linked to psychosocial factors, including acute and chronic life stressors, low socioeconomic status, mental health disorders, depression, and inadequate sleep patterns. These factors are associated with the development and prognosis of CAD [52].

They exert their influence through a range of underlying mechanisms. Individuals struggling with compromised psychosocial well-being are more prone to adopting detrimental habits, such as smoking, alcohol/substance abuse, unhealthy diet, sedentary lifestyle, and inadequate adherence to prescribed medical regimens. This is all compounded by the fact that they often face limited access to health care resources. A large body of evidence indicates that stress triggers the activation of the inflammatory and neurohormonal systems, an elevation in blood pressure (BP), and a dysregulation of glucose metabolism. These effects can lead to clinical consequences, like myocardial ischemia, cardiac arrhythmias, atherosclerosis development, and the formation of more vulnerable coronary plaques [52,53]. Psychological factors have a significantly higher prevalence in certain demographic subgroups, including women, lower socioeconomic groups, and black individuals, contributing to disparities in CAD development and associated morbidity and mortality [54]. To improve the outcomes for CCS patients, it is imperative to systematically assess psychosocial risk factors and facilitate effective behavioral and pharmacological interventions by mental health professionals. These interventions are also critical in reducing social disparities in cardiovascular health [54–56].

3.2.3. Blood Pressure Targets

Hypertension is the most common CV risk factor in CCS patients. Several studies have underscored the importance of anti-hypertensive treatment in CV secondary prevention, demonstrating that each 10 mmHg reduction in systolic BP is associated with an approximately 17% reduction in the rate of MACE [57,58]. Current ESC guidelines recommend a systolic BP target value of 120–130 mmHg in general CCS population and a target value of 130–140 mmHg in the elderly (Class I, LoE A) [59].

In symptomatic CCS patients, beta-blockers and calcium antagonists (CCBs) should be the drugs of choice, whereas in post-MI patients, beta-blockers and renin-angiotensin system (RAS) blockers should be used (Class I, LoE A). Treatment with both angiotensin-converting enzyme (ACE) inhibitors and angiotensin receptor blockers (ARBs) for hypertension is not recommended because it is linked with a higher incidence of major kidney adverse events (Class III, LoE A) [60].

3.2.4. Residual Thrombotic Risk

For several decades, aspirin has been considered the basic component of antithrombotic therapy in patients with CCS. However, based on recent evidence, the latest ESC guidelines recommend a more potent antithrombotic approach in individuals exhibiting clinical, anatomic, and/or procedural features of high thrombotic risk without high bleeding risk (HBR) (Class II, LoE A) [1,61].

Two distinct and more intensive antithrombotic approaches have been demonstrated to significantly reduce recurrent MACE in this population: prolonged DAPT, which combines P2Y12 receptor antagonists, preferably ticagrelor 60 mg with aspirin [13], or a dual-pathway inhibition (DPI) approach, which combines a low-dose of rivaroxaban (2.5 mg) and aspirin [15]. Although the aforementioned guidelines do not indicate when one of the two strategies should be preferred over the other, a careful analysis of the trials testing these strategies allows us to identify the ideal candidates for the two pharmacological approaches. The best candidates for prolonged DAPT (>12 months) are non-HBR post-MI patients (within 2 years) with a moderate-high residual ischemic risk, who have not stopped DAPT for more than one year and who have tolerated DAPT for 12 months. Instead, CCS patients eligible for the DPI approach are non-HBR patients at any time after a MI with an additional ischemic risk factor, including those who have stopped DAPT for over one year, are high-risk patients without a prior MI, are patients with a prior stroke, or are patients with peripheral arterial disease (PAD) [62].

The Effect of Ticagrelor on Health Outcomes in Diabetes Mellitus Patients Intervention Study (THEMIS) evaluated DAPT with aspirin plus ticagrelor in stable diabetic patients without previous ischemic event. This study did not show a greater net clinical benefit of DAPT in these patients. Specifically, patients in the aspirin plus ticagrelor group exhibited a lower rate of MACE but a higher incidence of major bleeding compared to patients in the aspirin plus placebo group [63]. In THEMIS-PCI, which included only stable diabetic patients with previous PCI, the investigators demonstrated a lower incidence of MACE in the ticagrelor plus aspirin group. Major bleeding was significantly higher in the treatment arm, but fatal bleeding and intracranial hemorrhage were not significantly different between the two groups [64].

More recently, a new antithrombotic strategy involving long-term monotherapy with ticagrelor, after a short-term DAPT, has been tested in a population at high ischemic risk [65]. Although this so-called aspirin-free strategy is currently not yet recommended by the guidelines, it may become a valid pharmacological alternative in the future to achieve greater anti-ischemic efficacy without the trade-off of increased bleeding complications, particularly in HBR post-PCI patients who are not eligible for more intensive antithrombotic approaches.

In patients with CCS and atrial fibrillation (AF) who underwent PCI, dual antithrombotic therapy with an oral anticoagulant (OAC), preferably Direct Oral Anticoagulants (DOACs), and clopidogrel is the default strategy recommended, with aspirin limited to the periprocedural phase, whereas only in the case of patients with additional clinical risk factors (diabetes, CKD, PAD, recurrent MI, etc.) and/or who have undergone complex PCI, triple antithrombotic therapy (TAT), which includes an OAC, clopidogrel, and ASA, should be continued for up to one month. Six months after elective PCI and lifelong in CCS patients, OAC alone is the recommended strategy [66]. For specific high-risk patients, dual antithrombotic therapy with OAC in combination with either clopidogrel or aspirin should be considered.

3.2.5. Residual Metabolic Risk

- LDL:

In accordance with the ESC/EAS guidelines for the management of dyslipidaemias, the target of LDL-C levels should be lower than <1.4 mmol/L (<55 mg/dL) with a reduction of at least 50% from baseline (Class I, LoE A).

Moreover, an LDL-C target of <1.0 mmol/L (<40 mg/dL) may be considered for patients with CV disease who had a recurrent event within 2 years (Class IIb, LoE B) [67]. Management of dyslipidaemias includes lifestyle changes and LLT. Today, we have a broad therapeutic armamentarium to achieve these ambitious therapeutic goals, including high-intensity statins, ezetimibe, bempedoic acid, PSCK9i, and inclisiran. A high-intensity statin at the maximum tolerated dose represents the first-line therapy in CCS patients [68,69]. If statins fail to achieve LDL-C targets, a stepwise approach with ezetimibe first and then PSCK9i/inclisiran in combination with statins is recommended. For patients with intolerance to statins, the ESC guidelines [67] also recommend ezetimibe, bempedoic acid, and PSCK9i/inclisiran alone or in combination.

- Triglycerides (TG):

Hypertriglyceridemia is also linked with CV disease. Statin therapy is recommended in CCS patients with hypertriglyceridemia [triglycerides—TG—levels >2.3 mmol/L (>200 mg/dL)] (Class I, LoE B) [67]. Moreover, high-dose eicosapentaenoic acid (EPA) (2 g) taken b.i.d should be considered in high-risk individuals with persistent high TG levels (135–499 mg/dL) on statin treatment (Class IIa, LoE B). The Reduction of Cardiovascular Events with Icosapent Ethyl–Intervention (REDUCE-IT) trial, in fact, showed that in statin-treated patients with CAD or diabetes and mild–moderate hypertriglyceridemia (TG levels of 135 to 499 mg/dL) a high-dose EPA significantly reduced the incidence of ischemic events over a follow-up of 4.9 years. Indeed, the interventional group had a 25% relative risk reduction in the primary endpoint, a composite of CV death, MI, stroke, unstable angina, and coronary revascularization [70].

Despite this evidence, in contrast to LDL, current guidelines do not recommend a target for triglycerides [67].

- Lipoprotein(a) (Lp(a)):

Lp(a) is a genetically determined LDL variant that contains cholesterol, triglycerides, and an apolipoprotein(a) unit. Elevated Lp(a) levels are significantly linked to an increased risk of atherosclerotic CV diseases [71]. To date, there are no approved therapies specifically targeting Lp(a). Nevertheless, several agents aimed at lowering Lp(a), such as pelacarsen, olpasiran, and SLN360, are currently being evaluated in clinical outcome trials (Lp(a)-HORIZON; NCT04270760; NCT04606602). If proven effective, Lp(a) will soon become a new therapeutic target for reducing residual metabolic risk in CCS patients.

- Diabetes:

Individuals with CCS and diabetes represent a very high-risk population; therefore, ESC guidelines recommend a close monitoring of risk factors. For diabetic patients, BP should be 130/80 mmHg or below, whereas LDL-C < 1.4 mmol/L (<55 mg/dL) and reduced by at least 50% from the baseline. Additionally, a target glycated HbA1c level of less than 7% (<53 mmol/L) is recommended (Class I, LoE A) [72].

Until recently, none of the antidiabetic drugs could be shown to reduce MACE in diabetic patients, thus the results of randomized clinical trials (RCTs), which assessed the efficacy of two novel classes of glucose-lowering drugs, the sodium–glucose co-transporter-2 inhibitors (SGLT-2i) and the glucagon-like peptide-1 receptor agonists (GLP1-RA) marked a "new era" in diabetes treatment [73–77]. Notably, in these RCTs, these drugs provided additive benefits to GDMT (ACEi/ARB statins, statins, etc.). For these reasons, the ESC guidelines include strong recommendations for the use of SGLT2i and GLP-1 RA in patients with CCS and diabetes (Class I, LoE A) [72] and the new ADA guidelines recommend SGLT-2i and/or GLP1-RA for initial therapy, with or without metformin based on glycemic needs, in diabetic patients with high-risk features or established CV disease [78].

- Non-alcoholic fatty liver disease (NAFLD):

Nearly one-third of the adult population worldwide is affected by non-alcoholic fatty liver disease (NAFLD), which encompasses a broad spectrum of liver conditions. These range from simple steatosis to severe manifestations, such as non-alcoholic steatohepatitis (NASH). In some cases, NAFLD can progress into fibrosis and cirrhosis [79]. NAFLD, which is recognized as the hepatic component of the metabolic syndrome and closely associated with both obesity and diabetes, represents an emerging contemporary CV risk factor according to several studies [80–82]. There are a number of underlying mechanisms by which NAFLD may contribute to CAD development. These include insulin resistance, enhanced hepatic gluconeogenesis, atherogenic dyslipidemia, increased oxidative stress, and a prothrombotic state.

To date, specific treatments for NAFLD are lacking, and lifestyle interventions involving dietary modification, weight loss, increased physical activity and smoking/alcohol cessation are the primary recommended therapeutic strategies for patients with NAFLD [83]. A risk reduction in MACE as well as a modest improved NAFLD was shown in recent studies through the use of GLP1-Ras, improving glycemic control and supporting weight loss [84,85]. In addition, the ESSENTIAL study demonstrated the safety and efficacy of combination treatment with ezetimibe and rosuvastatin in reducing liver fat in patients with NAFLD [86]. Promising drug therapies targeting different stages of NAFLD are currently under investigation. However, many of these treatments have shown only moderate efficacy and, in some cases, their utility has been hampered by potential side effects and concerns about toxicity.

3.2.6. Residual Inflammatory Risk

Systemic inflammation has emerged as an important player in the progression and destabilization of CV disease [87–89]. However, since the degree of inflammation as part of the residual ischemic risk varies among patients, it is important to have specific biomarkers and therapeutic targets to identify and treat patients at a high residual inflammatory risk to provide more personalized CCS care. As previously described, hs-CRP is the most extensively researched inflammatory marker linked to an elevated ischemic risk, independently of LDL levels. [87]. Statins can decrease hs-CRP (a pleiotropic effect), with the greater reduction in CV events observed in those who reached both the lowest LDL-C and hs-CRP levels (<2 mg/L) [90]. This effect has also been demonstrated when non-statin treatments, such as ezetimibe [91] or PCSK9i, were combined with statins [92].

The hypothesis that inflammation plays a key role in the pathogenesis of atherosclerosis was first demonstrated by the Canakinumab Anti-Inflammatory Thrombosis Outcome Study (CANTOS). In the CANTOS trial, 10,061 subjects with a history of MI, optimal LDL-C levels, and hs-CRP $\geq$ 2 mg/L were randomly assigned to receive OMT plus placebo or OMT plus canakinumab, an interleukin-1 beta blocker (IL-1β) without effect on LDL-C, BP, or platelets. Canakinumab (150 mg every 3 months) led to a significantly lower rate of CV events than placebo, but with a higher incidence of thrombocytopenia, neutropenia, and life-threatening infection [93]. However, the Food and Drug Administration (FDA), has not approved the use of canakinumab in patients with CAD. In contrast to CANTOS, the Cardiovascular Inflammation Reduction Trial (CIRT) demonstrated that low-dose methotrexate failed to reduce CV events in secondary prevention [94]. Recently, the Low-dose Colchicine 2 (LoDoCo2) trial showed that the anti-inflammatory drug colchicine in low doses (0.5 mg once daily) safely reduced CV events, including MI and the need for coronary revascularization in CCS patients on top of LDL-C lowering and antithrombotic treatments [95].

At present, despite the evidence supporting the role of inflammation in the development of atherosclerotic CV disease, effectively targeting inflammatory pathways in patients with CCS has proven challenging. Consequently, current guidelines do not recommend anti-inflammatory drugs for secondary CV prevention.

Novel anti-inflammatory interventions, including neutralization of IL-6 and the inflammasome, are still under investigation in several clinical trials.

4. Diagnostic Tests: What, When, and to Whom, with a View to Appropriateness and Rationalization of Resources

In CCS patients, the annual CV mortality rate describes the risk of an event. Thus, a CV mortality rate >3% per year identifies high-risk patients whereas a CV mortality rate <1% per year identifies low-risk patients [96]. In addition, an annual risk assessment is warranted, even if the patient is asymptomatic. Several diagnostic tests may be useful for the diagnosis of CCS patients [1]. The main challenge in daily clinical practice is to ensure the right test for the right patient at the right time for an individualized diagnostic-therapeutic pathway in the context of healthcare resources rationalization.

4.1. Pre-Test Probability (PTP)

The effectiveness of available diagnostic tests in diagnosing obstructive CAD depends on the prevalence of CAD in the population being studied. A simple predictive model, which includes only age, sex, and symptoms, can be routinely used to evaluate the pre-test probability (PTP) of obstructive CAD [97]. Based on more contemporary data [98,99], the new ESC guidelines on CCS have updated the method for estimating the PTP of obstructive CAD by significantly reducing the absolute values of the PTP [1]. The new PTP method increases the proportion of patients for whom diagnostic testing is not recommended. In fact, more patients fall into the PTP <15% category, where the estimated CV mortality or MI rate per year is <1%, substantially reducing unnecessary diagnostic tests and costs. In addition, several PTP modifiers, such as CV risk factors, resting or exercise ECG abnormalities, LV dysfunction, and the presence of coronary calcium, have been introduced to better identify the clinical probability of CAD, particularly in patients with low PTP (5–15%) [1]. It should be kept in mind that each test has its own peculiarities to rule in or rule out CAD; therefore, clinicians should tailor the appropriate test according to patient's PTP categories. Notably, stress ECG has limited diagnostic value across all levels of PTP; non-invasive stress imaging tests, in particular positron emission tomography (PET) and stress nuclear cardiac magnetic resonance (CMR), have better performance and may be preferred in patients with high PTP, whereas coronary computed tomography angiography

(CTA) is the ideal technique to accurately exclude anatomic CAD in patients with a lower range of clinical likelihood of CAD [96,100].

4.2. Invasive Coronary Angiography (ICA)

The current gold standard test for the diagnosis of CAD is invasive coronary angiography (ICA). However, due to its invasive nature, ICA is associated with risks; therefore, it should be performed in patients who are likely to require coronary revascularization (patients with a high clinical probability or with severe symptoms despite OMT) [1]. Invasive functional test imaging, including fractional flow reserve (FFR) and instantaneous wave-free ratio (iFR), should be available to improve the diagnostic power of ICA and should be used to confirm or exclude uncertain diagnoses on non-invasive tests or to better assess stenosis severity before revascularization [101,102]. Therefore, current guidelines recommend non-invasive ischemia testing as a gatekeeper to ICA in individuals at low and intermediate risk for significant coronary stenosis [1].

4.3. Stress ECG

Stress ECG detects myocardial ischemia according to the electrocardiographic changes induced by exercise. However, its diagnostic power in detecting obstructive CAD is lower than that of other diagnostic imaging tests [96,103]. The prevalence of inconclusive stress ECG results is notably high, underscoring its limited efficacy in detecting myocardial ischemia. A stress ECG test should be avoided in patients with preexcitation, paced rhythm, and a left bundle branch block in whom ST-segment variations cannot be evaluated. Therefore, the dependence of the test on the patient's physical fitness poses a significant limitation, potentially excluding individuals who are unable to undergo the procedure [104]. Stress ECG alone may be used as an alternative to detect ischemia if other imaging exams are unavailable, but caution is needed due to the risk of false-negative and false-positive results. Current guidelines recommend performing a non-invasive imaging or an anatomical test as the exam of choice for the diagnosis and for the follow-up of CCS patients after revascularization (IIa, LoE B) [1,2,103].

4.4. Non-Invasive Stress Imaging Tests

Stress echocardiography, in which the stressor may be represented by physical exercise or by pharmacological agents, is a useful non-invasive test for CAD diagnosis by detecting new or worsening ischemia-induced wall-motion abnormalities. Developments in contrast agents, image acquisition, and strain imaging have improved the diagnostic accuracy of this test. However, as stress echocardiography is an operator-dependent exam, its accuracy is highly dependent on the training and expertise of professionals performing the test to correctly interpret the results obtained.

The limitations of echocardiography in detecting exercise-induced kinetic abnormalities can be largely overcome, where available, using CMR. Conversely, both single-photon emission computed tomography (SPECT) and PET can identify myocardial ischemia by imaging regional myocardial tracer uptake, allowing the assessment of relative myocardial blood flow at rest and during stress. Overall, non-invasive functional tests exhibit a high sensibility and specificity for detecting flow-limiting obstructive CAD and are more accurate than ECG testing in defining the site of ischemia and in providing prognostic information [1,96,100]. The choice of non-invasive diagnostic exams is strictly dependent on patient characteristics (e.g., any contraindication to the administration of contrast medium), professional skills, and availability of such tests.

4.5. Coronary Computed Tomography Angiography (CCTA)

Coronary computed tomography angiography (CCTA) is a non-invasive imaging technique that uses an intravenous contrast agent to the visualize coronary artery wall with a high accuracy for the assessment of obstructive CAD. This diagnostic exam is not recommended (Class III, LoE C) for patients with high or irregular heart rates, extensive coronary calcification, severe obesity, or difficulty complying with breath-hold instructions that may interfere with the acquisition of high-quality images [1].

In cases of uncertain CCTA results or when CCTA is inconclusive, integrating functional data is advised. It is important to note that CCTA should not be used as a stand-alone follow-up test for patients with known CAD unless accompanied by functional information regarding myocardial ischemia. Recent technological developments have allowed the integration of three-dimensional CT-derived anatomical reconstructions with techniques able to predict FFR through computational fluid dynamics or machine learning. Although some studies have demonstrated a high diagnostic value of CCTA-based FFR [105], there are contrast data regarding its predictive value to detect CAD. A recent study of 2298 patients who underwent a CCTA-based FFR, reported a low positive predictive value (49%) [106]. Furthermore, Mittal et al. also highlighted the increased costs associated with CCTA-based FFR strategy compared with that of other stress imaging tests. The diagnostic landscape for CCS is characterized by the availability of multiple imaging modalities. However, the optimal selection of the most appropriate approach remains a challenge for most clinicians. Careful, case-by-case evaluation is essential to achieve optimal results and to rationalize the use of available resources. Several cost-effectiveness studies have been conducted to address this issue. In low-risk patients, anatomical analysis using CCTA has been shown to be cost-effective; functional strategy based on an echo stress test has shown comparable cost-effectiveness, whereas SPECT showed lower cost-effectiveness [107–109]. In contrast, in patients with an intermediate risk of CAD, functional tests, such as SPECT and stress echocardiography, seem to be the most cost-effective [109,110].

5. Pharmacological Management of Symptoms

Ideally, optimal treatment of CCS patients will not only improve prognosis but also symptoms and quality of life (QoL). Therefore, OMT must include effective antianginal drugs in combination with event prevention drugs. Current guidelines advocate for a tailored, stepwise approach in which antianginal therapy should be personalized, taking into account patient characteristics (such as BP, heart rate, LVEF, etc.), comorbidities, potential drug interactions, and specific underlying pathogenic mechanisms of angina [1].

Beta-adrenergic blockers (BBs) and/or calcium channel blockers (CCBs) represent the first-line treatment. The anti-ischemic effect of these classes of drugs is due to a reduction in heart rate, BP, and contractility, resulting in a reduced myocardial oxygen requirement. To optimize their efficacy, long-acting formulations should be preferred, and drugs should be carefully titrated. Beta-blockers and non-dihydropyridine CCBs are contraindicated in patients with sick sinus syndrome, severe bradycardia, advanced heart block, hypotension, and acute HF. If BBs and/or CCBs fail to successfully control angina symptoms, or if contraindications occur for these agents, several second-line drugs are available. These include long-acting nitrates and nicorandil, ivabradine, ranolazine, and trimetazidine. The addition of long-acting nitrates is a reasonable therapeutic option for patients who continue to experience symptoms despite taking BBs and CCBs, while short-acting nitrates can be used for the management of acute symptoms. Nitrates are contraindicated in patients taking phosphodiesterase inhibitors and in patients with hypertrophic obstructive cardiomyopathy (Class III, LoE B) [1]. Ivabradine and ranolazine are suitable therapeutic options for patients who develop low BP with usual anti-anginal drugs, as they do not exert vasoactive actions. Regardless of the type of initial treatment used, the patient's response to therapy should be evaluated promptly.

6. Revascularization Strategy

In contrast to the clear data supporting the advantage of timely revascularization in reducing MACE and mortality in ACS patients [111,112], it is still controversial whether the revascularization strategy offers a prognostic benefit over OMT in the management of CCS patients.

The Clinical Outcomes Utilizing Revascularization and Aggressive Drug Evaluation (COURAGE) trial involved 2287 patients with CCS and was the first trial to demonstrate that PCI plus OMT did not improve CV outcomes compared to OMT alone in patients with stable CAD. However, patients who underwent PCI were symptom-free and had an improved QoL after the intervention, though this difference was not maintained at 36 months [113].

Subsequently, in the 2nd Bypass Angioplasty Revascularization Investigation in Diabetes (BARI 2D) trial, which included 2368 diabetic patients with stable CAD, a revascularization strategy (PCI or Coronary Artery Bypass Graft-CABG) plus OMT was not superior to intensive OMT alone in reducing all-cause mortality at 5 years. However, in the CABG stratum, the incidence of MACE was significantly lower than in the OMT group, driven predominantly by a reduction in non-fatal MI [114].

The fractional flow reserve versus Angiography for Multivessel Evaluation 2 (FAME 2) trial showed that in CCS patients with angiographically documented coronary atherosclerosis, and at least one functionally significant stenosis (fractional flow reserve (FFR) $\leq$ 0.80), FFR-guided PCI with DES resulted in a significantly lower rate of death, non-fatal MI, or urgent revascularization compared to OMT alone. The benefit of FFR-guided PCI over OMT was driven by a significantly lower need for urgent revascularization in the PCI group and was sustained at 5 years of follow-up. This strategy has also shown a significant improvement in symptoms and QoL [115]. The FAME 2 trial established that the detection of significant ischemia, identified by a positive FFR test, allows a better risk stratification of patients with CCS before performing a PCI. Of note, in the subsequent FAME 3 trial, FFR-guided PCI with currently used DES failed to meet noninferiority compared with CABG among patients with three-vessel CAD.

The Objective Randomized Blinded Investigation with Optimal Medical Therapy of Angioplasty in Stable Angina (ORBITA) trial showed no significant improvement in exercise time at 6 weeks in patients with stable CAD undergoing PCI compared to the placebo procedure [116]. Although the scientific debate generated by this study underlines the importance of the indication for PCI in CCS patients, its impact on clinical practice and guidelines does not appear to be significant considering the important limitations of this study. These limitations include inadequate statistical power to demonstrate clinical endpoints, a small sample size, and a short follow-up period.

Finally, the International Study of Comparative Health Effectiveness with Medical and Invasive Approaches (ISCHEMIA) trial was designed to overcome the limitations of previous trials. None of the previous trials were blinded; they enrolled patients with only mild ischemia whose coronary anatomy was known prior to randomization, raising the possibility of selection and referral bias. Moreover, patients in most of these trials were not treated with the current standard of care, which includes aggressive OMT, FFR-guided PCI, and the use of the latest generation of DES. The ISCHEMIA trial enrolled 5179 patients with moderate to severe ischemia at baseline prior to ICA. Coronary CTA was performed in all patients without renal dysfunction to exclude left main disease and non-obstructive CAD. Patients were randomized to receive OMT or invasive strategy plus OMT (revascularization by PCI or CABG, as clinically determined). This trial failed to demonstrate significant differences between the conservative and invasive strategy in the primary endpoint (a combination of CV death, MI, hospitalization for UA, hospitalization for HF, or resuscitated cardiac arrest). However, the invasive treatment strategy is associated with improved symptom control and QoL at the end of the trial [117].

More recently, an interim analysis of the ISCHEMIA EXTENDED, an observational study, including 4825 of the original ISCHEMIA trial participants, showed no difference in all-cause mortality between the two approaches. However, the invasive strategy demonstrated a lower CV mortality rate but a higher non-CV mortality rate during the 5.7 years of follow-up [118]. Table 3 shows the key characteristics and results of studies assessing OMT versus revascularization strategy in patients with CCS.

Table 3. Principal contemporary studies assessing OMT versus the revascularization strategy in patients with CCS.

	COURAGE [113]	BARI 2D [114]	FAME 2 [115]	ISCHEMIA [117]
Publication year	2007	2009	2014	2020
N° pts	2287	2368	1220	5279
Follow-up (yrs)	4.6	5	2	3.2
Documentation of ischemia required?	No	No	No	Yes, >10%
CTA performed before enrollment?	No	No	No	Yes
Enrollment before ICA?	No	No	No	Yes
Contemporary conservative strategy?	No	No	Yes	Yes
Contemporary invasive strategy?	No, only PCI, no DES	No, only 35% DES, 10% no stent	Yes, DES, FFR	Yes, DES, FFR
Main Results	Neutral QoL improvement	Neutral Less CV events in CABG arm	Neutral Less need for urgent revascularization	Neutral QoL improvement

° in patients with previous abnormal rest echo; OMT: optimal medical therapy; CTA: computed tomography angiography; ICA: invasive coronary angiography; DES: drug-eluting stent; FFR: fractional flow reserve.

The decision to perform complete coronary revascularization in patients with ACS and evidence of multivessel CAD remains a matter of debate. Complete revascularization appears to be associated with a better outcome, with a reduction in both new revascularizations and hard clinical events [119].

Current ACC/SCAI/AHA guidelines for coronary artery revascularization suggest the use of FFR or iFR to assess angiographic, intermediate coronary lesions only in the presence of stable CAD (Class I, level of evidence A), but their role in ACS patients has not been clearly addressed [120]. The FLOWER-MI (FLOW Evaluation to Guide Revascularization in Multi-vessel ST-elevation Myocardial Infarction) trial compared angiography-guided and FFR-guided complete revascularization in STEMI patients with multivessel disease. The authors demonstrated that an FFR-guided strategy had no significant advantage over an angiography-guided strategy with respect to the primary endpoint (composite of death, MI, and urgent revascularization at 1 year) [121]. More recently, a comprehensive network meta-analysis of 11 RCTs comparing FFR and angiography in this setting concluded that complete revascularization of non-culprit stenosis was associated with a lower incidence of adverse events compared with culprit-only revascularization, but FFR guidance was not superior to angiography guidance in reducing MACE [122].

Some studies have investigated the best strategy in CCS patients with reduced LVEF. In the Surgical Treatment for Ischemic Heart Failure (STICH) trial, patients with extensive CAD and LV systolic dysfunction were randomly assigned to initial OMT or CABG. At the 10-year follow-up, CABG plus OMT demonstrated a prognostic benefit versus OMT alone [123]. The REVascularization for Ischemic VEntricular Dysfunction (REVIVED)-BCIS2 trial, the first powered trial to assess the efficacy and safety of PCI in patients with severe ischemic cardiomyopathy and evidence of myocardial viability, did not show a significant benefit of multivessel PCI versus OMT over 3.4 years of follow-up [124]. However, the failure of an invasive strategy in this setting may have been due to less extensive CAD, small sample size, and shorter follow-up.

Based on this evidence, the management of patients with CCS should always start with an aggressive contemporary OMT, and only after functional assessment of CAD should an individualized revascularization strategy be considered if the conservative strategy fails or is in subgroups of patients in whom a prognostic benefit has been demonstrated. Current guidelines suggest a tailored approach in which the decision to revascularize each individual patient by PCI or CABG should be established based on symptoms and QoL despite OMT, prognostic indicators (ischemic area >10% LV or ischemic cardiomyopathy with

LVEF $\leq$ 35%), evidence of ischemia, and invasive assessment of CAD severity (FFR $\leq$ 0.80 or iwFR $\leq$ 0.89 in a major coronary vessel) [1].

While the prognostic significance of invasive methods for functionally assessing coronary lesions in ACS patients remains uncertain, recent years have seen growing evidence supporting the prognostic value of the use of intracoronary imaging techniques in complex PCI, regardless of clinical CAD presentation (ACS or CCS). In particular, various studies and meta-analyses have shown that IVUS-guided complex PCI, when compared to conventional angiography-guided PCI, leads to a significantly reduced rate of long-term MACE [125–128].

Regarding antiplatelet therapy in CCS patients undergoing elective PCI, the DAPT with clopidogrel plus aspirin remains the standard of care. In fact, trials testing the more potent P2Y12 inhibitors, such as prasugrel or ticagrelor, have not demonstrated their superiority over clopidogrel in this specific patient population [129,130].

7. Follow-Up Strategies and Care Pathways: From the Hospital to the Community Care

In clinical practice, even asymptomatic CCS patients require a regular clinical follow-up by a CV professional to evaluate any change in the patient's residual CV risk, adherence to lifestyle recommendations and pharmacological therapy, or the occurrence of comorbidities that may affect therapy and CV outcomes. Identifying the patient's clinical risk is also important to ensure that the right patient receives the right instrumental follow-up modality. Resting echocardiography should be performed annually if previously abnormal or every 3/5 years if previously normal. In patients who have undergone revascularization, an early echocardiographic assessment may be useful 1-3 months after the procedure [1]. In general, the routine use of inductive ischemia tests is not advised, regardless of the presence or absence of symptoms, even in cases of previous revascularization. Non-invasive stress exams may be considered 1 year after PCI and 5 years after CABG or every 3/5 years to assess silent ischemia, preferably using non-invasive stress-imaging techniques (Class IIb, LoE C) [1]. Among high-risk post-PCI patients with incomplete or suboptimal revascularization, early evaluation (3 months after the procedure), preferably with an imaging stress test, could be useful. In addition, an early evaluation (1-3 months after the procedure) has been suggested, in particular, in clinical settings of CCS to establish a reference for subsequent follow-up. A model for the management of CCS patients, tailoring examinations and follow-up visits according to CCS categories and their level of risk is shown in Figure 2.

Coronary CTA should not be used as a routine follow-up test for CCS patients, whereas ICA, with FFR/iFR when necessary, is the test of choice for high-risk patients according to non-invasive test results and for patients with severe symptoms despite OMT.

It is critical that after hospitalization for ACS or elective PCI, the follow-up modality is established at the time of discharge based on the patient's risk level.

To reduce the recurrence of CV events, the ESC guidelines recommend that patients with CAD be discharged according to a structured modality for the optimal management of the post-discharge pathway (Class IIa, LoE B) [49]. In addition, a recent Cochrane analysis demonstrated that discharge planning can reduce unplanned readmissions and improve the coordination of post-discharge services [131]. To this end, the discharge letter is a key component of the transition between hospital and community care.

Recent CCS diagnosis or Elective Revascularization

	CV visit	Risk stratification	Rest ECG	Rest Echo	Stress Test
Baseline	✓	✓	✓	✓	
1-3 months				✓	✓†
6 months	✓*	✓	✓		
12 months	✓**	✓	✓	✓°	
Yearly	✓	✓	✓	✓	
Every 3-5 yrs				✓	✓

CCS Pts with previous ACS (> 1 year)

	CV visit	Risk stratification	Rest ECG	Rest Echo	Stress Test
Baseline	✓**	✓	✓	✓	
1-3 months				✓	✓†
6 months					
12 months	✓**	✓	✓	✓	
Yearly	✓**	✓			
Every 3-5 yrs					✓

Long-standing diagnosis of CCS (> 1 year)

	CV visit	Risk stratification	Rest ECG	Rest Echo	Stress Test
Baseline	✓	✓	✓	✓	
Yearly	✓	✓	✓	✓	
Every 3-5 yrs					✓†

Figure 2. Model for the management of CCS patients. Modified from Knuuti J et al., EHJ 2020 [1]. * Time for decision-making on DAPT/SAPT in post-PCI patients; ** time for decision-making on long term antithrombotic therapy according clinical and procedural residual ischemic risk; † at any time to investigate changes in symptoms and/or functional status; invasive coronary angiography only for patients with symptoms despite OMT or with moderate/severe ischemia on non-invasive stress tests. ° In pts with previous abnormal rest echo. CV: cardiovascular; ECG: electrocardiogram; Echo: echocardiography.

8. Multidisciplinary and Multi-Professional Management Aspects

Modern secondary prevention of CV is evolving into a partnership between CCS patients and healthcare professionals to improve prognosis through appropriate medications, interventions, and lifelong healthy lifestyle behaviors. This collaborative approach requires an integrated, multidisciplinary team approach, including (in both hospital and community settings) cardiologists, nurses, dieticians, physiotherapists, psychologists, general physicians, diabetologists, nephrologists, geriatricians, and others, who can provide holistic and personalized care to patients. To achieve this, professionals should have sufficient knowledge, expertise, and tools to manage the complex, specialized cardiac needs of a patient who often has multiple comorbidities. Today, digital medicine through new telemedicine and telemonitoring technologies can help improve an integrated, patient-centered approach among the different professionals involved in managing CCS patients, optimizing the use of healthcare resources, and improving the prognosis of this patient population.

It is also essential that national core components of cardiac support and secondary prevention are structured to ensure that CCS patients have equal access to the best evidence-based care. This requires an integrated network between hospitals and the community on a regional basis to guarantee continuity of care and patient empowerment.

9. Conclusions

The management of patients with CCS remains a diagnostic and therapeutic challenge. Despite significant therapeutic advances in recent years, patients with CCS continue to experience a high rate of recurrent CV events [132]. As a result, the concept of stable CAD has been reevaluated and the notion of residual CV risk has been introduced. This risk persists despite the use of the best available evidence-based secondary prevention strategies [133]. To significantly reduce this risk, comprehensive strategies should be employed, including: (a) a selection of the most appropriate diagnostic tools; (b) a personalized assessment of residual risk, taking into account contemporary, non-traditional risk factors and their evolution over time; (c) tailoring of therapeutic approaches, both pharmacological and non-pharmacological, to individual risk profiles; (d) an establishment of optimal and individualized follow-up protocols according to the CCS categories and their risk level; (e) implementing a multidisciplinary patient-centered approach to care that can incorporate innovative telemedicine and telemonitoring technologies; (f) promoting integrated management between hospital and community care; (g) incorporating non-pharmacological interventions to improve CV health education.

Author Contributions: Conceptualization, S.G., F.L., M.G.A., L.G., C.M.R., N.I., F.A., R.R., G.C., S.C., I.D.M., C.D.N., S.F., A.P. (Anna Pilleri), A.P. (Andrea Pozzi), P.L.T., M.Z., A.F.A., C.R., M.G., F.C., F.O. and M.M.G.; writing—original draft preparation: S.G., F.L., M.G.A., L.G., C.M.R., N.I., F.A., R.R., G.C., S.C., I.D.M., C.D.N., S.F., A.P. (Anna Pilleri), A.P. (Andrea Pozzi), P.L.T., M.Z., A.F.A., C.R., M.G., F.C., F.O. and M.M.G.; writing—review and editing: S.G., F.L., M.G.A., L.G., C.M.R., N.I., F.A., R.R., G.C., S.C., I.D.M., C.D.N., S.F., A.P. (Anna Pilleri), A.P. (Andrea Pozzi), P.L.T., M.Z., A.F.A., C.R., M.G., F.C., F.O. and M.M.G. All authors have read and agreed to the published version of the manuscript.

Funding: This research received no external funding.

Institutional Review Board Statement: Not applicable.

Informed Consent Statement: Not applicable.

Data Availability Statement: Data sharing is not applicable to this article as no new data were created or analyzed in this study.

Conflicts of Interest: The authors declare no conflict of interest.

References

1. Knuuti, J.; Wijns, W.; Saraste, A.; Capodanno, D.; Barbato, E.; Funck-Brentano, C.; Prescott, E.; Storey, R.F.; Deaton, C.; Cuisset, T.; et al. 2019 ESC Guidelines for the diagnosis and management of chronic coronary syndromes. *Eur. Heart J.* **2020**, *41*, 407–477. [CrossRef]
2. Winchester, D.E.; Maron, D.J.; Blankstein, R.; Chang, I.C.; Kirtane, A.J.; Kwong, R.Y.; Pellikka, P.A.; Prutkin, J.M.; Russell, R.; Sandhu, A.T. ACC/AHA/ASE/ASNC/ASPC/HFSA/HRS/SCAI/SCCT/SCMR/STS 2023 Multimodality Appropriate Use Criteria for the Detection and Risk Assessment of Chronic Coronary Disease. *J. Am. Coll. Cardiol.* **2023**, *81*, 2445–2467. [CrossRef]
3. Roth, G.A.; Mensah, G.A.; Johnson, C.O.; Addolorato, G.; Ammirati, E.; Baddour, L.M.; Barengo, N.C.; Beaton, A.Z.; Benjamin, E.J.; Benziger, C.P.; et al. Global Burden of Cardiovascular Diseases and Risk Factors, 1990–2019: Update from the GBD 2019 Study. *J. Am. Coll. Cardiol.* **2020**, *76*, 2982–3021. [CrossRef]
4. Sorbets, E.; Fox, K.M.; Elbez, Y.; Danchin, N.; Dorian, P.; Ferrari, R.; Ford, I.; Greenlaw, N.; Kalra, P.R.; Parma, Z.; et al. Long-term outcomes of chronic coronary syndrome worldwide: Insights from the international CLARIFY registry. *Eur. Heart J.* **2020**, *41*, 347–356. [CrossRef] [PubMed]
5. Mozaffarian, D.; Benjamin, E.J.; Go, A.S.; Arnett, D.K.; Blaha, M.J.; Cushman, M.; Das, S.R.; De Ferranti, S.; Després, J.P.; Fullerton, H.J.; et al. Heart Disease and Stroke Statistics-2016 Update: A Report from the American Heart Association. *Circulation* **2016**, *133*, e38–e360. [CrossRef] [PubMed]
6. Komajda, M.; Cosentino, F.; Ferrari, R.; Laroche, C.; Maggioni, A.; Steg, P.G.; Tavazzi, L.; Kerneis, M.; Valgimigli, M.; Gale, C.P.; et al. The ESC-EORP Chronic Ischaemic Cardiovascular Disease Long Term (CICD LT) registry. *Eur. Heart J.—Qual. Care Clin. Outcomes* **2019**, *7*, 28–33. [CrossRef] [PubMed]
7. Kerneis, M.; Cosentino, F.; Ferrari, R.; Georges, J.L.; Kosmachova, E.; Laroche, C.; Maggioni, A.P.; Rittger, H.; Steg, P.G.; Maczynska, J.; et al. Impact of chronic coronary syndromes on cardiovascular hospitalization and mortality: The ESC-EORP CICD-LT registry. *Eur. J. Prev. Cardiol.* **2022**, *29*, 1945–1954. [CrossRef]
8. Steg, P.G.; Greenlaw, N.; Tardif, J.C.; Tendera, M.; Ford, I.; Kääb, S.; Abergel, H.; Fox, K.M.; Ferrari, R.; CLARIFY Registry Investigators. Women and men with stable coronary artery disease have similar clinical outcomes: Insights from the international prospective CLARIFY registry. *Eur. Heart J.* **2012**, *33*, 2831–2840. [CrossRef]
9. Tran, C.T.; Laupacis, A.; Mamdani, M.M.; Tu, J.V. Effect of age on the use of evidence-based therapies for acute myocardial infarction. *Am. Heart J.* **2004**, *148*, 834–841. [CrossRef]
10. Olesen, K.K.W.; Jensen, E.S.; Gyldenkerne, C.; Würtz, M.; Mortensen, M.B.; Nørgaard, B.L.; Sørensen, H.T.; Bøtker, H.E.; Maeng, M. Thirteen-year trends in cardiovascular risk in men and women with chronic coronary syndrome. *Eur. Heart J.—Qual. Care Clin. Outcomes* **2022**, *8*, 437–446. [CrossRef]
11. Szummer, K.; Wallentin, L.; Lindhagen, L.; Alfredsson, J.; Erlinge, D.; Held, C.; James, S.; Kellerth, T.; Lindahl, B.; Ravn-Fischer, A.; et al. Improved outcomes in patients with ST-elevation myocardial infarction during the last 20 years are related to implementation of evidence-based treatments: Experiences from the SWEDEHEART registry 1995–2014. *Eur. Heart J.* **2017**, *38*, 3056–3065. [CrossRef] [PubMed]
12. Szummer, K.; Wallentin, L.; Lindhagen, L.; Alfredsson, J.; Erlinge, D.; Held, C.; James, S.; Kellerth, T.; Lindahl, B.; Ravn-Fischer, A.; et al. Relations between implementation of new treatments and improved outcomes in patients with non-ST-elevation myocardial infarction during the last 20 years: Experiences from SWEDEHEART registry 1995 to 2014. *Eur. Heart J.* **2018**, *39*, 3766–3776. [CrossRef] [PubMed]
13. Bonaca, M.P.; Bhatt, D.L.; Cohen, M.; Steg, P.G.; Storey, R.F.; Jensen, E.C.; Magnani, G.; Bansilal, S.; Fish, M.P.; Im, K.; et al. Long-term use of ticagrelor in patients with prior myocardial infarction. *N. Engl. J. Med.* **2015**, *372*, 1791–1800. [CrossRef] [PubMed]
14. Mauri, L.; Kereiakes, D.J.; Yeh, R.W.; Driscoll-Shempp, P.; Cutlip, D.E.; Steg, P.G.; Normand, S.-L.T.; Braunwald, E.; Wiviott, S.D.; Cohen, D.J.; et al. Twelve or 30 Months of Dual Antiplatelet Therapy after Drug-Eluting Stents. *N. Engl. J. Med.* **2014**, *371*, 2155–2166. [CrossRef]
15. Eikelboom, J.W.; Connolly, S.J.; Bosch, J.; Dagenais, G.R.; Hart, R.G.; Shestakovska, O.; Diaz, R.; Alings, M.; Lonn, E.M.; Anand, S.S.; et al. Rivaroxaban with or without aspirin in stable cardiovascular disease. *N. Engl. J. Med.* **2017**, *377*, 1319–1330. [CrossRef] [PubMed]
16. Sabatine, M.S.; Giugliano, R.P.; Keech, A.C.; Honarpour, N.; Wiviott, S.D.; Murphy, S.A.; Kuder, J.F.; Wang, H.; Liu, T.; Wasserman, S.M.; et al. Evolocumab and Clinical Outcomes in Patients with Cardiovascular Disease. *N. Engl. J. Med.* **2017**, *376*, 1713–1722. [CrossRef] [PubMed]
17. Schwartz, G.G.; Steg, P.G.; Szarek, M.; Bhatt, D.L.; Bittner, V.A.; Diaz, R.; Edelberg, J.M.; Goodman, S.G.; Hanotin, C.; Harrington, R.A.; et al. Alirocumab and Cardiovascular Outcomes after Acute Coronary Syndrome. *N. Engl. J. Med.* **2018**, *379*, 2097–2107. [CrossRef]
18. Steg, P.G.; Bhatt, D.L.; Wilson, P.W.F.; D'agostino, R.; Ohman, E.M.; Röther, J.; Liau, C.-S.; Hirsch, A.T.; Mas, J.-L.; Ikeda, Y.; et al. One-Year Cardiovascular Event Rates in Outpatients with Atherothrombosis. *JAMA* **2007**, *297*, 1197–1206. [CrossRef]
19. Jernberg, T.; Hasvold, P.; Henriksson, M.; Hjelm, H.; Thuresson, M.; Janzon, M. Cardiovascular risk in post-myocardial infarction patients: Nationwide real world data demonstrate the importance of a long-term perspective. *Eur. Heart J.* **2015**, *36*, 1163–1170. [CrossRef]

20. Fox, K.A.; Carruthers, K.F.; Dunbar, D.R.; Graham, C.; Manning, J.R.; De Raedt, H.; Buysschaert, I.; Lambrechts, D.; Van de Werf, F. Underestimated and under-recognized: The late consequences of acute coronary syndrome (GRACE UK-Belgian Study). *Eur. Heart J.* **2010**, *31*, 2755–2764. [CrossRef]
21. Jespersen, L.; Hvelplund, A.; Abildstrøm, S.Z.; Pedersen, F.; Galatius, S.; Madsen, J.K.; Jørgensen, E.; Kelbaek, H.; Prescott, E. Stable angina pectoris with no obstructive coronary artery disease is associated with increased risks of major adverse cardiovascular events. *Eur. Heart J.* **2012**, *33*, 734–744. [CrossRef] [PubMed]
22. Sedlak, T.L.; Lee, M.; Izadnegahdar, M.; Merz, C.N.B.; Gao, M.; Humphries, K.H. Sex differences in clinical outcomes in patients with stable angina and no obstructive coronary artery disease. *Am. Heart J.* **2013**, *166*, 38–44. [CrossRef]
23. Lee, J.M.; Choi, K.H.; Hwang, D.; Park, J.; Jung, J.-H.; Kim, H.Y.; Jung, H.W.; Cho, Y.-K.; Yoon, H.-J.; Bin Song, Y.; et al. Prognostic Implication of Thermodilution Coronary Flow Reserve in Patients Undergoing Fractional Flow Reserve Measurement. *JACC Cardiovasc. Interv.* **2018**, *11*, 1423–1433. [CrossRef] [PubMed]
24. Pepine, C.J.; Anderson, R.D.; Sharaf, B.L.; Reis, S.E.; Smith, K.M.; Handberg, E.M.; Johnson, B.D.; Sopko, G.; Bairey Merz, C.N. Coronary microvascular reactivity to adenosine predicts adverse outcome in women evaluated for suspected ischemia results from the National Heart, Lung and Blood Institute WISE (Women s Ischemia. Syndrome Evaluation) study. *J. Am. Coll. Cardiol.* **2010**, *55*, 2825–2832. [CrossRef] [PubMed]
25. Murthy, V.L.; Naya, M.; Foster, C.R.; Gaber, M.; Hainer, J.; Klein, J.; Dorbala, S.; Blankstein, R.; Di Carli, M.F. Association between coronary vascular dysfunction and cardiac mortality in patients with and without diabetes mellitus. *Circulation* **2012**, *126*, 1858–1868. [CrossRef] [PubMed]
26. Del Buono, M.G.; La Vecchia, G.; Rinaldi, R.; Sanna, T.; Crea, F.; Montone, R.A. Myocardial infarction with nonobstructive coronary arteries: The need for precision medicine. *Curr. Opin. Cardiol.* **2022**, *37*, 481–487. [CrossRef]
27. Bryniarski, K.; Gasior, P.; Legutko, J.; Makowicz, D.; Kedziora, A.; Szolc, P.; Bryniarski, L.; Kleczynski, P.; Jang, I.-K. OCT Findings in MINOCA. *J. Clin. Med.* **2021**, *10*, 2759. [CrossRef]
28. Borzillo, I.; De Filippo, O.; Manai, R.; Bruno, F.; Ravetti, E.; Galanti, A.A.; Vergallo, R.; Porto, I.; De Ferrari, G.M.; D'ascenzo, F. Role of Intracoronary Imaging in Myocardial Infarction with Non-Obstructive Coronary Disease (MINOCA): A Review. *J. Clin. Med.* **2023**, *12*, 2129. [CrossRef]
29. Gudigar, A.; Nayak, S.; Samanth, J.; Raghavendra, U.A.J.A.; Barua, P.D.; Hasan, N.; Ciaccio, E.J.; Tan, R.-S.; Acharya, U.R. Recent Trends in Artificial Intelligence-Assisted Coronary Atherosclerotic Plaque Characterization. *Int. J. Environ. Res. Public Health* **2021**, *18*, 10003. [CrossRef]
30. Lewis, E.F.; Moye, L.A.; Rouleau, J.L.; Sacks, F.M.; Arnold, J.M.O.; Warnica, J.W.; Flaker, G.C.; Braunwald, E.; Pfeffer, M.A. Predictors of late development of heart failure in stable survivors of myocardial infarction: The CARE study. *J. Am. Coll. Cardiol.* **2003**, *42*, 1446–1453. [CrossRef]
31. Lewis, E.F.; Solomon, S.D.; Jablonski, K.A.; Rice, M.M.; Clemenza, F.; Hsia, J.; Maggioni, A.P.; Zabalgoitia, M.; Huynh, T.; Cuddy, T.E.; et al. Predictors of heart failure in patients with stable coronary artery disease: A PEACE study. *Circ. Heart Fail.* **2009**, *2*, 209–216. [CrossRef] [PubMed]
32. Bauters, C.; Deneve, M.; Tricot, O.; Meurice, T.; Lamblin, N.; CORONOR Investigators. Prognosis of patients with stable coronary artery disease (from the CORONOR study). *Am. J. Cardiol.* **2014**, *113*, 1142–1145. [CrossRef] [PubMed]
33. Lamblin, N.; Meurice, T.; Tricot, O.; de Groote, P.; Lemesle, G.; Bauters, C. First Hospitalization for Heart Failure in Outpatients with Stable Coronary Artery Disease: Determinants, Role of Incident Myocardial Infarction, and Prognosis. *J. Card. Fail.* **2018**, *24*, 815–822. [CrossRef]
34. Dhindsa, D.S.; Sandesara, P.B.; Shapiro, M.D.; Wong, N.D. The Evolving Understanding and Approach to Residual Cardiovascular Risk Management. *Front. Cardiovasc. Med.* **2020**, *7*, 88. [CrossRef] [PubMed]
35. Varenhorst, C.; Hasvold, P.; Johansson, S.; Janzon, M.; Albertsson, P.; Leosdottir, M.; Hambraeus, K.; James, S.; Jernberg, T.; Svennblad, B.; et al. Culprit and Nonculprit Recurrent Ischemic Events in Patients with Myocardial Infarction: Data From SWEDEHEART (Swedish Web System for Enhancement and Development of Evidence-Based Care in Heart Disease Evaluated According to Recommended Therapies). *J. Am. Heart Assoc.* **2018**, *7*, e007174. [CrossRef]
36. Yeh, R.W.; Secemsky, E.A.; Kereiakes, D.J.; Normand, S.-L.T.; Gershlick, A.H.; Cohen, D.J.; Spertus, J.A.; Steg, P.G.; Cutlip, D.E.; Rinaldi, M.J.; et al. Development and Validation of a Prediction Rule for Benefit and Harm of Dual Antiplatelet Therapy Beyond 1 Year after Percutaneous Coronary Intervention. *JAMA* **2016**, *315*, 1735–1749. [CrossRef]
37. Chichareon, P.; Modolo, R.; Kawashima, H.; Takahashi, K.; Kogame, N.; Chang, C.-C.; Tomaniak, M.; Ono, M.; Walsh, S.; Suryapranata, H.; et al. DAPT Score and the Impact of Ticagrelor Monotherapy During the Second Year after PCI. *JACC Cardiovasc. Interv.* **2020**, *13*, 634–646. [CrossRef]
38. Ueda, P.; Jernberg, T.; James, S.; Alfredsson, J.; Erlinge, D.; Omerovic, E.; Persson, J.; Ravn-Fischer, A.; Tornvall, P.; Svennblad, B.; et al. External Validation of the DAPT Score in a Nationwide Population. *J. Am. Coll. Cardiol.* **2018**, *72*, 1069–1078. [CrossRef]
39. Montalto, C.; Ferlini, M.; Casula, M.; Mandurino-Mirizzi, A.; Costa, F.; Leonardi, S.; Visconti, L.O. DAPT Score to Stratify Ischemic and Bleeding Risk after Percutaneous Coronary Intervention: An Updated Systematic Review, Meta-Analysis, and Meta-Regression of 100,211 Patients. *Thromb. Haemost.* **2021**, *121*, 687–689. [CrossRef]

40. Costa, F.; van Klaveren, D.; James, S.; Heg, D.; Räber, L.; Feres, F.; Pilgrim, T.; Hong, M.-K.; Kim, H.-S.; Colombo, A.; et al. Derivation and validation of the predicting bleeding complications in patients undergoing stent implantation and subsequent dual antiplatelet therapy (PRECISE-DAPT) score: A pooled analysis of individual-patient datasets from clinical trials. *Lancet* **2017**, *389*, 1025–1034. [CrossRef]
41. Clifford, C.R.; Boudreau, R.; Visintini, S.; Orr, N.; Fu, A.Y.N.; Malhotra, N.; Barry, Q.; So, D.Y.F. The association of PRECISE-DAPT score with ischaemic outcomes in patients taking dual antiplatelet therapy following percutaneous coronary intervention: A meta-analysis. *Eur. Heart J.—Cardiovasc. Pharmacother.* **2022**, *8*, 511–518. [CrossRef] [PubMed]
42. Lindholm, D.; Sarno, G.; Erlinge, D.; Svennblad, B.; Hasvold, L.P.; Janzon, M.; Jernberg, T.; James, S.K. Combined association of key risk factors on ischaemic outcomes and bleeding in patients with myocardial infarction. *Heart* **2019**, *105*, 1175–1181. [CrossRef] [PubMed]
43. Bhatt, D.L.; Eagle, K.A.; Ohman, E.M.; Hirsch, A.T.; Goto, S.; Mahoney, E.M.; Wilson, P.W.; Alberts, M.J.; D'Agostino, R.; Liau, C.S.; et al. Comparative determinants of 4-year cardiovascular event rates in stable outpatients at risk of or with atherothrombosis. *JAMA* **2010**, *304*, 1350–1357. [CrossRef] [PubMed]
44. Stone, G.W.; Maehara, A.; Lansky, A.J.; de Bruyne, B.; Cristea, E.; Mintz, G.S.; Mehran, R.; McPherson, J.; Farhat, N.; Marso, S.P.; et al. A Prospective Natural-History Study of Coronary Atherosclerosis. *N. Engl. J. Med.* **2011**, *364*, 226–235. [CrossRef]
45. Prati, F.; Romagnoli, E.; Gatto, L.; La Manna, A.; Burzotta, F.; Ozaki, Y.; Marco, V.; Boi, A.; Fineschi, M.; Fabbiocchi, F.; et al. Relationship between coronary plaque morphology of the left anterior descending artery and 12 months clinical outcome: The CLIMA study. *Eur. Heart J.* **2020**, *41*, 383–391. [CrossRef]
46. Chow, C.K.; Jolly, S.; Rao-Melacini, P.; Fox, K.A.; Anand, S.S.; Yusuf, S. Association of Diet, Exercise, and Smoking Modification with Risk of Early Cardiovascular Events after Acute Coronary Syndromes. *Circulation* **2010**, *121*, 750–758. [CrossRef]
47. Booth, J.N.; Levitan, E.B.; Brown, T.M.; Farkouh, M.E.; Safford, M.M.; Muntner, P. Effect of Sustaining Lifestyle Modifications (Nonsmoking, Weight Reduction, Physical Activity, and Mediterranean Diet) after Healing of Myocardial Infarction, Percutaneous Intervention, or Coronary Bypass (from the REasons for Geographic and Racial Differences in Stroke Study). *Am. J. Cardiol.* **2014**, *113*, 1933–1940.
48. Giannuzzi, P.; Temporelli, P.L.; Marchioli, R.; Maggioni, A.P.; Balestroni, G.; Ceci, V.; Chieffo, C.; Gattone, M.; Griffo, R.; Schweiger, C.; et al. Global secondary prevention strategies to limit event recurrence after myocardial infarction: Results of the GOSPEL study, a multicenter, randomized controlled trial from the Italian Cardiac Rehabilitation Network. *Arch. Intern. Med.* **2008**, *168*, 21942204. [CrossRef]
49. Visseren, F.L.J.; Mach, F.; Smulders, Y.M.; Carballo, D.; Koskinas, K.C.; Bäck, M.; Benetos, A.; Biffi, A.; Boavida, J.M.; Capodanno, D.; et al. 2021 ESC Guidelines on cardiovascular disease prevention in clinical practice. *Eur. Heart J.* **2021**, *42*, 3227–3337. [CrossRef]
50. Wood, D.; Kotseva, K.; Connolly, S.; Jennings, C.; Mead, A.; Jones, J.; Holden, A.; De Bacquer, D.; Collier, T.; De Backer, G.; et al. Nurse-coordinated multidisciplinary, family-based cardiovascular disease prevention programme (EUROACTION) for patients with coronary heart disease and asymptomatic individuals at high risk of cardiovascular disease: A paired, cluster-randomised controlled trial. *Lancet* **2008**, *371*, 1999–2012. [CrossRef]
51. Clar, C.; Oseni, Z.; Flowers, N.; Keshtkar-Jahromi, M.; Rees, K. Influenza vaccines for preventing cardiovascular disease. *Cochrane Database Syst. Rev.* **2015**, *5*, CD005050.
52. Peterson, P.N. *JAHA* Spotlight on Psychosocial Factors and Cardiovascular Disease. *J. Am. Heart Assoc.* **2020**, *9*, e017112. [CrossRef] [PubMed]
53. Rozanski, A.; Blumenthal, J.A.; Kaplan, J. Impact of Psychological Factors on the Pathogenesis of Cardiovascular Disease and Implications for Therapy. *Circulation* **1999**, *99*, 2192–2217. [CrossRef] [PubMed]
54. Powell-Wiley, T.M.; Baumer, Y.; Baah, F.O.; Baez, A.S.; Farmer, N.; Mahlobo, C.T.; Pita, M.A.; Potharaju, K.A.; Tamura, K.; Wallen, G.R. Social Determinants of Cardiovascular Disease. *Circ. Res.* **2022**, *130*, 782–799. [CrossRef]
55. Richards, S.H.; Anderson, L.; Jenkinson, C.E.; Whalley, B.; Rees, K.; Davies, P.; Bennett, P.; Liu, Z.; West, R.; Thompson, D.R.; et al. Psychological interventions for coronary heart disease: Cochrane systematic review and meta-analysis. *Eur. J. Prev. Cardiol.* **2018**, *25*, 247–259. [CrossRef]
56. Rutledge, T.; Redwine, L.S.; Linke, S.E.; Mills, P.J. A Meta-Analysis of Mental Health Treatments and Cardiac Rehabilitation for Improving Clinical Outcomes and Depression among Patients with Coronary Heart Disease. *Psychosom. Med.* **2013**, *75*, 335–349. [CrossRef]
57. Rahimi, K.; MacMahon, S. Blood pressure management in the 21st century: Maximizing gains and minimizing waste. *Circulation* **2013**, *128*, 2283–2285. [CrossRef]
58. Ettehad, D.; Emdin, C.A.; Kiran, A.; Anderson, S.G.; Callender, T.; Emberson, J.; Chalmers, J.; Rodgers, A.; Rahimi, K. Blood pressure lowering for prevention of cardiovascular disease and death: A systematic review and meta-analysis. *Lancet* **2016**, *387*, 957–967. [CrossRef]
59. Williams, B.; Mancia, G.; Spiering, W.; Agabiti Rosei, E.; Azizi, M.; Burnier, M.; Clement, D.L.; Coca, A.; de Simone, G.; Dominiczak, A.; et al. 2018 ESC/ESH Guidelines for the management of arterial hypertension. *Eur. Heart J.* **2018**, *39*, 3021–3104. [CrossRef]
60. Fried, L.F.; Emanuele, N.; Zhang, J.H.; Brophy, M.; Conner, T.A.; Duckworth, W.; Leehey, D.J.; McCullough, P.A.; O'Connor, T.; Palevsky, P.M.; et al. Combined Angiotensin Inhibition for the Treatment of Diabetic Nephropathy. *N. Engl. J. Med.* **2013**, *369*, 1892–1903. [CrossRef]

61. Collet, J.P.; Thiele, H.; Barbato, E.; Barthélémy, O.; Bauersachs, J.; Bhatt, D.L.; Dendale, P.; Dorobantu, M.; Edvardsen, T.; Folliguet, T.; et al. 2020 ESC Guidelines for the management of acute coronary syndromes in patients presenting without persistent ST-segment elevation. *Eur. Heart J.* **2021**, *42*, 1289–1367. [CrossRef] [PubMed]
62. Capodanno, D.; Bhatt, D.L.; Eikelboom, J.W.; Fox, K.A.A.; Geisler, T.; Gibson, C.M.; Gonzalez-Juanatey, J.R.; James, S.; Lopes, R.D.; Mehran, R.; et al. Dual-pathway inhibition for secondary and tertiary antithrombotic prevention in cardiovascular disease. *Nat. Rev. Cardiol.* **2020**, *17*, 242–257. [CrossRef] [PubMed]
63. Steg, P.G.; Bhatt, D.L.; Simon, T.; Fox, K.; Mehta, S.R.; Harrington, R.A.; Held, C.; Andersson, M.; Himmelmann, A.; Ridderstråle, W.; et al. Ticagrelor in Patients with Stable Coronary Disease and Diabetes. *N. Engl. J. Med.* **2019**, *381*, 1309–1320. [CrossRef]
64. Bhatt, D.L.; Steg, P.G.; Mehta, S.R.; Leiter, L.A.; Simon, T.; Fox, K.; Held, C.; Andersson, M.; Himmelmann, A.; Ridderstråle, W.; et al. Ticagrelor in patients with diabetes and stable coronary artery disease with a history of previous percutaneous coronary intervention (THEMIS-PCI): A phase 3, placebo-controlled, randomised trial. *Lancet* **2019**, *394*, 1169–1180. [CrossRef] [PubMed]
65. Vranckx, P.; Valgimigli, M.; Jüni, P.; Hamm, C.; Steg, P.G.; Heg, D.; van Es, G.A.; McFadden, E.P.; Onuma, Y.; van Meijeren, C.; et al. Ticagrelor plus aspirin for 1 month, followed by ticagrelor monotherapy for 23 months vs aspirin plus clopidogrel or ticagrelor for 12 months, followed by aspirin monotherapy for 12 months after implantation of a drug-eluting stent: A multicentre, open-label, randomised superiority trial. *Lancet* **2018**, *392*, 940–949. [CrossRef]
66. Hindricks, G.; Potpara, T.; Dagres, N.; Arbelo, E.; Bax, J.J.; Blomström-Lundqvist, C.; Boriani, G.; Castella, M.; Dan, G.A.; Dilaveris, P.E.; et al. 2020 ESC Guidelines for the diagnosis and management of atrial fibrillation developed in collaboration with the European Association for Cardio-Thoracic Surgery (EACTS): The Task Force for the diagnosis and management of atrial fibrillation of the European Society of Cardiology (ESC) Developed with the special contribution of the European Heart Rhythm Association (EHRA) of the ESC. *Eur. Heart J.* **2021**, *42*, 373–498.
67. Mach, F.; Baigent, C.; Catapano, A.L.; Koskinas, K.C.; Casula, M.; Badimon, L.; Chapman, M.J.; De Backer, G.G.; Delgado, V.; Ference, B.A.; et al. 2019 ESC/EAS Guidelines for the management of dyslipidaemias: Lipid modification to reduce cardiovascular risk. *Eur. Heart J.* **2020**, *41*, 111–188. [CrossRef]
68. Baigent, C.; Keech, A.; Kearney, P.M.; Blackwell, L.; Buck, G.; Pollicino, C.; Kirby, A.; Sourjina, T.; Peto, R.; Collins, R.; et al. Efficacy and safety of cholesterol-lowering treatment: Prospective meta-analysis of data from 90,056 participants in 14 randomised trials of statins. *Lancet* **2005**, *366*, 1267–1278.
69. Cholesterol Treatment Trialists' (CTT) Collaboration; Baigent, C.; Blackwell, L.; Emberson, J.; Holland, L.E.; Reith, C.; Bhala, N.; Peto, R.; Barnes, E.H.; Keech, A.; et al. Efficacy and safety of more intensive lowering of LDL cholesterol: A meta-analysis of data from 170,000 participants in 26 randomised trials. *Lancet* **2010**, *376*, 16701681. [CrossRef]
70. Bhatt, D.L.; Steg, P.G.; Miller, M.; Brinton, E.A.; Jacobson, T.A.; Ketchum, S.B.; Doyle, R.T., Jr.; Juliano, R.A.; Jiao, L.; Granowitz, C.; et al. Cardiovascular Risk Reduction with Icosapent Ethyl for Hypertriglyceridemia. *N. Engl. J. Med.* **2019**, *380*, 11–22. [CrossRef]
71. Kronenberg, F.; Mora, S.; Stroes, E.S.G.; Ference, B.A.; Arsenault, B.J.; Berglund, L.; Dweck, M.R.; Koschinsky, M.; Lambert, G.; Mach, F.; et al. Lipoprotein(a) in atherosclerotic cardiovascular disease and aortic stenosis: A European Atherosclerosis Society consensus statement. *Eur. Heart J.* **2022**, *43*, 3925–3946. [CrossRef] [PubMed]
72. Cosentino, F.; Grant, P.J.; Aboyans, V.; Bailey, C.J.; Ceriello, A.; Delgado, V.; Federici, M.; Filippatos, G.; Grobbee, D.E.; Hansen, T.B.; et al. 2019 ESC Guidelines on diabetes, pre-diabetes, and cardiovascular diseases developed in collaboration with the EASD. *Eur. Heart J.* **2020**, *41*, 255–323. [CrossRef] [PubMed]
73. Perkovic, V.; Jardine, M.J.; Neal, B.; Bompoint, S.; Heerspink, H.J.L.; Charytan, D.M.; Edwards, R.; Agarwal, R.; Bakris, G.; Bull, S.; et al. Canagliflozin and Renal Outcomes in Type 2 Diabetes and Nephropathy. *N. Engl. J. Med.* **2019**, *380*, 2295–2306. [CrossRef] [PubMed]
74. Wiviott, S.D.; Raz, I.; Bonaca, M.P.; Mosenzon, O.; Kato, E.T.; Cahn, A.; Silverman, M.G.; Zelniker, T.A.; Kuder, J.F.; Murphy, S.A.; et al. Dapagliflozin and Cardiovascular Outcomes in Type 2 Diabetes. *N. Engl. J. Med.* **2019**, *380*, 347–357. [CrossRef] [PubMed]
75. Marso, S.P.; Daniels, G.H.; Brown-Frandsen, K.; Kristensen, P.; Mann, J.F.E.; Nauck, M.A.; Nissen, S.E.; Pocock, S.; Poulter, N.R.; Ravn, L.S.; et al. Liraglutide and Cardiovascular Outcomes in Type 2 Diabetes. *N. Engl. J. Med.* **2016**, *375*, 311–322. [CrossRef] [PubMed]
76. Marso, S.P.; Bain, S.C.; Consoli, A.; Eliaschewitz, F.G.; Jódar, E.; Leiter, L.A.; Lingvay, I.; Rosenstock, J.; Seufert, J.; Warren, M.L.; et al. Semaglutide and Cardiovascular Outcomes in Patients with Type 2 Diabetes. *N. Engl. J. Med.* **2016**, *375*, 1834–1844. [CrossRef]
77. Hernandez, A.F.; Green, J.B.; Janmohamed, S.; D'Agostino, R.B.; Granger, C.B.; Jones, N.P.; Leiter, L.A.; Rosenberg, A.E.; Sigmon, K.N.; Somerville, M.C.; et al. Albiglutide and cardiovascular outcomes in patients with type 2 diabetes and cardiovascular disease (Harmony Outcomes): A double-blind, randomised placebo-controlled trial. *Lancet* **2018**, *392*, 1519–1529. [CrossRef]
78. ElSayed, N.A.; Aleppo, G.; Aroda, V.R.; Bannuru, R.R.; Brown, F.M.; Bruemmer, D.; Collins, B.S.; Hilliard, M.E.; Isaacs, D.; Johnson, E.L.; et al. 9. Pharmacologic Approaches to Glycemic Treatment: Standards of Care in Diabetes—2023. *Diabetes Care* **2023**, *46*, S140–S157. [CrossRef]
79. Younossi, Z.M.; Anstee, Q.M.; Marietti, M.; Hardy, T.; Henry, L.; Eslam, M.; George, J.; Bugianesi, E. Global burden of NAFLD and NASH: Trends, predictions, risk factors and prevention. *Nat. Rev. Gastroenterol. Hepatol.* **2018**, *15*, 11–20. [CrossRef]
80. Alon, L.; Corica, B.; Raparelli, V.; Cangemi, R.; Basili, S.; Proietti, M.; Romiti, G.F. Risk of cardiovascular events in patients with non-alcoholic fatty liver disease: A systematic review and meta-analysis. *Eur. J. Prev. Cardiol.* **2022**, *29*, 938–946. [CrossRef]

81. Hassen, G.; Singh, A.; Belete, G.; Jain, N.; De la Hoz, I.; Camacho-Leon, G.P.; Dargie, N.K.; Carrera, K.G.; Alemu, T.; Jhaveri, S.; et al. Nonalcoholic Fatty Liver Disease: An Emerging Modern-Day Risk Factor for Cardiovascular Disease. *Cureus* **2022**, *14*, e25495. [CrossRef] [PubMed]
82. Duell, P.B.; Welty, F.K.; Miller, M.; Chait, A.; Hammond, G.; Ahmad, Z.; Cohen, D.E.; Horton, J.D.; Pressman, G.S.; Toth, P.P.; et al. Nonalcoholic Fatty Liver Disease and Cardiovascular Risk: A Scientific Statement from the American Heart Association. *Arterioscler. Thromb. Vasc. Biol.* **2022**, *42*, e168–e185. [CrossRef] [PubMed]
83. Chalasani, N.; Younossi, Z.; LaVine, J.E.; Charlton, M.; Cusi, K.; Rinella, M.; Harrison, S.A.; Brunt, E.M.; Sanyal, A.J. The diagnosis and management of nonalcoholic fatty liver disease: Practice guidance from the American Association for the Study of Liver Diseases. *Hepatology* **2018**, *67*, 328–357. [CrossRef]
84. Armstrong, M.J.; Gaunt, P.; Aithal, G.P.; Barton, D.; Hull, D.; Parker, R.; Hazlehurst, J.M.; Guo, K.; Abouda, G.; Aldersley, M.A.; et al. Liraglutide safety and efficacy in patients with non-alcoholic steatohepatitis (LEAN): A multicentre, double-blind, randomised, placebo-controlled phase 2 study. *Lancet* **2016**, *387*, 679–690. [CrossRef]
85. Newsome, P.N.; Buchholtz, K.; Cusi, K.; Linder, M.; Okanoue, T.; Ratziu, V.; Sanyal, A.J.; Sejling, A.-S.; Harrison, S.A. A Placebo-Controlled Trial of Subcutaneous Semaglutide in Nonalcoholic Steatohepatitis. *N. Engl. J. Med.* **2021**, *384*, 1113–1124. [CrossRef] [PubMed]
86. Cho, Y.; Rhee, H.; Kim, Y.-E.; Lee, M.; Lee, B.-W.; Kang, E.S.; Cha, B.-S.; Choi, J.-Y.; Lee, Y.-H. Ezetimibe combination therapy with statin for non-alcoholic fatty liver disease: An open-label randomized controlled trial (ESSENTIAL study). *BMC Med.* **2022**, *20*, 93. [CrossRef] [PubMed]
87. Arroyo-Espliguero, R.; Avanzas, P.; Quiles, J.; Kaski, J.C. Predictive value of coronary artery stenoses and C-reactive protein levels in patients with stable coronary artery disease. *Atherosclerosis* **2009**, *204*, 239–243. [CrossRef]
88. Libby, P. Inflammation in Atherosclerosis—No Longer a Theory. *Clin. Chem.* **2021**, *67*, 131–142. [CrossRef]
89. Lawler, P.R.; Bhatt, D.L.; Godoy, L.C.; Lüscher, T.F.; Bonow, R.O.; Verma, S.; Ridker, P.M. Targeting cardiovascular inflammation: Next steps in clinical translation. *Eur. Heart J.* **2021**, *42*, 113–131. [CrossRef]
90. Koenig, W. High-sensitivity C-reactive protein and atherosclerotic disease: From improved risk prediction to risk-guided therapy. *Int. J. Cardiol.* **2013**, *168*, 5126–5134. [CrossRef]
91. Bohula, E.A.; Giugliano, R.P.; Cannon, C.P.; Zhou, J.; Murphy, S.A.; White, J.A.; Tershakovec, A.M.; Blazing, M.A.; Braunwald, E. Achievement of dual low-density lipo- protein cholesterol and high-sensitivity C-reactive protein targets more frequent with the addition of ezetimibe to simvastatin and associated with better outcomes in IMPROVE-IT. *Circulation* **2015**, *132*, 1224–1233. [CrossRef] [PubMed]
92. Bohula, E.A.; Giugliano, R.P.; Leiter, L.A.; Verma, S.; Park, J.G.; Sever, P.S.; Lira Pineda, A.; Honarpour, N.; Wang, H.; Murphy, S.A.; et al. Inflammatory and cholesterol risk in the FOURIER trial. *Circulation* **2018**, *138*, 131–140. [CrossRef] [PubMed]
93. Ridker, P.M.; MacFadyen, J.G.; Thuren, T.; Everett, B.M.; Libby, P.; Glynn, R.J.; Ridker, P.; Lorenzatti, A.; Krum, H.; Varigos, J.; et al. Effect of interleukin-1beta inhibition with canakinumab on incident lung cancer in patients with atherosclerosis: Exploratory results from a randomised, double-blind, placebo-controlled trial. *Lancet* **2017**, *390*, 1833–1842. [CrossRef] [PubMed]
94. Ridker, P.M.; Everett, B.M.; Pradhan, A.; MacFadyen, J.G.; Solomon, D.H.; Zaharris, E.; Mam, V.; Hasan, A.; Rosenberg, Y.; Iturriaga, E.; et al. Low-Dose Methotrexate for the Prevention of Atherosclerotic Events. *N. Engl. J. Med.* **2018**, *380*, 752–762. [CrossRef] [PubMed]
95. Nidorf, S.M.; Fiolet, A.T.L.; Mosterd, A.; Eikelboom, J.W.; Schut, A.; Opstal, T.S.J.; The, S.H.K.; Xu, X.-F.; Ireland, M.A.; Lenderink, T.; et al. Colchicine in Patients with Chronic Coronary Disease. *N. Engl. J. Med.* **2020**, *383*, 1838–1847. [CrossRef]
96. Knuuti, J.; Ballo, H.; Juarez-Orozco, L.E.; Saraste, A.; Kolh, P.; Rutjes, A.W.S.; Jüni, P.; Windecker, S.; Bax, J.J.; Wijns, W. The performance of non-invasive tests to rule-in and rule-out significant coronary artery stenosis in patients with stable angina: A meta-analysis focused on post-test disease probability. *Eur. Heart J.* **2018**, *39*, 3322–3330. [CrossRef]
97. Diamond, G.A.; Forrester, J.S. Analysis of Probability as an Aid in the Clinical Diagnosis of Coronary-Artery Disease. *N. Engl. J. Med.* **1979**, *300*, 1350–1358. [CrossRef]
98. Foldyna, B.; Udelson, J.E.; Karady, J.; Banerji, D.; Lu, M.T.; Mayrhofer, T.; Bittner, D.O.; Meyersohn, N.M.; Emami, H.; Genders, T.S.S.; et al. Pretest probability for patients with suspected obstructive coronary artery disease: Re-evaluating Diamond-Forrester for the contemporary era and clinical implications: Insights from the PROMISE trial. *Eur. Heart J. Cardiovasc. Imaging* **2018**, *20*, 574–581. [CrossRef]
99. Adamson, P.D.; Newby, D.E.; Hill, C.L.; Coles, A.; Douglas, P.S.; Fordyce, C.B. Comparison of International Guidelines for Assessment of Suspected Stable Angina: Insights from the PROMISE and SCOT-HEART. *JACC Cardiovasc. Imaging* **2018**, *11*, 1301–1310. [CrossRef]
100. Juarez-Orozco, L.E.; Saraste, A.; Capodanno, D.; Prescott, E.; Ballo, H.; Bax, J.J.; Wijns, W.; Knuuti, J. Impact of a decreasing pre-test probability on the performance of diagnostic tests for coronary artery disease. *Eur. Heart J.—Cardiovasc. Imaging* **2019**, *20*, 1198–1207. [CrossRef]
101. Tonino, P.A.L.; De Bruyne, B.; Pijls, N.H.J.; Siebert, U.; Ikeno, F.; van't Veer, M.; Klauss, V.; Manoharan, G.; Engstrøm, T.; Oldroyd, K.G.; et al. Fractional flow reserve versus angiography for guiding percutaneous coronary intervention. *N. Engl. J. Med.* **2009**, *360*, 213–224. [CrossRef]

102. De Maria, G.L.; Garcia-Garcia, H.M.; Scarsini, R.; Hideo-Kajita, A.; López, N.G.; Leone, A.M.; Sarno, G.; Daemen, J.; Shlofmitz, E.; Jeremias, A.; et al. Novel Indices of Coronary Physiology: Do We Need Alternatives to Fractional Flow Reserve? *Circ. Cardiovasc. Interv.* **2020**, *13*, e008487. [CrossRef]
103. Neumann, F.J.; Sousa-Uva, M.; Ahlsson, A.; Alfonso, F.; Banning, A.P.; Benedetto, U.; Byrne, R.A.; Collet, J.P.; Falk, V.; Head, S.J.; et al. 2018 ESC/EACTS Guidelines on myocardial revascularization. *Eur. Heart J.* **2019**, *40*, 87–165. [CrossRef]
104. Committee Members; Gibbons, R.J.; Balady, G.J.; Bricker, J.T.; Chaitman, B.R.; Fletcher, G.F.; Froelicher, V.F.; Mark, D.B.; McCallister, B.D.; Mooss, A.N.; et al. ACC/AHA 2002 guideline update for exercise testing: Summary article: A report of the American College of Cardiology/American Heart Association Task Force on Practice Guidelines (Committee to Update the 1997 Exercise Testing Guidelines). *Circulation* **2002**, *106*, 1883–1892. [CrossRef]
105. Hecht, H.S.; Narula, J.; Fearon, W.F. Fractional Flow Reserve and Coronary Computed Tomographic Angiography: A Review and Critical Analysis. *Circ. Res.* **2016**, *119*, 300–316. [CrossRef] [PubMed]
106. Mittal, T.K.; Hothi, S.S.; Venugopal, V.; Taleyratne, J.; O'brien, D.; Adnan, K.; Sehmi, J.; Daskalopoulos, G.; Deshpande, A.; Elfawal, S.; et al. The Use and Efficacy of FFR-CT: Real-World Multicenter Audit of Clinical Data with Cost Analysis. *JACC Cardiovasc Imaging.* **2023**, *16*, 1056–1065. [CrossRef] [PubMed]
107. Bertoldi, E.G.; Stella, S.F.; Rohde, L.E.P.; Polanczyk, C.A. Cost-effectiveness of anatomical and functional test strategies for stable chest pain: Public health perspective from a middle-income country. *BMJ Open* **2017**, *7*, e012652. [CrossRef]
108. Karády, J.; Mayrhofer, T.; Ivanov, A.; Foldyna, B.; Lu, M.T.; Ferencik, M.; Pursnani, A.; Salerno, M.; Udelson, J.E.; Mark, D.B.; et al. Cost-effectiveness Analysis of Anatomic vs Functional Index Testing in Patients with Low-Risk Stable Chest Pain. *JAMA Netw. Open* **2020**, *3*, e2028312. [CrossRef] [PubMed]
109. van Waardhuizen, C.N.; Khanji, M.Y.; Genders, T.S.; Ferket, B.S.; Fleischmann, K.E.; Hunink, M.M.; Petersen, S.E. Comparative cost-effectiveness of non-invasive imaging tests in patients presenting with chronic stable chest pain with suspected coronary artery disease: A systematic review. *Eur. Heart J.—Qual. Care Clin. Outcomes* **2016**, *2*, 245–260. [CrossRef]
110. Nazir, M.S.; Rodriguez-Guadarrama, Y.; Rua, T.; Bui, K.H.; Gola, A.B.; Chiribiri, A.; McCrone, P.; Plein, S.; Pennington, M. Cost-effectiveness in diagnosis of stable angina patients: A decision-analytical modelling approach. *Open Heart* **2022**, *9*, e001700. [CrossRef]
111. Fox, K.A.; Clayton, T.C.; Damman, P.; Pocock, S.J.; de Winter, R.J.; Tijssen, J.G.; Lagerqvist, B.; Wallentin, L. Long-Term Outcome of a Routine versus Selective Invasive Strategy in Patients with Non–ST-Segment Elevation Acute Coronary Syndrome: A Meta-Analysis of Individual Patient Data. *J. Am. Coll. Cardiol.* **2010**, *55*, 2435–2445. [CrossRef] [PubMed]
112. Bavry, A.A.; Kumbhani, D.J.; Rassi, A.N.; Bhatt, D.L.; Askari, A.T. Benefit of Early Invasive Therapy in Acute Coronary Syndromes: A Meta-Analysis of Contemporary Randomized Clinical Trials. *J. Am. Coll. Cardiol.* **2006**, *48*, 1319–1325. [CrossRef] [PubMed]
113. Boden, W.E.; O'Rourke, R.A.; Teo, K.K.; Hartigan, P.M.; Maron, D.J.; Kostuk, W.J.; Knudtson, M.; Dada, M.; Casperson, P.; Harris, C.L.; et al. Optimal Medical Therapy with or without PCI for Stable Coronary Disease. *N. Engl. J. Med.* **2007**, *356*, 1503–1516. [CrossRef] [PubMed]
114. BARI 2D Study Group; Frye, R.L.; August, P.; Brooks, M.M.; Hardison, R.M.; Kelsey, S.F.; MacGregor, J.M.; Orchard, T.J.; Chaitman, B.R.; Genuth, S.M.; et al. A Randomized Trial of Therapies for Type 2 Diabetes and Coronary Artery Disease. *N. Engl. J. Med.* **2009**, *360*, 2503–2515. [CrossRef]
115. De Bruyne, B.; Pijls, N.H.; Kalesan, B.; Barbato, E.; Tonino, P.A.; Piroth, Z.; Jagic, N.; Mobius-Winckler, S.; Rioufol, G.; Witt, N.; et al. Fractional Flow Reserve–Guided PCI versus Medical Therapy in Stable Coronary Disease. *N. Engl. J. Med.* **2012**, *367*, 991–1001. [CrossRef]
116. Al-Lamee, R.; Thompson, D.; Dehbi, H.-M.; Sen, S.; Tang, K.; Davies, J.; Keeble, T.; Mielewczik, M.; Kaprielian, R.; Malik, I.S.; et al. Percutaneous coronary intervention in stable angina (ORBITA): A double-blind, randomised controlled trial. *Lancet* **2018**, *391*, 31–40. [CrossRef]
117. Maron, D.J.; Hochman, J.S.; Reynolds, H.R.; Bangalore, S.; O'Brien, S.M.; Boden, W.E.; Chaitman, B.R.; Senior, R.; López-Sendón, J.; Alexander, K.P.; et al. Initial invasive or conservative strategy for stable coronary disease. *N. Engl. J. Med.* **2020**, *382*, 1395–1407. [CrossRef]
118. Hochman, J.S.; Anthopolos, R.; Reynolds, H.R.; Bangalore, S.; Xu, Y.; O'brien, S.M.; Mavromichalis, S.; Chang, M.; Contreras, A.; Rosenberg, Y.; et al. Survival after Invasive or Conservative Management of Stable Coronary Disease. *Circulation* **2023**, *147*, 8–19. [CrossRef]
119. Bainey, K.R.; Engstrøm, T.; Smits, P.C.; Gershlick, A.H.; James, S.K.; Storey, R.F.; Wood, D.A.; Mehran, R.; Cairns, J.A.; Mehta, S.R. Complete vs culprit-lesion-only revascularization for ST-segment elevation myocardial infarction: A systematic review and meta-analysis. *JAMA Cardiol.* **2020**, *5*, 881–888. [CrossRef]
120. Writing Committee Members; Lawton, J.S.; Tamis-Holland, J.E.; Bangalore, S.; Bates, E.R.; Beckie, T.M.; Bischoff, J.M.; Bittl, J.A.; Cohen, M.G.; DiMaio, J.M.; et al. 2021 ACC/AHA/SCAI Guideline for Coronary Artery Revascularization: A Report of the American College of Cardiology/American Heart Association Joint Committee on Clinical Practice Guidelines. *J. Am. Coll. Cardiol.* **2022**, *79*, e21–e129.
121. Puymirat, E.; Cayla, G.; Simon, T.; Steg, P.G.; Montalescot, G.; Durand-Zaleski, I.; le Bras, A.; Gallet, R.; Khalife, K.; Morelle, J.-F.; et al. Multivessel PCI Guided by FFR or Angiography for Myocardial Infarction. *N. Engl. J. Med.* **2021**, *385*, 297–308. [CrossRef] [PubMed]

122. Elbadawi, A.; Dang, A.T.; Hamed, M.; Eid, M.; Prakash Hiriyur Prakash, M.; Saleh, M.; Gad, M.; Mamas, M.A. FFR-Versus Angiography-Guided Revascularization for Nonculprit Stenosis in STEMI and Multivessel Disease. A Network Meta-Analysis. *J. Am. Coll. Cardiovasc. Interv.* **2022**, *15*, 656–666. [CrossRef] [PubMed]
123. Velazquez, E.J.; Lee, K.L.; Deja, M.A.; Jain, A.; Sopko, G.; Marchenko, A.; Ali, I.S.; Pohost, G.; Gradinac, S.; Abraham, W.T.; et al. Coronary-Artery Bypass Surgery in Patients with Left Ventricular Dysfunction. *N. Engl. J. Med.* **2011**, *364*, 1607–1616. [CrossRef] [PubMed]
124. Perera, D.; Clayton, T.; O'kane, P.D.; Greenwood, J.P.; Weerackody, R.; Ryan, M.; Morgan, H.P.; Dodd, M.; Evans, R.; Canter, R.; et al. Percutaneous Revascularization for Ischemic Left Ventricular Dysfunction. *N. Engl. J. Med.* **2022**, *387*, 1351–1360. [CrossRef] [PubMed]
125. Hong, S.-J.; Mintz, G.S.; Ahn, C.-M.; Kim, J.-S.; Kim, B.-K.; Ko, Y.-G.; Kang, T.-S.; Kang, W.-C.; Kim, Y.H.; Hur, S.-H.; et al. Effect of Intravascular Ultrasound–Guided Drug-Eluting Stent Implantation: 5-Year Follow-Up of the IVUS-XPL Randomized Trial. *JACC Cardiovasc. Interv.* **2020**, *13*, 62–71. [CrossRef]
126. Gao, X.-F.; Ge, Z.; Kong, X.-Q.; Kan, J.; Han, L.; Lu, S.; Tian, N.-L.; Lin, S.; Lu, Q.-H.; Wang, X.-Y.; et al. 3-Year Outcomes of the ULTIMATE Trial Comparing Intravascular Ultrasound Versus Angiography-Guided Drug-Eluting Stent Implantation. *JACC Cardiovasc. Interv.* **2021**, *14*, 247–257. [CrossRef]
127. Jakabčin, J.; Špaček, R.; Bystroň, M.; Kvašňák, M.; Jager, J.; Veselka, J.; Kala, P.; Červinka, P. Long term health outcome and mortality evaluation after invasive coronary treatment using drug eluting stents with or without the IVUS guidance. *Randomized control trial*. HOME DES IVUS. *Catheter. Cardiovasc. Interv.* **2010**, *75*, 578–583. [CrossRef]
128. Chieffo, A.; Latib, A.; Caussin, C.; Presbitero, P.; Galli, S.; Menozzi, A.; Varbella, F.; Mauri, F.; Valgimigli, M.; Arampatzis, C.; et al. A prospective, randomized trial of intravascular-ultrasound guided compared to angiography guided stent implantation in complex coronary lesions: The AVIO trial. *Am. Heart J.* **2013**, *165*, 65–72. [CrossRef]
129. Silvain, J.; Lattuca, B.; Beygui, F.; Motovska, Z.; Dillinger, J.-G.; Boueri, Z.; Brunel, P.; Lhermusier, T.; Pouillot, C.; Larrieu-Ardilouze, E.; et al. Ticagrelor versus clopidogrel in elective percutaneous coronary intervention (ALPHEUS): A randomised, open-label, phase 3b trial. *Lancet* **2020**, *396*, 1737–1744. [CrossRef]
130. Mehilli, J.; Baquet, M.; Hochholzer, W.; Mayer, K.; Tesche, C.; Aradi, D.; Xu, Y.; Thienel, M.; Gschwendtner, S.; Zadrozny, M.; et al. Randomized Comparison of Intensified and Standard P2Y12-Receptor-Inhibition Before Elective Percutaneous Coronary Intervention: The SASSICAIA Trial. *Circ. Cardiovasc. Interv.* **2020**, *13*, e008649. [CrossRef]
131. Shepperd, S.; Lannin, N.A.; Clemson, L.M.; McCluskey, A.; Cameron, I.D.; Barras, S.L. Discharge planning from hospital to home. *Cochrane Database Syst. Rev.* **2013**. [CrossRef]
132. Lucà, F.; Oliva, F.; Rao, C.M.; Abrignani, M.G.; Amico, A.F.; Di Fusco, S.A.; Caretta, G.; Di Matteo, I.; Di Nora, C.; Pilleri, A.; et al. Management and Quality, Cronicity, Cardiovascular Prevention Working Groups of the Italian Association of Hospital Cardiologists (ANMCO). Appropriateness of Dyslipidemia Management Strategies in Post-Acute Coronary Syndrome: A 2023 Update. *Metabolites* **2023**, *13*, 916. [CrossRef] [PubMed]
133. Siniawski, D.; Masson, G.; Masson, W.; Barbagelata, L.; Destaville, J.; Lynch, S.; Vitagliano, L.; Parodi, J.B.; Berton, F.; Indavere, A.; et al. Residual cardiovascular risk, use of standard care treatments, and achievement of treatment goals in patients with cardiovascular disease. *Int. J. Cardiol. Cardiovasc. Risk Prev.* **2023**, *18*, 200198. [CrossRef] [PubMed]

Disclaimer/Publisher's Note: The statements, opinions and data contained in all publications are solely those of the individual author(s) and contributor(s) and not of MDPI and/or the editor(s). MDPI and/or the editor(s) disclaim responsibility for any injury to people or property resulting from any ideas, methods, instructions or products referred to in the content.

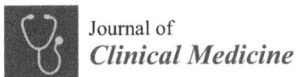 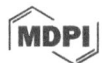

Opinion

Blood Pressure Variability as a Risk Factor for Cardiovascular Disease: Which Antihypertensive Agents Are More Effective?

Alejandro de la Sierra

Hospital Mutua Terrassa, University of Barcelona, 08221-Terrassa, Spain; adelasierra@mutuaterrassa.cat

Abstract: Blood pressure oscillations during different time scales, known as blood pressure variability (BPV), have become a focus of growing scientific interest. BPV can be measured at long-term (seasonal variability or visit-to-visit), at mid-term (differences in consecutive days or weeks) or at short-term (day-night differences or changes induced by other daily activities and conditions). An increased BPV, either at long, mid or short-term is associated with a poor cardiovascular prognosis independently of the amount of blood pressure elevation. There is scarce evidence on the effect of different antihypertensive treatments on BPV, but some observational and interventional studies suggest that calcium channel blockers in general, and particularly amlodipine, either in monotherapy or combined with renin-angiotensin system blockers, can reduce BPV more efficiently than other antihypertensive drugs or combinations. Nevertheless, there are several aspects of the relationship between BPV, antihypertensive treatment, and clinical outcomes that are still unknown, and more work should be performed before considering BPV as a therapeutical target in clinical practice.

Keywords: blood pressure variability; antihypertensive treatment; cardiovascular disease; cardiovascular risk; ambulatory blood pressure monitoring

1. Introduction

High blood pressure (BP) is one of the most powerful determinants of cardiovascular risk [1]. BP estimates, obtained punctually in the clinic or through measurements in different hours, days or weeks, are associated with the risk of cardiovascular events and mortality [2]. However, BP is not a static component, and fluctuates due to a large number of internal and external influences. Blood pressure variability (BPV) is defined as the BP variation over different time scales, ranging from beat-to-beat to years [3].

The importance of BPV is that such fluctuations are related with the development of organ damage, cardiovascular events and mortality, independently of the absolute degree of BP elevation. Such circumstances have created a great interest in the understanding of mechanisms responsible for BPV, the different types of variability and the methods of assessment, as well as possible therapeutical interventions modifying several aspects of BPV.

2. Types of Blood Pressure Variability, Physiological Regulation, and Methods of Assessment

The types of BPV, their physiological regulation, and methods of assessment depend on the time scale contemplated. It ranges from very short periods of time, such as beat-to-beat or even intra-beat variability, short-term variability, usually defined as variations occurring in a 24 h period of time, day-to-day, week-to-week, or long-term variability, including variations occurring among visits, in different seasons of the year, or even through several years [3,4].

The physiological regulation of BP variations, as well as its derangements, are complex and poorly understood. They constitute a mixture of cardiovascular regulatory mechanisms, as well as behavioral and environmental factors [4]. In addition, several treatments, and both cardiovascular drugs and non-cardiovascular drugs, influence BPV. Among the intrinsic mechanisms regulating BPV, baroreflex activity and arterial stiffness are possibly the most

---

Citation: de la Sierra, A. Blood Pressure Variability as a Risk Factor for Cardiovascular Disease: Which Antihypertensive Agents Are More Effective?. *J. Clin. Med.* **2023**, *12*, 6167. https://doi.org/10.3390/jcm12196167

Academic Editor: Anna Kabłak-Ziembicka

Received: 28 July 2023
Revised: 22 September 2023
Accepted: 22 September 2023
Published: 24 September 2023

Copyright: © 2023 by the author. Licensee MDPI, Basel, Switzerland. This article is an open access article distributed under the terms and conditions of the Creative Commons Attribution (CC BY) license (https://creativecommons.org/licenses/by/4.0/).

important. Short-term variability is highly dependent on the circadian rhythm of activity and sleep and, during sleep, is particularly affected by sleep disturbances. The adherence to antihypertensive treatment and the duration of action of different antihypertensive drugs clearly influence day-to-day, week-to-week, as well as visit-to-visit variability. Changes in weather and outdoor temperature are the main influencers of seasonal variability.

The assessment of very-short-term BPV requires continuous monitoring. This can be achieved by intra-arterial recording, or with the use of some non-invasive devices. Its use is usually restricted to monitor patients in intensive care units, emergencies or operation rooms. Continuous ambulatory non-invasive devices using finger plethysmography were developed several years ago, but were impractical for its use in ambulatory patients [5,6]. Short-term BPV is usually assessed by Ambulatory Blood Pressure Monitoring (ABPM) with oscillometric validated cuff devices, measuring BP at repeated intervals, usually from 15 to 30 min [7]. Home Blood Pressure Monitoring (HBPM) is the method of choice for assessing mid-term BPV, such as day-to-day or week-to-week changes. It is usually recommended to proceed to a 7-day period of measurement, twice per day, three repeated measurements each [8]. The results of this schedule are very close to daytime BP obtained through ABPM. Finally, office BP is usually the method of assessment of visit-to-visit variability or seasonal variability. It is necessary to strictly adhere to a protocol of measurement, which should be always the same. Minor deviations can cause important differences in BP, which are not necessarily patient-dependent [3].

3. Blood Pressure Variability Indices

The standard deviation (SD) and the coefficient of variation (the ratio between standard deviation and absolute BP value) are the most commonly used indices for all types of BPV. Variability independent of the mean has been also proposed for the assessment of visit-to-visit variability, and it is calculated by dividing SD by the mean powered to a value obtained by non-linear regression analysis of population values [9].

Several other indices are also commonly used for short-term BPV. Among them, the most important are weighted SD and average real variability (AVR). The first is obtained by the average of daytime and nighttime SD weighted for the duration of each period [10]. Its main advantage over the classic 24 h SD is that is not affected by the amount of nocturnal BP decline. ARV is obtained by calculating the average of the differences (in absolute value) between consecutive measures [11]. It better reflects within subject variability, although is more affected by poor quality of the data.

4. Prognostic Value of Blood Pressure Variability

The first and most consistent data regarding the prognostic influence of BPV refers to long-term or visit-to-visit variability. A post hoc analysis of four large clinical trials, including a large cohort of patients with a history of transient ischemic attacks (UK-TIA Aspirin Trial) and a large population of patients with hypertension and added risk factors (ASCOT-BPLA) demonstrated that intervisit BP variability and peak BP values were strong predictors of stroke independently of mean SBP and, albeit to a lesser extent, equally associated with coronary risk [12]. Since then, these findings have been reproduced in both cohort studies [13] and post hoc analyses of other clinical trials, especially in subjects at high risk for the development of cardiovascular diseases [14–16]. In contrast, other studies in hypertensive patients without added risk or in the general population have not been able to determine a significant contribution of long-term variability between visits to cardiovascular morbidity and mortality, which would suggest that the association between BP variability between visits and cardiovascular outcomes could be significantly influenced by the individual's baseline cardiovascular risk level. These discrepancies were also revealed in a meta-analysis of 23 studies in which, although the variability between visits was associated with the development of coronary and cerebrovascular events, as well as with the number of total and cardiovascular deaths, the degree of association in all cases was modest and did not exceed a 20% increase in risk [17].

Regarding mid-term BPV and cardiovascular prognosis, two population studies have confirmed the prognostic value of BP variability in the medium term. In the Ohasama study [18], increased variability values in home SBP, measured over a total of 26 days, was associated with a higher composite risk of cardiac death and stroke. Moreover, in the HOME-BP study in Finland, carried out in a cohort of adults from the general population, increased variability in systolic and diastolic BP measurements for seven consecutive days was associated with an increased risk of cardiovascular events after almost 8 years of follow-up, which remained significant even after adjusting for age and mean HT levels, thus supporting the additional value of home BP variability in predicting cardiovascular prognosis [19]. This has been recently confirmed using the multinational IDHOCO database [20]. In contrast to these results, a study with 12-year follow-up in a Belgian population did not show any predictive value for BP variability when adjusting for mean BP values [21]. However, in this latter study, BPV was estimated from only two home visits.

With regard to short-term BPV, as measured through ABPM, the relationship has been established both with the standard deviation estimators, night pressure fall and with the morning surge. An increase in the standard deviation both during the day [22] and at night [23] has been related to a worse cardiovascular prognosis in prospective studies. This relationship is even more evident when the aforementioned estimators of weighted standard deviation [24] or average real variability [25] are calculated.

The nocturnal fall in BP also has an important impact on cardiovascular prognosis. The first studies already suggested that a lack of nocturnal decrease in BP was associated with a worse cardiovascular prognosis [26]. The data from the Spanish ABPM Registry [27] have revealed that the prevalence of these "deleterious" patterns is very high, and that they are close to 50% in untreated patients and exceed this figure in those who are under treatment. Advanced age, female sex, obesity, diabetes, and a history of previous cardiovascular disease are associated with inadequate decline in both treated and untreated patients. In the former, the number of drugs also intervenes in a greater probability of presenting a "nondipper" or "riser" pattern.

The main problem in assessing the prognostic value of circadian pattern alterations is the association of both nocturnal BP fall with nocturnal BP levels, a very well known factor for a higher risk of mortality and cardiovascular events [28].

Not only the nocturnal decrease in BP, but also the increase that occurs upon awakening may be important from the prognostic point of view. Thus, in the Japanese population or those of other Asian countries, an excessive increase in the morning has been associated with a greater risk of events, especially cerebral vascular accidents of hemorrhagic etiology [29]. However, the actual prognostic significance of this morning rise remains a matter of debate, given the significant positive correlation between the degree of morning BP rise (a potentially deleterious phenomenon) and the degree of nighttime BP fall (a potentially protective phenomenon). In addition, the morning increase that occurs in Caucasian populations appears to be clearly less than that in Asian populations. In the former, when both elements are analyzed in the same group, the importance of the lack of nocturnal decrease seems to be greater than the excess of morning increase [30].

5. Blood Pressure Variability and Antihypertensive Treatment

Meta-analyses of clinical trials in hypertension with different classes of antihypertensive drugs have strongly supported that mean BP reduction is essential to achieve cardiovascular protection [31]. Moreover, it has been suggested that the reduction in long-term variability provided by some drug classes may confer additional benefits in addition to lowering mean BP levels. In support of this concept, a meta-analysis comparing the calcium antagonist amlodipine against other antihypertensives suggested a favorable impact of the former on blood pressure variability between visits [32]. In the ASCOT study, there was also a parallelism between the greater impact of amlodipine compared to atenolol on long-term variability and protection against stroke [9], although it should be recognized that other advantages of amlodipine with respect to atenolol, such as a greater impact on central BP reduction, were also present in this study [33]. This favorable effect of amlodipine on visit-to-visit variability was also observed in the SPRINT study [34], and it could possibly be related to the long half-life of this drug, of about 30 h. It has also been hypothesized that certain drug combinations might be more effective than others in reducing long-term variability. In this sense, the combination of an angiotensin receptor antagonist with a calcium antagonist was capable to promote a greater reduction in blood pressure variability between visits compared to the same receptor antagonist combined with a diuretic, regardless of the reductions in mean BP levels [35].

With respect to mid-term BPV, studies on the effect of antihypertensive treatment are few and quite inconsistent. Only one comparative study evaluating the effects of two types of antihypertensive combinations found that a combination of an angiotensin receptor antagonist with a calcium antagonist was more effective in reducing home SBP variability than the combination of the same receptor antagonist with a thiazide diuretic [36]. Finally, a non-randomized analysis of a population of diabetic subjects who received different classes of antihypertensive drugs found lower morning BP variability values in the subjects who received calcium antagonists, compared to those treated with angiotensin converting enzyme (ACE) inhibitors or angiotensin-receptor blockers (ARB) [37].

With respect to short-term BPV, again studies have shown a beneficial effect of calcium channel blockers, particularly amlodipine. The X-CELLENT study [38] showed a greater reduction in short-term variability in patients treated with amlodipine, or the diuretic indapamide in comparison to the angiotensin receptor antagonist candesartan. Another study in treated hypertensive patients showed that subjects who received calcium antagonists or diuretics, alone or associated with other groups, had significantly lower SBP standard deviations compared with those who received angiotensin-converting enzyme inhibitors, receptor antagonists or beta-blockers [39].

In the Spanish ABPM Registry, we looked at short-term BPV in a very large number of patients under different types of antihypertensive therapies, including monotherapies and different combinations [40]. A total of 38,188 patients were included. BPV indices, including daytime and nighttime SD, weighted SD and average real variability increased as the number of antihypertensive drugs increased, being statistically significant when compared the group receiving three or more drugs with those on monotherapy.

In this latter group of patients treated with monotherapy, the comparison among the major drug classes revealed lower BPV indices in those treated with calcium channel blockers or diuretics, in comparison with beta blockers, ACE inhibitors or ARB. When looking at the different compounds inside each therapeutic class, there were no differences in BPV among diuretics (hydrochlorothiazide, chlorthalidone or indapamide), while in the calcium channel blocker group, amlodipine was associated with lower values of BPV, in comparison to other dihydropyridines, diltiazem or verapamil. Finally, this favorable effect of calcium channel blockers, particularly amlodipine, was also observed in patients treated with a two-drug or a three-drug combination, with those including a calcium channel blocker being associated with lower values of BPV indices.

It has recently been suggested that new non-pharmacological treatments for resistant AHT, such as renal denervation, could have a beneficial effect on short-term variability. In this regard, in a clinical trial comparing treatment with spironolactone versus renal sympathetic denervation, the latter procedure had a greater effect on the short-term variability of diastolic pressure, measured by the 24 h weighted standard deviation or by the average real variability [41]. A recent meta-analysis has also concluded that renal denervation favorably affects short-term BPV in patients with resistant hypertension [42].

6. Clinical Significance, Practical Recommendations and Future Directions

There is considerable theoretical evidence that abnormalities in BPV are associated with the cardiovascular prognosis. However, BPV is a general term including several possible abnormalities, which in fact may have different pathogenetic mechanisms. It is difficult to admit that differences in BP among long-term visits or seasonal variations have any relation with day–night changes or other changes in shorter periods of time. They are all considered BPV, but mechanisms responsible are obviously different. Moreover, it is still a matter of debate if increased BPV is a true risk factor influencing the prognosis or merely a marker of other alterations. In addition, all the evidence regarding the impact of therapeutical maneuvers on BPV are based on post hoc analyses of clinical trials, in which the primary objective was the cardiovascular prevention through the achievement of an absolute BP reduction.

Considering these limitations, it can be hypothesized that the impact of different antihypertensive treatments, in reducing BPV in addition to their effect on absolute BP, might be an advantage in terms of protection. Results from clinical observations suggest that long-acting calcium channel blockers have an advantage over other types of drugs. However, if this advantage is related to the mechanism of action or to their pharmacokinetic properties is still unknown. New drugs under development include some possible changes in the way antihypertensive treatment is currently administered. The possibility of using drugs administered once per month or even once or twice per year will open different perspective in the assessment and the role of BPV.

Not only possible changes in antihypertensive treatment, but future changes in BP measurement and monitoring will also impact in the study of BPV. The growing use of wearable BP devices represents a unique opportunity, and may change the way BP is measured in the future. They have obvious advantages, as the possibility of monitoring BP very frequently, almost continuously, without interfering individual activities and without tolerability issues is clearly promising. These aspects are of particular relevance in the evaluation of BPV, and can serve for future studies. However, as it has been recently stated [43], the accuracy of such wearable devices has not been unequivocally demonstrated, and this is an obvious previous requirement before they can be ready for clinical use.

7. Conclusions

It is possible that the different classes of antihypertensives may have a different impact on blood pressure variability, at short, mid or long terms. If this could be translated to a greater cardiovascular protection, independently or added to the decrease in mean BP values will need specific clinical trials to be assessed. It is also possible that not only the antihypertensive drug class, through its mechanism of action, but also the pharmacokinetics of each compound would impact BPV, with drugs with longer duration of action reducing more efficiently BPV.

Funding: This research received no external funding.

Conflicts of Interest: The author declares no conflict of interest.

References

1. Zhou, B.; Perel, P.; Mensah, G.A.; Ezzati, M. Global epidemiology, health burden and effective interventions for elevated blood pressure and hypertension. *Nat. Rev. Cardiol.* **2021**, *18*, 785–802. [CrossRef] [PubMed]
2. Mancia, G.; Kreutz, R.; Brunström, M.; Burnier, M.; Grassi, G.; Januszewicz, A. 2023 ESH Guidelines for the management of arterial hypertension. *J. Hypertens.* **2023**, *online ahead of print*.
3. Parati, G.; Bilo, G.; Kollias, A.; Pengo, M.; Ochoa, J.E.; Castiglioni, P.; Stergiou, G.S.; Mancia, G.; Asayama, K.; Asmar, R.; et al. Blood pressure variability: Methodological aspects, clinical relevance and practical indications for management—A European Society of Hypertension position paper. *J. Hypertens.* **2023**, *41*, 527–544. [CrossRef] [PubMed]
4. Parati, G.; Ochoa, J.E.; Lombardi, C.; Bilo, G. Assessment and management of blood-pressure variability. *Nat. Rev. Cardiol.* **2013**, *10*, 143–155. [CrossRef] [PubMed]
5. Omboni, S.; Parati, G.; Castiglioni, P.; Di Rienzo, M.; Imholz, B.P.; Langewouters, G.J.; Wesseling, K.H.; Mancia, G. Estimation of blood pressure variability from 24-hour ambulatory finger blood pressure. *Hypertension* **1998**, *32*, 52–58. [CrossRef] [PubMed]
6. Gómez-Angelats, E.; De La Sierra, A.; Sierra, C.; Parati, G.; Mancia, G.; Coca, A. Blood pressure variability and silent cerebral damage in essential hypertension. *Am. J. Hypertens.* **2004**, *17*, 696–700. [CrossRef]
7. O'Brien, E.; Parati, G.; Stergiou, G.; Asmar, R.; Beilin, L.; Bilo, G.; Clement, D.; De La Sierra, A.; De Leeuw, P.; Dolan, E.; et al. European Society of Hypertension position paper on ambulatory blood pressure monitoring. *J. Hypertens.* **2013**, *31*, 1731–1768. [CrossRef]

8. Parati, G.; Stergiou, G.S.; Bilo, G.; Kollias, A.; Pengo, M.; Ochoa, J.E.; Agarwal, R.; Asayama, K.; Asmar, R.; Burnier, M.; et al. Home blood pressure monitoring: Methodology, clinical relevance and practical application: A 2021 position paper by the Working Group on Blood Pressure Monitoring and Cardiovascular Variability of the European Society of Hypertension. *J. Hypertens.* **2021**, *39*, 1742–1767. [CrossRef]
9. Rothwell, P.M.; Howard, S.C.; Dolan, E.; O'Brien, E.; Dobson, J.E.; Dahlöf, B.; Poulter, N.R.; Sever, P.S. Effects of beta blockers and calcium-channel blockers on within-individual variability in blood pressure and risk of stroke. *Lancet Neurol.* **2010**, *9*, 469–480. [CrossRef]
10. Bilo, G.; Giglio, A.; Styczkiewicz, K.; Caldara, G.; Maronati, A.; Kawecka-Jaszcz, K.; Mancia, G.; Parati, G. A new method for assessing 24-h blood pressure variability after excluding the contribution of nocturnal blood pressure fall. *J. Hypertens.* **2007**, *25*, 2058–2066. [CrossRef]
11. Mena, L.; Pintos, S.; Queipo, N.V.; Aizpúrua, J.A.; Maestre, G.; Sulbarán, T. A reliable index for the prognostic significance of blood pressure variability. *J. Hypertens.* **2005**, *23*, 505–511. [CrossRef] [PubMed]
12. Rothwell, P.M.; Howard, S.C.; Dolan, E.; O'Brien, E.; Dobson, J.E.; Dahlöf, B.; Sever, P.S.; Poulter, N.R. Prognostic significance of visit-to-visit variability, maximum systolic blood pressure, and episodic hypertension. *Lancet* **2010**, *375*, 895–905. [CrossRef] [PubMed]
13. Shimbo, D.; Newman, J.D.; Aragaki, A.K.; LaMonte, M.J.; Bavry, A.A.; Allison, M.; Manson, J.E.; Wassertheil-Smoller, S. Association between annual visit-to-visit blood pressure variability and stroke in postmenopausal women: Data from the Women's Health Initiative. *Hypertension* **2012**, *60*, 625–630. [CrossRef] [PubMed]
14. Chowdhury, E.K.; Owen, A.; Krum, H.; Wing, L.M.; Nelson, M.R.; Reid, C.M. Second Australian National Blood Pressure Study Management Committee. Systolic blood pressure variability is an important predictor of cardiovascular outcomes in elderly hypertensive patients. *J. Hypertens.* **2014**, *32*, 525–533. [CrossRef]
15. Muntner, P.; Whittle, J.; Lynch, A.I.; Colantonio, L.D.; Simpson, L.M.; Einhorn, P.T.; Levitan, E.B.; Whelton, P.K.; Cushman, W.C.; Louis, G.T.; et al. Visit-to-visit variability of blood pressure and coronary heart disease, stroke, heart failure, and mortality: A cohort study. *Ann. Intern. Med.* **2015**, *163*, 329–338. [CrossRef]
16. Ohkuma, T.; Woodward, M.; Jun, M.; Muntner, P.; Hata, J.; Colagiuri, S.; Harrap, S.; Mancia, G.; Poulter, N.; Williams, B.; et al. ADVANCE Collaborative Group. Prognostic value of variability in systolic blood pressure related to vascular events and premature death in type 2 diabetes mellitus: The ADVANCE-ON Study. *Hypertension* **2017**, *70*, 461–468. [CrossRef]
17. Wang, J.; Shi, X.; Ma, C.; Zheng, H.; Xiao, J.; Bian, H.; Ma, Z.; Gong, L. Visit-to-visit blood pressure variability is a risk factor for all-cause mortality and cardiovascular disease: A systematic review and meta-analysis. *J. Hypertens.* **2017**, *35*, 10–17. [CrossRef]
18. Kikuya, M.; Ohkubo, T.; Metoki, H.; Asayama, K.; Hara, A.; Obara, T.; Inoue, R.; Hoshi, H.; Hashimoto, J.; Totsune, K.; et al. Day-by-day variability of blood pressure and heart rate at home as a novel predictor of prognosis: The Ohasama study. *Hypertension* **2008**, *52*, 1045–1050. [CrossRef]
19. Johansson, J.K.; Niiranen, T.J.; Puukka, P.J.; Jula, A.M. Prognostic value of the variability in home-measured blood pressure and heart rate: The Finn-Home Study. *Hypertension* **2012**, *59*, 212–218. [CrossRef]
20. Juhanoja, E.P.; Niiranen, T.J.; Johansson, J.K.; Puukka, P.J.; Thijs, L.; Asayama, K.; Langén, V.L.; Hozawa, A.; Aparicio, L.S.; Ohkubo, T.; et al. Outcome-driven thresholds for increased home blood pressure variability. *Hypertension* **2017**, *69*, 599–607. [CrossRef]
21. Schutte, R.; Thijs, L.; Liu, Y.P.; Asayama, K.; Jin, Y.; Odili, A.; Gu, Y.M.; Kuznetsova, T.; Jacobs, L.; Staessen, J.A. Within-subject blood pressure level—Not variability—Predicts fatal and nonfatal outcomes in a general population. *Hypertension* **2012**, *60*, 1138–1147. [CrossRef] [PubMed]
22. Bilo, G.; Dolan, E.; O'Brien, E.; Facchetti, R.; Soranna, D.; Zambon, A.; Mancia, G.; Parati, G. The impact of systolic and diastolic blood pressure variability on mortality is age dependent: Data from the Dublin Outcome Study. *Eur. J. Prev. Cardiol.* **2020**, *27*, 355–364. [CrossRef] [PubMed]
23. Palatini, P.; Reboldi, G.; Beilin, L.J.; Casiglia, E.; Eguchi, K.; Imai, Y.; Kario, K.; Ohkubo, T.; Pierdomenico, S.D.; Schwartz, J.E.; et al. Added predictive value of night-time blood pressure variability for cardiovascular events and mortality: The Ambulatory Blood Pressure-International Study. *Hypertension* **2014**, *64*, 487–493. [CrossRef] [PubMed]
24. Stevens, S.L.; Wood, S.; Koshiaris, C.; Law, K.; Glasziou, P.; Stevens, R.J.; McManus, R.J. Blood pressure variability and cardiovascular disease: Systematic review and meta-analysis. *BMJ* **2016**, *354*, i4098. [CrossRef] [PubMed]
25. Hansen, T.W.; Thijs, L.; Li, Y.; Boggia, J.; Kikuya, M.; Björklund-Bodegård, K.; Richart, T.; Ohkubo, T.; Jeppesen, J.; Torp-Pedersen, C.; et al. Prognostic value of reading-to-reading blood pressure variability over 24 hours in 8938 subjects from 11 populations. *Hypertension* **2010**, *55*, 1049–1057. [CrossRef]
26. O'Brien, E.; Sheridan, J.; O'Malley, K. Dippers and non-dippers. *Lancet* **1988**, *2*, 397. [CrossRef]
27. De La Sierra, A.; Redon, J.; Banegas, J.R.; Segura, J.; Parati, G.; Gorostidi, M.; de la Cruz, J.J.; Sobrino, J.; Llisterri, J.L.; Alonso, J.; et al. Prevalence and factors associated with circadian blood pressure patterns in hypertensive patients. *Hypertension* **2009**, *53*, 466–472. [CrossRef]
28. Banegas, J.R.; Ruilope, L.M.; de la Sierra, A.; Vinyoles, E.; Gorostidi, M.; de la Cruz, J.J.; Ruiz-Hurtado, G.; Segura, J.; Rodríguez-Artalejo, F.; Williams, B. Relationship between clinic and ambulatory blood pressure and mortality. An observational cohort study in 59,124 patients. *Lancet* **2023**, *401*, 2041–2050.

29. Kario, K.; Pickering, T.G.; Umeda, Y.; Hoshide, S.; Hoshide, Y.; Morinari, M.; Murata, M.; Kuroda, T.; Schwartz, J.E.; Shimada, K. Morning surge in blood pressure as a predictor of silent and clinical cerebrovascular disease in elderly hypertensives: A prospective study. *Circulation* **2003**, *107*, 1401–1406. [CrossRef]
30. Hoshide, S.; Kario, K.; de la Sierra, A.; Bilo, G.; Schillaci, G.; Banegas, J.R.; Gorostidi, M.; Segura, J.; Lombardi, C.; Omboni, S.; et al. Ethnic differences in the degree of morning blood pressure surge and in its determinants between Japanese and European hypertensive subjects: Data from the ARTEMIS study. *Hypertension* **2015**, *66*, 750–756. [CrossRef]
31. Ettehad, D.; Emdin, C.A.; Kiran, A.; Anderson, S.G.; Callender, T.; Emberson, J.; Chalmers, J.; Rodgers, A.; Rahimi, K. Blood pressure lowering for prevention of cardiovascular disease and death: A systematic review and meta-analysis. *Lancet* **2016**, *387*, 957–967. [CrossRef] [PubMed]
32. Wang, J.G.; Yan, P.; Jeffers, B.W. Effects of amlodipine and other classes of antihypertensive drugs on long-term blood pressure variability: Evidence from randomized controlled trials. *J. Am. Soc. Hypertens.* **2014**, *8*, 340–349. [CrossRef] [PubMed]
33. Williams, B.; Lacy, P.S.; Thom, S.M.; Cruickshank, K.; Stanton, A.; Collier, D.; Hughes, A.D.; Thurston, H.; O'Rourke, M. Differential impact of blood pressure-lowering drugs on central aortic pressure and clinical outcomes: Principal results of the Conduit Artery Function Evaluation (CAFE) study. *Circulation* **2006**, *113*, 1213–1225. [CrossRef] [PubMed]
34. De Havenon, A.; Petersen, N.; Wolcott, Z.; Goldstein, E.; Delic, A.; Sheibani, N.; Anadani, M.; Sheth, K.N.; Lansberg, M.; Turan, T.; et al. Effect of dihydropyridine calcium channel blockers on blood pressure variability in the SPRINT trial: A treatment effects approach. *J. Hypertens.* **2022**, *40*, 462–469. [CrossRef]
35. Sato, N.; Saijo, Y.; Sasagawa, Y.; Morimoto, H.; Takeuchi, T.; Sano, H.; Koyama, S.; Takehara, N.; Morita, K.; Sumitomo, K.; et al. Visit-to-visit variability and seasonal variation in blood pressure: Combination of Antihypertensive Therapy in the Elderly, Multicenter Investigation (CAMUI) Trial subanalysis. *Clin. Exp. Hypertens.* **2015**, *37*, 411–419. [CrossRef]
36. Matsui, Y.; O'Rourke, M.F.; Hoshide, S.; Ishikawa, J.; Shimada, K.; Kario, K. Combined effect of angiotensin II receptor blocker and either a calcium channel blocker or diuretic on day-by-day variability of home blood pressure: The Japan Combined Treatment with Olmesartan and a Calcium-Channel Blocker Versus Olmesartan and Diuretics Randomized Efficacy Study. *Hypertension* **2012**, *59*, 1132–1138.
37. Ushigome, E.; Fukui, M.; Hamaguchi, M.; Tanaka, T.; Atsuta, H.; Ohnishi, M.; Oda, Y.; Yamazaki, M.; Hasegawa, G.; Nakamura, N. Beneficial effect of calcium channel blockers on home blood pressure variability in the morning in patients with type 2 diabetes. *J. Diabetes Investig.* **2013**, *8*, 399–404. [CrossRef]
38. Zhang, Y.; Agnoletti, D.; Safar, M.E.; Blacher, J. Effect of antihypertensive agents on blood pressure variability: The Natrilix SR versus candesartan and amlodipine in the reduction of systolic blood pressure in hypertensive patients (X-CELLENT) study. *Hypertension* **2011**, *58*, 155–160. [CrossRef]
39. Levi-Marpillat, N.; Macquin-Mavier, I.; Tropeano, A.I.; Parati, G.; Maison, P. Antihypertensive drug classes have different effects on short-term blood pressure variability in essential hypertension. *Hypertens. Res.* **2014**, *37*, 585–590. [CrossRef]
40. De la Sierra, A.; Mateu, A.; Gorostidi, M.; Vinyoles, E.; Segura, J.; Ruilope, L.M. Antihypertensive therapy and short-term blood pressure variability. *J. Hypertens.* **2021**, *39*, 349–355. [CrossRef]
41. De La Sierra, A.; Pareja, J.; Armario, P.; Barrera, Á.; Yun, S.; Vázquez, S.; Sans, L.; Pascual, J.; Oliveras, A. Renal Denervation vs. Spironolactone in Resistant Hypertension: Effects on Circadian Patterns and Blood Pressure Variability. *Am. J. Hypertens.* **2017**, *30*, 37–41. [CrossRef] [PubMed]
42. Persu, A.; Gordin, D.; Jacobs, L.; Thijs, L.; Bots, M.L.; Spiering, W.; Miroslawska, A.; Spaak, J.; Rosa, J.; De Jong, M.R.; et al. Blood pressure response to renal denervation is correlated with baseline blood pressure variability: A patient-level meta-analysis. *J. Hypertens.* **2018**, *36*, 221–229. [CrossRef] [PubMed]
43. Stergiou, G.S.; Avolio, A.P.; Palatini, P.; Kyriakoulis, K.G.; Schutte, A.E.; Mieke, S.; Kollias, A.; Parati, G.; Asmar, R.; Pantazis, N.; et al. European Society of Hypertension recommendations for the validation of cuffless blood pressure measuring devices: European Society of Hypertension Working Group on Blood Pressure Monitoring and Cardiovascular Variability. *J. Hypertens.* **2022**, *40*, 1449–1460. [CrossRef] [PubMed]

Disclaimer/Publisher's Note: The statements, opinions and data contained in all publications are solely those of the individual author(s) and contributor(s) and not of MDPI and/or the editor(s). MDPI and/or the editor(s) disclaim responsibility for any injury to people or property resulting from any ideas, methods, instructions or products referred to in the content.

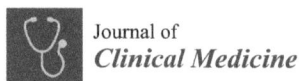 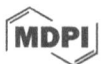

Review

Polypill Therapy for Cardiovascular Disease Prevention and Combination Medication Therapy for Hypertension Management

Keisuke Narita, Satoshi Hoshide and Kazuomi Kario *

Division of Cardiovascular Medicine, Department of Internal Medicine, Jichi Medical University School of Medicine, Shimotsuke 329-0498, Japan
* Correspondence: kkario@jichi.ac.jp

Abstract: Although various guidelines for cardiovascular disease prevention have been established, the optimal drug therapy is often not implemented due to poor medication adherence and the clinical inertia of healthcare practitioners. Polypill strategies are one solution to this problem. Previous studies have established the usefulness of polypills, i.e., combination tablets including three or more medications, for the prevention of cardiovascular disease. For this purpose, the polypills generally contain an antiplatelet medication, an antihypertensive medication, and a statin. For the specific management of hypertension, combination therapy including more than two classes of antihypertensive medications is recommended by most international guidelines. Combination tablets including two classes of antihypertensive medications, such as renin-angiotensin system (RAS) inhibitors (angiotensin-converting enzyme inhibitors [ACEIs] and angiotensin receptor blockers [ARBs]) and Ca-channel blockers or thiazide diuretics, have been reported to be useful for cardiovascular disease prevention and lowering blood pressure (BP) levels. The use of RAS inhibitors is recommended for a wide range of complications, including diabetes, chronic heart failure, and chronic kidney disease. The combination of an RAS inhibitor and diuretic or Ca-channel blocker is thus recommended for the management of hypertension. Finally, we expect that novel medications such as angiotensin receptor neprilysin inhibitors (ARNIs) and sodium glucose cotransporter 2 inhibitors (SGLT2i), which have a more diverse range of effects in hypertension, heart failure, or diabetes, may be a solution to the problem of polypharmacy. Evidence is accumulating on the benefits of polypill strategies in cardiovascular disease prevention. Combination tablets are also effective for the treatment of hypertension.

Keywords: polypill strategy; combination medication therapy; cardiovascular prevention; blood pressure; hypertension

Citation: Narita, K.; Hoshide, S.; Kario, K. Polypill Therapy for Cardiovascular Disease Prevention and Combination Medication Therapy for Hypertension Management. *J. Clin. Med.* **2023**, *12*, 7226. https://doi.org/10.3390/jcm12237226

Academic Editor: Carlos Escobar

Received: 10 October 2023
Revised: 17 November 2023
Accepted: 17 November 2023
Published: 22 November 2023

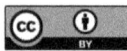

Copyright: © 2023 by the authors. Licensee MDPI, Basel, Switzerland. This article is an open access article distributed under the terms and conditions of the Creative Commons Attribution (CC BY) license (https://creativecommons.org/licenses/by/4.0/).

1. Introduction

Cardiovascular disease (CVD) is one of the most common causes of disability and death worldwide. Many guidelines for the prevention of CVD have been established in Asia, Europe, and the United States. However, the optimal drug therapy recommended in the guidelines is not being implemented in all patients due to poor adherence to treatment medications and a lack of prescribing due to clinical inertia in healthcare practitioners [1–4].

One major obstacle to the implementation of optimal therapy is poor medication compliance, and one major reason for poor medication compliance is the number of pills in the therapeutic regimen. In the case of CVD, complications that place patients at high risk include hypertension, diabetes, and dyslipidemia, and these diseases often co-occur and require multidrug therapy. Combination pills, which combine two or more drugs into a single pill, are a possible solution to this problem [3,5,6].

In the field of hypertension management, a substantial population of untreated hypertensive patients exists not only in Japan but also in other developed countries, including the United States and Europe. Moreover, the persistently low success rate in reaching treatment objectives poses a significant challenge in hypertension management. The Japanese Hypertension Guidelines refer to this issue as the "hypertension paradox" and view it as a concern, despite the relatively straightforward diagnostic methods available for hypertension, such as blood pressure measurement, and the availability of numerous highly effective antihypertensive medications [2]. Poor medication adherence and healthcare provider inertia are frequently cited as reasons for the suboptimal achievement of target BP levels in the treatment of hypertension. Utilizing combination tablets for hypertension therapy could potentially offer a viable solution to address these challenges.

In this review, the usefulness of polypills in CVD prevention and medication adherence is presented. We also present the evidence and our opinion on the usefulness of the combination therapy of antihypertensive medications in the management of hypertension.

2. Polypill Strategies for the Cardiovascular Disease Prevention

Several previous studies have established the usefulness of polypill treatment for the prevention of CVD [5–11]. With regard to the benefit of combination therapy with aspirin, statins and antihypertensives, polypills have been shown to be more effective than usual care. [12,13]. Table 1 shows a summary of the major clinical trials designed to assess the effect of polypill strategies for medication adherence and the prevention of CVD events. In terms of the effects of polypills on the primary and secondary prevention of CVD, Huffman et al. summarized 13 polypill trials and concluded that polypill therapy could be one of the most scalable strategies to reduce the risk of premature cardiac death, resulting in a 25% reduction in premature cardiac death by 2025 through an improvement in medication adherence and access [8]. The recent PolyIran study, a pragmatic, cluster-randomized trial conducted as part of the Golestan Cohort Study, found that polypills that included aspirin, atorvastatin, hydrochlorothiazide, and either enalapril or valsartan were useful for achieving the high adherence of medications and noted a reduction in the risk of major CVD events compared to those of patients receiving minimal care (HR 0.66, 95% CI 0.55–0.80) [9]. Merat et al. conducted a randomized controlled trial as a sub-study of the PolyIran-Liver trial in order to assess the effects of polypills including an angiotensin receptor blocker (ARB), a thiazide diuretic, a statin, and aspirin in patients with non-alcoholic steatohepatitis, and they demonstrated that the polypill is more useful for the prevention of CVD events compared to multiple tablets administered separately [14].

Table 1. Major clinical trials designed to compare between polypill and usual care (multiple tablets administered separately) for medication adherence and cardiovascular outcome.

Trial	Year	Confirmation of Polypill	Primary or Secondary Prevention	Number of Patients	Findings
CRUCIAL	2011	amlodipine, atorvastatin	-	1461	Lower BP and cholesterol with polypill than usual care (UC). Framingham 10-year CHD risk 13% with polypill vs. 16% in usual care.
UMPIRE	2013	aspirin, simvastatin, lisinopril, atenolol or hydrochlorothiazide	Primary and secondary	2004	Lower BP and cholesterol with polypill than UC. There is no difference in major CVD events at median 15 mo. follow-up: 50 (5%) with polypill vs. 35 (3.5%) in UC, RR 1.45, 95%CI 0.94–2.29, $p = 0.09$ (NS)
IMPACT	2014	aspirin, simvastatin, lisinopril, atenolol or hydrochlorothiazide	Primary and secondary	513	Improved adherence with polypill. No difference in BP and LDL-cholesterol between polypill and UC. There is no difference major CVD events at 12 mo. follow-up: 16 with polypill vs. 18 in UC, $p = 0.73$ (NS)
Kanyini GAP	2014	aspirin, simvastatin, lisinopril, atenolol or hydrochlorothiazide	Primary and secondary	623	Improved adherence with polypill. No difference in BP and LDL-cholesterol between polypill and UC.
FOCUS	2014	aspirin, simvastatin. ramipril	Secondary	2118	Improved adherence with polypill. No difference in BP and LDL-cholesterol between polypill and UC
SPACE	2016	aspirin, simvastatin, lisinopril, atenolol or hydrochlorothiazide	Primary and secondary	3140	Combination of three trials (UMPIRE, Kyayini GAP, and IMPACT) for polypill. Improved adherence with polypill. Lower BP and cholesterol with polypill than UC.
PolyIran	2022	aspirin, atorvastatin, hydrochlorothiazide, enalapril or valsartan	Primary and secondary	6838	Polypill is associated with reduced major CVD events at 60 mo. follow-up: 202 (5.9%) with polypill vs. 301 (8.8%) in UC, HR 0.66, 95%CI 0.55–0.80. Improved adherence with polypill.
SECURE	2022	aspirin, ramipril, atorvastatin	Secondary	2499	Polypill is associated with reduced major CVD events at 36 mo. follow-up: 118 (9.5%) with polypill vs. 156 (12.7%) in UC, HR 0.76, 95%CI 0.60–0.96, $p = 0.02$.

CRUCIAL, Cluster Randomized Usual Care vs. Caduet Investigation Assessing Long-Term-Risk; FOCUS, Fixed-Dose Combination Drug for Secondary Cardiovascular Prevention; IMPACT, IMProving Adherence using Combination Therapy; Kanyini GAP, Kanyini Guidelines Adherence to Polypill; SECURE, Secondary Prevention of Cardiovascular Disease in Elderly; SPACE, Single Pill to Avert Cardiovascular Events; UMPIRE, Use of a Multidrug Pill in Reducing Cardiovascular Events.

Previous studies have suggested the benefit of including aspirin in polypill therapy. Yusuf et al. examined the effect of adding aspirin to polypill therapy on the prevention of cardiovascular events in patients without cardiovascular disease by using a two-by-two-by-two factorial design that included a double placebo, aspirin, a polypill (simvastatin, atenolol, hydrochlorothiazide, and ramipril), and a polypill-plus-aspirin. In participants without cardiovascular disease and at intermediate risk for cardiovascular disease, the polypill-plus-aspirin therapy reduced the incidence of cardiovascular events compared with the double placebo group [15]. Moreover, Joseph et al. conducted an individual patient-level meta-analysis of three large, controlled trials (TIPS-3, HOPE-3, and PolyIran: n = 18,162). With a median follow-up of 5 years, a primary outcome benefit, including cardiovascular death, myocardial infarction, and stroke, of the polypill strategy was observed (HR: 0.62). Sub-analysis with and without aspirin showed a greater risk reduction with the aspirin-containing strategy [16]. From these findings, the polypill strategy is useful for the prevention of CVD incidence [17–19]. Secondarily, these combination drugs used for the secondary prevention of CVD also include beta-blockers such as atenolol, metoprolol, and others [15,20]. Although beta-blockers are useful in the secondary prevention of coronary artery disease and the treatment of heart failure and have cardiovascular protective effects, adverse effects such as bradycardia and syncope should be considered [21].

2.1. Polypill Therapy for Secondary Prevention of Cardiovascular Disease

To assess the usefulness of polypills for the secondary prevention of CVD, the randomized controlled Secondary Prevention of Cardiovascular Disease in Elderly (SECURE) trial was conducted in 2499 patients in Europe. This study demonstrated that a polypill including an angiotensin-converting enzyme inhibitor (ACEI), a statin, and aspirin significantly improved CVD outcomes compared to the usual care (HR 0.76, 95% CI 0.60–0.96 for composite CVD events including CVD death) [10]. In terms of the secondary prevention of CVD, polypill treatment is acceptable for use in clinical practice. In addition, studies of polypill treatment strategies for acute coronary syndromes have recently been underway. These studies have employed polypill therapy, i.e., combination tablets, containing antiplatelet agents and statins. It is anticipated that evidence will continue to accumulate regarding the utility of polypills in the treatment of acute coronary syndromes.

2.2. Polypill Therapy and Medication Adherence

Many previous studies have established evidence regarding the usefulness of the polypill strategy for the improvement of medication adherence [9,22–25]. In the Use of a Multidrug Pill in Reducing Cardiovascular Events (UMPIRE) trial, a randomized control trial designed to assess the effectiveness of fixed-dose combinations (polypills), combination drug treatment was shown to achieve greater reductions in BP, cholesterol, and platelet control compared to multiple tablets administered separately [22]. In addition, many healthcare providers consider the polypill beneficial in terms of improving patient adherence and reducing drug costs [26–29]. A polypill strategy is also important for preventing CVD events in low-to-medium-income countries and communities [30]. Polypill treatments were reported to realize greater reductions in systolic blood pressure (BP) and LDL cholesterol levels than the usual care in a socioeconomically vulnerable minority population in the United States. Muñoz, et al. conducted an interventional trial to assess the efficacy of a polypill (atorvastatin, amlodipine, losartan, and hydrochlorothiazide) treatment group compared to a usual treatment group in 303 patients in low-income regions [31]. From these results of previous studies, polypill therapy is useful in reducing the costs of treatment and preventing primary and secondary CVD events in lower- or middle-income regions.

3. Combination Therapy of Antihypertensive Medications in the Management of Hypertension

Compared to monotherapy, combination tablets have gained rapid popularity in recent years due to their superior antihypertensive effects, improved patient adherence, and health economic benefits. Furthermore, not only are combination tablets of antihypertensive drugs utilized but combination formulations with diabetes drugs and other types of medications are also employed in clinical practice. Hypertensive patients often present with additional cardiovascular risk factors, including a history of cardiovascular disease, lipid abnormalities, diabetes, and obesity. In these cases, the number and variety of oral medications can be substantial, resulting in challenges related to reduced patient adherence and increased healthcare costs. Combination tablets of antihypertensive drugs are expected to offer a solution to these issues. Most international guidelines for the management of hypertension recommend a combination therapy of renin-angiotensin system (RAS) inhibitors (ACEIs and ARBs), Ca-channel blockers, and diuretics [2,32,33]. The World Health Organization (WHO) guideline for the pharmacological treatment of hypertension recommends combination therapy chosen from the above-mentioned three classes of antihypertensive medications, such as thiazide diuretics, ACEIs/ARBs, and Ca-channel blockers [34]. In this WHO guideline, it is mentioned that combination medication therapy may be especially valuable when the baseline BP is more than SBP 20 mmHg higher than the target BP level, and single-pill combination therapy improves medication-taking adherence and persistence and BP control [34].

Many interventional trials have provided evidence of the usefulness of combination therapy with antihypertensive medications for lowering BP levels and preventing CVD events. The combination of RAS inhibitors (ACEIs or ARBs) and diuretics has been shown to be useful for preventing CVD events in randomized control trials [35]. In the ADVANCE trial, Patel, et al. demonstrated that a fixed combination of ACEI (perindopril) and thiazide diuretic (indapamide) treatment reduced major cardiovascular events by 9% compared to placebo (HR 0.91, 95% CI 0.83–1.00, $p = 0.04$) [36]. In addition, the combination of RAS inhibitors and Ca-channel blockers was also reported to be useful for the prevention of CVD [37–39]. Based on the findings from these studies, RAS inhibitors (ACEIs or ARBs) and diuretics or Ca-channel blockers are a reasonable choice for a combination of antihypertensive medications. European guidelines also recommend this combination [33]. RAS inhibitors are recommended for use in a wide range of diseases, such as diabetes, left ventricular hypertrophy, chronic heart failure, and chronic kidney disease. There are some advantages to using RAS inhibitors with diuretics, such as a decreased risk of diuretic-induced hypokalemia. However, side effects and patient tolerability should be noted.

Recently, a polypill strategy using a quad-pill including an RAS inhibitor, a Ca-channel blocker, a diuretic, and a beta-blocker has been reported. Chow et al. conducted an interventional trial to assess the effect of a quad-pill containing irbesartan, amlodipine, indapamide, and bisoprolol for lowering BP and observed significantly better BP control in the quad-pill group compared to the monotherapy group (relative risk 1.30, 95% CI 1.15–1.47), with no difference in adverse events between the two groups [20].

The WHO guidelines emphasize the significance of treating hypertension in developing countries and non-urban areas characterized by remote and impoverished economic conditions [40]. The polypill treatment strategy has proven to be effective in cardiovascular prevention within regions marked by economic hardship, particularly in terms of improving drug adherence. Similarly, a two-drug combination for hypertension treatment may offer benefits in regions with limited economic resources and low health literacy.

4. Combination Therapy of Renin-Angiotensin System (RAS) Inhibitors and Ca-Channel Blockers or Thiazide Diuretics

RAS inhibitors (ACEIs or ARBs), along with diuretics or calcium channel blockers, constitute a rational choice for a combination of antihypertensive medications. European guidelines also advocate for this particular combination [33]. RAS inhibitors are recommended for application in a broad spectrum of conditions including diabetes, left ventricular hypertrophy, chronic heart failure, and chronic kidney disease, further emphasizing their versatility in the management of hypertension. Figure 1 shows recommendation of antihypertensive medications for each comorbidity. Subsequently, many studies assessing the effectiveness of combination therapy of antihypertensive medications have not incorporated out-of-office blood pressure measurements, such as ambulatory BP monitoring (ABPM) and home BP monitoring, in their evaluation of BP control. These out-of-office BP measurements including ABPM and home BP monitoring have been recognized as more valuable than office BP measurements for stratifying cardiovascular risk and are recommended in clinical guidelines [2,32,33]. Therefore, the evaluation of combination therapy with antihypertensive drugs should also include an assessment of their antihypertensive efficacy using out-of-office BP measurements.

The usefulness of combination tablets including RAS inhibitors and diuretics or Ca-channel blockers has been reported (Figure 2) [33,41,42]. It has been reported that the standard-dose combination of ARB and Ca-channel blockers is superior to high-dose Ca-channel blocker monotherapy for lowering BP and reducing adverse events in hypertensive patients [43]. Moreover, Filipova et al. have reported that the combination tablet of ARB and hydrochlorothiazide showed a greater reduction in BP compared with ARB in a meta-analysis [44]. In the J-CORE study, it has been reported that a combination tablet containing the ARB olmesartan and the Ca-channel blocker azelnidipine has achieved a greater reduction in central BP and measured pulse wave velocity (PWV) compared to olmesartan and hydrochlorothiazide tablets. In addition, the same study has reported that the olmesartan and azelnidipine combination tablet has also achieved a greater reduction in home BP variability compared to the olmesartan and hydrochlorothiazide combination tablet [45]. On the other hand, olmesartan and hydrochlorothiazide tablets reduced nighttime BP and albuminuria more strongly than the olmesartan and azelnidipine combination tablet [46]. Nighttime BP is related to hypertensive target organ damage such as renal dysfunction and is an important treatment target in the management of hypertension since it is a better predictor of CVD compared to daytime BP [47]. In addition, it has been reported that for patients with poorly controlled BP on ARBs, the addition of mineralocorticoid receptor antagonist (MRA) (eplerenone) significantly reduced nighttime BP levels [48]. Previous studies have suggested that the combination therapy of RAS inhibitors (ACEIs or ARBs) and Ca-channel blockers or diuretics may be useful for lowering BP levels and conferring protection against hypertensive organ damage. A recent meta-analysis has reported that combination tablets of ARBs and Ca-channel blockers show superior cardiovascular disease prevention compared with combination tablets of ARBs and diuretics [49]. However, more evidence needs to be accumulated through new intervention studies. Internists should use a combination tablet of an ARB and Ca-channel blockers or a combination tablet of an ARB and diuretics, depending on the individual pathological condition of the hypertensive patient. Combination therapy with RAS inhibitors as the main axis and CCB or diuretics added as recommended in the guidelines is a reasonable choice for hypertension management [42].

	RAS inhibitors		CCB	Diuretics	Beta-blockers	MRA	Note
	ARB	ACEI					
Resistant HT							MRA is recommended for resistant HT.
CAD, angina							
CAD, post-MI							Polypill containing an ACEI, beta-blocker, statin, and aspirin is available for secondary prevention of MI
Heart Failure							MRA and SGLT2i are also recommended for patients with HFrEF
LVH							
Diabetes							RAS inhibitors are recommended for diabetes or CKD with albuminuria
CKD							
COPD or asthma							Beta-1 selective blockers are available in patients with COPD (beta-blockers are contraindicated in patients with asthma) ACEIs are not recommended for patients with asthma because of cough.

Figure 1. Strategy for combination therapy of antihypertensive medications. The international guidelines recommend the combination: renin angiotensin system (RAS) inhibitors and Ca-channel blockers or diuretics. RAS inhibitors are recommended for use in a wide range of conditions, such as diabetes, left ventricular hypertrophy, chronic heart failure, and chronic kidney disease. Red colour, highly recommended; Beige colour, recommended.

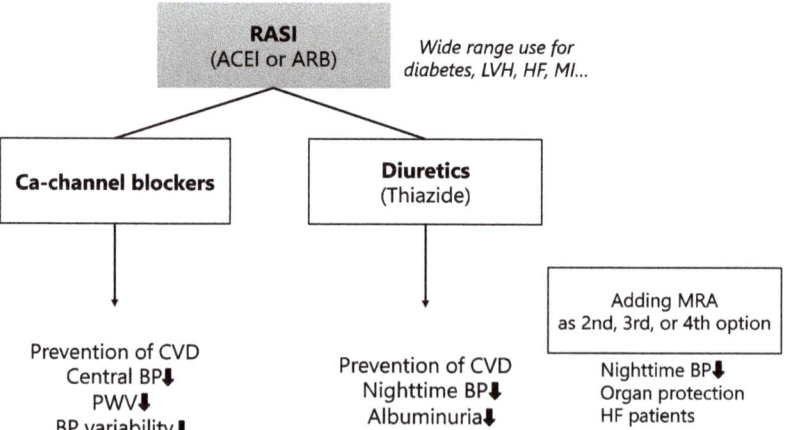

Figure 2. Strategy for combination therapy of antihypertensive medications. The international guidelines recommend the combination: renin angiotensin system (RAS) inhibitors and Ca-channel blockers or diuretics. RAS inhibitors are recommended for use in a wide range of conditions, such as diabetes, left ventricular hypertrophy, chronic heart failure, and chronic kidney disease.

5. Novel Medications with Diverse Effects

The goal of polypill therapy is to improve medication adherence and quality of treatment by reducing the number of tablets. In recent years, novel medications have become available that exert more effects via a single tablet compared to conventional medications for the treatment of hypertension, heart failure, or diabetes. Angiotensin receptor neprilysin inhibitor (ARNI) and sodium glucose cotransporter 2 inhibitor (SGLT2i) are two promising examples [50–53]. These drugs have the potential to combine the effects of two drugs into a single drug and may be a solution to the problem of polypharmacy in recent clinical practice.

5.1. Angiotensin Receptor Neprilysin Inhibitors (ARNI)

ARNI was developed primarily for the treatment of heart failure and is applied for the treatment of heart failure in Europe and the U.S. and the treatment of hypertension in Japan. ARNI has (1) an inhibitory effect on angiotensin and (2) an inhibitory effect on neprilysin, which is the enzyme that degrades b-type natriuretic peptide (BNP). Thus, ARNI has been reported to have a variety of effects, such as suppressing excessive sympathetic nerve activity and vasoconstriction and decreasing fluid retention. These multiple effects of ARNI are useful in the pathogenesis of nocturnal hypertension, structural hypertension, and treatment-resistant hypertension (Figure 3). ARNI is useful in hypertensive organ disorders, including hypertensive heart disease [50]. Previous studies have documented the antihypertensive effects of ARNI. In an evaluation using ABPM, ARNI has also been reported to lower BP consistently over a 24 h period, during the daytime as well as the nighttime [51]. Moreover, ARNI (sacubitril/valsartan) has demonstrated superiority over ARB (valsartan) in reducing BP among patients with treatment-resistant hypertension. The reduction in systolic BP at week 16 was greater with sacubitril-valsartan vs. valsartan in patients with treatment-resistant hypertension (3.9 [−6.6 to −1.3] mmHg) and apparent MRA-resistant hypertension (−6.3 [−12.5 to −0.1] mmHg) [52].

5.2. Sodium Glucose Cotransporter 2 Inhibitor (SGLT2i)

SGLT2i has been shown to contribute to the prevention of CVD in patients with diabetes and heart failure [54–58]. SGLT2i can be used for two types of disease, such as diabetes and heart failure, via a single pill, which is considered a treatment consistent with the concept of polypill strategy. Furthermore, there is evidence to suggest that SGLT2 inhibitors may have a positive impact on the cardio-renal prognosis of patients with chronic renal failure in the context of hypertension research [59]. It has been reported that empagliflozin had the effect of lowering 24 h BP levels in patients with diabetes and uncontrolled nocturnal hypertension in a randomized controlled trial (after 12 weeks, 24 h ambulatory BP level was −7.7 mmHg in the interventional group versus the placebo group) [53]. In addition, canagliflozin has been reported to have the effect of lowering BP in patients with diabetes and chronic kidney disease [60]. From these study findings, SGLT2i is suggested to be appropriate for use in the treatment of diabetes and heart failure, and for the control of elevated BP [53,60,61]. The therapeutic effect of SGLT2i on many of these diseases may be considered as one possible polypill treatment strategy.

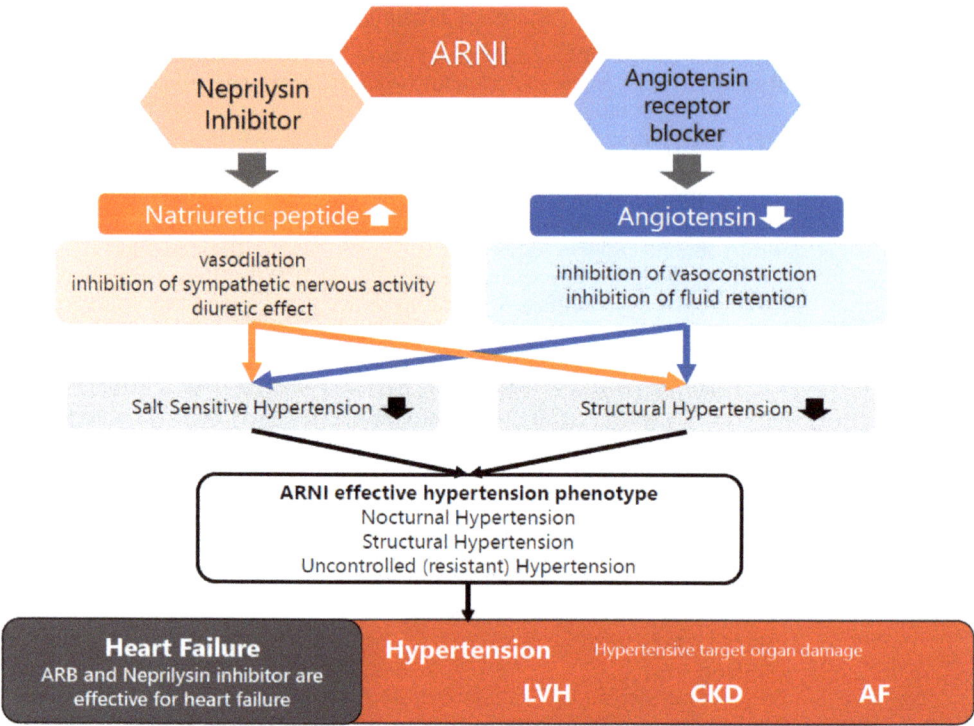

Figure 3. Mechanisms of the efficacy of ARNI for elevated BP and congestive heart failure. Angiotensin receptor neprilysin inhibitor (ARNI) has (1) an inhibitory effect on angiotensin and (2) an inhibitory effect on neprilysin. ARNI has been reported to have a variety of effects such as suppressing excessive sympathetic nerve activity and vasoconstriction and decreasing fluid retention. These multiple effects of ARNI are useful in the pathogenesis of nocturnal hypertension, structural hypertension, and treatment-resistant hypertension.

6. Problems and Limitations of Polypill Therapy

The advantages of a "one-size-fits-all" treatment strategy such as polypill therapy include (1) improved medication adherence, (2) a certain quality of treatment even in patients with low health literacy, and (3) effectiveness in preventing cardiovascular disease in low-income areas [3,62–64]. However, the recommendation of a "one-size-fits-all" treatment strategy for cardiovascular disease prevention, such as the polypill strategy, is inconsistent with the modern direction of precision medicine, which develops individualized treatment strategies based on a combination of clinical characteristics and genomic and lifestyle factors [65]. In the field of hypertension, the usefulness of artificial intelligence and machine learning for the early diagnosis of hypertension and the risk stratification of individual patients has been reported in recent years [66–68]. In addition, risk factors for nocturnal hypertension have been reported as a patient-specific pathophysiologic assessment [69]. Treatment management that takes into account the individual patient's pathophysiology is recommended [66,70]. In addition to traditional drug treatments, new therapies such as renal denervation and digital therapeutic applications for behavioral modification are being developed [68,71–73]. It is important to individualize treatment by combining these different treatment modalities, taking into account the response to each treatment. These treatment modalities are the opposite of one-size-fits-all polypill therapy. Clinical practitioners need to be aware of the advantages and disadvantages of polypill therapy.

7. Conclusions

Evidence is accumulating on the benefits of polypills in cardiovascular disease prevention. Novel therapeutic agents such as ARNI and SGLT2i with multimodal therapeutic effects may also be an avenue for polypill treatment strategies. Combination tablets are of particular importance in the field of hypertension treatment. Hypertension guidelines emphasize the use of combinations of multiple antihypertensive medications, and thus the use of combination forms is expected to improve medication compliance and provide stronger antihypertensive effects.

Author Contributions: K.N. wrote the entire paper and prepared the tables and figures; S.H. provided advice and edited the text; K.K. provided advice and edited the entire paper. All authors have read and agreed to the published version of the manuscript.

Funding: This research received no external funding.

Institutional Review Board Statement: Ethical review and approval were waived for this paper due to this is a review article.

Informed Consent Statement: Not applicable.

Data Availability Statement: As this is a review article, there is no data available on this paper.

Acknowledgments: We gratefully acknowledge A. Okura for editorial assistance.

Conflicts of Interest: K. Kario has received research grant from Daiichi Sankyo, MSD, Sumitomo Dainippon Pharma, Takeda Pharmaceutical, Mitsubishi Tanabe Pharma, Boehringer Ingelheim Japan, Mochida Pharmaceutical; Consulting fees from Kyowa Kirin, Sanwa Kagaku Kenkyusho, Mochida Pharmaceutical; Honoraria from Daiichi Sankyo, Novartis Pharma, Viatris; Participation in Advisory Board of Daiichi Sankyo, Novartis Pharma.

References

1. Lauder, L.; Mahfoud, F.; Azizi, M.; Bhatt, D.L.; Ewen, S.; Kario, K.; Parati, G.; Rossignol, P.; Schlaich, M.P.; Teo, K.K.; et al. Hypertension management in patients with cardiovascular comorbidities. *Eur. Heart J.* **2023**, *44*, 2066–2077. [CrossRef]
2. Umemura, S.; Arima, H.; Arima, S.; Asayama, K.; Dohi, Y.; Hirooka, Y.; Horio, T.; Hoshide, S.; Ikeda, S.; Ishimitsu, T.; et al. The Japanese Society of Hypertension Guidelines for the Management of Hypertension (JSH 2019). *Hypertens. Res.* **2019**, *42*, 1235–1481. [CrossRef]
3. Sukonthasarn, A.; Chia, Y.C.; Wang, J.; Nailes, J.G.; Buranakitjaroen, P.; Van Minh, H.; Verma, N.; Hoshide, S.; Shin, J.; Turana, Y.; et al. The feasibility of polypill for cardiovascular disease prevention in Asian Population. *J. Clin. Hypertens.* **2021**, *23*, 545–555. [CrossRef]
4. Kario, K.; Kai, H.; Nanto, S.; Yokoi, H. Anti-hypertensive medication adherence in the REQUIRE trial: Post-hoc exploratory evaluation. *Hypertens. Res.* **2023**, *46*, 2044–2047. [CrossRef]
5. Wald, N.J.; Law, M.R. A strategy to reduce cardiovascular disease by more than 80%. *BMJ* **2003**, *326*, 1419. [CrossRef]
6. Castellano, J.M.; Sanz, G.; Fuster, V. Evolution of the Polypill Concept and Ongoing Clinical Trials. *Can. J. Cardiol.* **2014**, *30*, 520–526. [CrossRef]
7. Zamorano, J.; Erdine, S.; Pavia, A.; Kim, J.-H.; Al-Khadra, A.; Westergaard, M.; Sutradhar, S.; Yunis, C. Proactive multiple cardiovascular risk factor management compared with usual care in patients with hypertension and additional risk factors: The CRUCIAL trial. *Curr. Med Res. Opin.* **2011**, *27*, 821–833. [CrossRef]
8. Huffman, M.D.; Xavier, D.; Perel, P. Uses of polypills for cardiovascular disease and evidence to date. *Lancet* **2017**, *389*, 1055–1065. [CrossRef]
9. Roshandel, G.; Khoshnia, M.; Poustchi, H.; Hemming, K.; Kamangar, F.; Gharavi, A.; Ostovaneh, M.R.; Nateghi, A.; Majed, M.; Navabakhsh, B.; et al. Effectiveness of polypill for primary and secondary prevention of cardiovascular diseases (PolyIran): A pragmatic, cluster-randomised trial. *Lancet* **2019**, *394*, 672–683. [CrossRef]
10. Castellano, J.M.; Pocock, S.J.; Bhatt, D.L.; Quesada, A.J.; Owen, R.; Fernandez-Ortiz, A.; Sanchez, P.L.; Marin Ortuño, F.; Vazquez Rodriguez, J.M.; Domingo-Fernández, A.; et al. Polypill Strategy in Secondary Cardiovascular Prevention. *N. Engl. J. Med.* **2022**, *387*, 967–977. [CrossRef]
11. Selak, V.; Webster, R.; Stepien, S.; Bullen, C.; Patel, A.; Thom, S.; Arroll, B.; Bots, M.L.; Brown, A.; Crengle, S.; et al. Reaching cardiovascular prevention guideline targets with a polypill-based approach: A meta-analysis of randomised clinical trials. *Heart* **2019**, *105*, 42–48. [CrossRef]
12. Wang, N.; Huffman, M.D.; Sundström, J.; Rodgers, A. Halving cardiovascular risk with combined blood pressure and cholesterol lowering – Why are we not there yet? *Int. J. Cardiol.* **2021**, *341*, 96–99. [CrossRef]

13. Grundy, S.M.; Stone, N.J.; Bailey, A.L.; Beam, C.; Birtcher, K.K.; Blumenthal, R.S.; Braun, L.T.; de Ferranti, S.; Faiella-Tommasino, J.; Forman, D.E.; et al. 2018 AHA/ACC/AACVPR/AAPA/ABC/ACPM/ADA/AGS/APhA/ASPC/NLA/PCNA Guideline on the Management of Blood Cholesterol: Executive Summary: A Report of the American College of Cardiology/American Heart Association Task Force on Clinical Practice Guidelines. *J. Am. Coll. Cardiol.* **2018**, *73*, 3168–3209. [CrossRef]
14. Merat, S.; Jafari, E.; Radmard, A.R.; Khoshnia, M.; Sharafkhah, M.; Baygi, A.N.; Marshall, T.; Khuzani, A.S.; Cheng, K.K.; Poustchi, H.; et al. Polypill for prevention of cardiovascular diseases with focus on non-alcoholic steatohepatitis: The PolyIran-Liver trial. *Eur. Heart J.* **2022**, *43*, 2023–2033. [CrossRef]
15. Yusuf, S.; Joseph, P.; Dans, A.; Gao, P.; Teo, K.; Xavier, D.; López-Jaramillo, P.; Yusoff, K.; Santoso, A.; Gamra, H.; et al. Polypill with or without Aspirin in Persons without Cardiovascular Disease. *N. Engl. J. Med.* **2021**, *384*, 216–228. [CrossRef]
16. Joseph, P.; Roshandel, G.; Gao, P.; Pais, P.; Lonn, E.; Xavier, D.; Avezum, A.; Zhu, J.; Liu, L.; Sliwa, K.; et al. Fixed-dose combination therapies with and without aspirin for primary prevention of cardiovascular disease: An individual participant data meta-analysis. *Lancet* **2021**, *398*, 1133–1146. [CrossRef]
17. Ibanez, B.; James, S.; Agewall, S.; Antunes, M.J.; Bucciarelli-Ducci, C.; Bueno, H.; Caforio, A.L.P.; Crea, F.; Goudevenos, J.A.; Halvorsen, S.; et al. 2017 ESC Guidelines for the management of acute myocardial infarction in patients presenting with ST-segment elevation: The Task Force for the management of acute myocardial infarction in patients presenting with ST-segment elevation of the European Society of Cardiology (ESC). *Eur. Heart J.* **2017**, *39*, 119–177. [CrossRef]
18. Collet, J.-P.; Thiele, H.; Barbato, E.; Barthélémy, O.; Bauersachs, J.; Bhatt, D.L.; Dendale, P.; Dorobantu, M.; Edvardsen, T.; Folliguet, T.; et al. 2020 ESC Guidelines for the management of acute coronary syndromes in patients presenting without persistent ST-segment elevation: The Task Force for the management of acute coronary syndromes in patients presenting without persistent ST-segment elevation of the European Society of Cardiology (ESC). *Eur. Heart J.* **2020**, *42*, 1289–1367. [CrossRef]
19. Visseren, F.L.J.; Mach, F.; Smulders, Y.M.; Carballo, D.; Koskinas, K.C.; Bäck, M.; Benetos, A.; Biffi, A.; Boavida, J.-M.; Capodanno, D.; et al. ESC Guidelines on cardiovascular disease prevention in clinical practice: Developed by the Task Force for cardiovascular disease prevention in clinical practice with representatives of the European Society of Cardiology and 12 medical societies With the special contribution of the European Association of Preventive Cardiology (EAPC). *Eur. Heart J.* **2021**, *42*, 3227–3337. [CrossRef]
20. Chow, C.K.; Atkins, E.R.; Hillis, G.S.; Nelson, M.R.; Reid, C.M.; Schlaich, M.P.; Hay, P.; Rogers, K.; Billot, L.; Burke, M.; et al. Initial treatment with a single pill containing quadruple combination of quarter doses of blood pressure medicines versus standard dose monotherapy in patients with hypertension (QUARTET): A phase 3, randomised, double-blind, active-controlled trial. *Lancet* **2021**, *398*, 1043–1052. [CrossRef]
21. Birla, S.; Angural, A.; Madathumchalil, A.; Shende, R.V.; Shastry, S.V.; Mahadevappa, M.; Shambhu, S.K.; Vishwanath, P.; Prashant, A. Redefining the polypill: Pros and cons in cardiovascular precision medicine. *Front. Pharmacol.* **2023**, *14*, 1268119. [CrossRef]
22. Thom, S.; Poulter, N.; Field, J.; Patel, A.; Prabhakaran, D.; Stanton, A.; Grobbee, D.E.; Bots, M.L.; Reddy, K.S.; Cidambi, R.; et al. Effects of a Fixed-Dose Combination Strategy on Adherence and Risk Factors in Patients with or at High Risk of CVD: The UMPIRE Randomized Clinical Trial. *JAMA* **2013**, *310*, 918–929. [CrossRef]
23. Selak, V.; Elley, C.R.; Bullen, C.; Crengle, S.; Wadham, A.; Rafter, N.; Parag, V.; Harwood, M.; Doughty, R.N.; Arroll, B.; et al. Effect of fixed dose combination treatment on adherence and risk factor control among patients at high risk of cardiovascular disease: Randomised controlled trial in primary care. *BMJ* **2014**, *348*, g3318. [CrossRef]
24. Castellano, J.M.; Sanz, G.; Peñalvo, J.L.; Bansilal, S.; Fernández-Ortiz, A.; Alvarez, L.; Guzmán, L.; Linares, J.C.; García, F.; D'aniello, F.; et al. A Polypill Strategy to Improve Adherence: Results from the FOCUS project. *J. Am. Coll. Cardiol.* **2014**, *64*, 2071–2082. [CrossRef]
25. Fuster, V.; Gambús, F.; Patriciello, A.; Hamrin, M.; Grobbee, D.E. The polypill approach – An innovative strategy to improve cardiovascular health in Europe. *BMC Pharmacol. Toxicol.* **2017**, *18*, 10. [CrossRef]
26. Castellano, J.M.; Sanz, G.; Ortiz, A.F.; Garrido, E.; Bansilal, S.; Fuster, V. A Polypill Strategy to Improve Global Secondary Cardiovascular Prevention: From concept to reality. *J. Am. Coll. Cardiol.* **2014**, *64*, 613–621. [CrossRef]
27. Webster, R.; Patel, A.; Selak, V.; Billot, L.; Bots, M.L.; Brown, A.; Bullen, C.; Cass, A.; Crengle, S.; Elley, C.R.; et al. Effectiveness of fixed dose combination medication ('polypills') compared with usual care in patients with cardiovascular disease or at high risk: A prospective, individual patient data meta-analysis of 3140 patients in six countries. *Int. J. Cardiol.* **2016**, *205*, 147–156. [CrossRef]
28. Liu, H.; Massi, L.; Laba, T.-L.; Peiris, D.; Usherwood, T.; Patel, A.; Cass, A.; Eades, A.-M.; Redfern, J.; Hayman, N.; et al. Patients' and Providers' Perspectives of a Polypill Strategy to Improve Cardiovascular Prevention in Australian Primary Health Care: A qualitative study set within a pragmatic randomized, controlled trial. *Circ. Cardiovasc. Qual. Outcomes* **2015**, *8*, 301–308. [CrossRef]
29. Patel, A.; Cass, A.; Peiris, D.; Usherwood, T.; Brown, A.; Jan, S.; Neal, B.; Hillis, G.S.; Rafter, N.; Tonkin, A.; et al. A pragmatic randomized trial of a polypill-based strategy to improve use of indicated preventive treatments in people at high cardiovascular disease risk. *Eur. J. Prev. Cardiol.* **2015**, *22*, 920–930. [CrossRef]
30. López-Jaramillo, P.; González-Gómez, S.; Zarate-Bernal, D.; Serrano, A.; Atuesta, L.; Clausen, C.; Castro-Valencia, C.; Camacho-Lopez, P.; Otero, J. Polypill: An affordable strategy for cardiovascular disease prevention in low–medium-income countries. *Ther. Adv. Cardiovasc. Dis.* **2018**, *12*, 169–174. [CrossRef]
31. Muñoz, D.; Uzoije, P.; Reynolds, C.; Miller, R.; Walkley, D.; Pappalardo, S.; Tousey, P.; Munro, H.; Gonzales, H.; Song, W.; et al. Polypill for Cardiovascular Disease Prevention in an Underserved Population. *N. Engl. J. Med.* **2019**, *381*, 1114–1123. [CrossRef]

32. Whelton, P.K.; Carey, R.M.; Aronow, W.S.; Casey, D.E., Jr.; Collins, K.J.; Himmelfarb, C.D.; DePalma, S.M.; Gidding, S.; Jamerson, K.A.; Jones, D.W.; et al. 2017 ACC/AHA/AAPA/ABC/ACPM/AGS/APhA/ASH/ASPC/NMA/PCNA Guideline for the Prevention, Detection, Evaluation, and Management of High Blood Pressure in Adults: A Report of the American College of Cardiology/American Heart Association Task Force on Clinical Practice Guidelines. *Hypertension* **2018**, *71*, e13–e115. [CrossRef]
33. Mancia Chairperson, G.; Kreutz Co-Chair, R.; Brunström, M.; Burnier, M.; Grassi, G.; Januszewicz, A.; Muiesan, M.L.; Tsioufis, K.; Agabiti-Rosei, E.; Algharably, E.A.E.; et al. 2023 ESH Guidelines for the management of arterial hypertension The Task Force for the management of arterial hypertension of the European Society of Hypertension Endorsed by the European Renal Association (ERA) and the International Society of Hypertension (ISH). *J. Hypertens.* **2023**, *41*, 1874–2071. [CrossRef]
34. World Health Organization. WHO Guideline for the Pharmacological Treatment of Hypertension in Adults. June 14, 2022. Available online: https://iris.who.int/bitstream/handle/10665/344424/9789240033986-eng.pdf?sequence=9789240033981 (accessed on 30 September 2023).
35. Lonn, E.M.; Bosch, J.; López-Jaramillo, P.; Zhu, J.; Liu, L.; Pais, P.; Diaz, R.; Xavier, D.; Sliwa, K.; Dans, A.; et al. Blood-Pressure Lowering in Intermediate-Risk Persons without Cardiovascular Disease. *N. Engl. J. Med.* **2016**, *374*, 2009–2020. [CrossRef]
36. Patel, A.; MacMahon, S.; Chalmers, J.; Neal, B.; Woodward, M.; Billot, L.; Harrap, S.; Poulter, N.; Marre, M.; Cooper, M.; et al. Effects of a fixed combination of perindopril and indapamide on macrovascular and microvascular outcomes in patients with type 2 diabetes mellitus (the ADVANCE trial): A randomised controlled trial. *Lancet* **2007**, *370*, 829–840. [CrossRef]
37. Staessen, J.A.; Fagard, R.; Thijs, L.; Celis, H.; Arabidze, G.G.; Birkenhäger, W.H.; Bulpitt, C.J.; de Leeuw, P.W.; Dollery, C.T.; Fletcher, A.E.; et al. Randomised double-blind comparison of placebo and active treatment for older patients with isolated systolic hypertension. The Systolic Hypertension in Europe (Syst-Eur) Trial Investigators. *Lancet* **1997**, *350*, 757–764. [CrossRef]
38. Wang, J.-G.; Staessen, J.A.; Gong, L.; Liu, L. Chinese Trial on Isolated Systolic Hypertension in the Elderly. Systolic Hypertension in China (Syst-China) Collaborative Group. *Arch. Intern. Med.* **2000**, *160*, 211–220. [CrossRef]
39. Ogawa, H.; Kim-Mitsuyama, S.; Matsui, K.; Jinnouchi, T.; Jinnouchi, H.; Arakawa, K. Angiotensin II Receptor Blocker-based Therapy in Japanese Elderly, High-risk, Hypertensive Patients. *Am. J. Med.* **2012**, *125*, 981–990. [CrossRef]
40. World Health Organization. WHO Global Report on Hypertension: The Race against a Silent Killer. September 19, 2023. Available online: https://www.who.int/publications/i/item/9789240081062 (accessed on 30 September 2023).
41. Weir, M.R.; Bakris, G.L. Combination Therapy With Renin-Angiotensin-Aldosterone Receptor Blockers for Hypertension: How Far Have We Come? *J. Clin. Hypertens.* **2008**, *10*, 146–152. [CrossRef]
42. Narita, K.; Hoshide, S.; Kario, K. The role of blood pressure management in stroke prevention: Current status and future prospects. *Expert Rev. Cardiovasc. Ther.* **2022**, *20*, 829–838. [CrossRef]
43. He, T.; Liu, X.; Li, Y.; Liu, X.Y.; Wu, Q.Y.; Liu, M.L.; Yuan, H. High-dose calcium channel blocker (CCB) monotherapy vs combination therapy of standard-dose CCBs and angiotensin receptor blockers for hypertension: A meta-analysis. *J. Hum. Hypertens.* **2017**, *31*, 79–88. [CrossRef]
44. Filipova, E.; Dineva, S.; Uzunova, K.; Pavlova, V.; Kalinov, K.; Vekov, T. Combining angiotensin receptor blockers with chlorthalidone or hydrochlorothiazide—which is the better alternative? A meta-analysis. *Syst. Rev.* **2020**, *9*, 195. [CrossRef]
45. Matsui, Y.; Eguchi, K.; O'Rourke, M.F.; Ishikawa, J.; Miyashita, H.; Shimada, K.; Kario, K. Differential Effects Between a Calcium Channel Blocker and a Diuretic When Used in Combination With Angiotensin II Receptor Blocker on Central Aortic Pressure in Hypertensive Patients. *Hypertension* **2009**, *54*, 716–723. [CrossRef]
46. Matsui, Y.; Eguchi, K.; Ishikawa, J.; Shimada, K.; Kario, K. Urinary Albumin Excretion During Angiotensin II Receptor Blockade: Comparison of Combination Treatment With a Diuretic or a Calcium-Channel Blocker. *Am. J. Hypertens.* **2011**, *24*, 466–473. [CrossRef]
47. Staplin, N.; de la Sierra, A.; Ruilope, L.M.; Emberson, J.R.; Vinyoles, E.; Gorostidi, M.; Ruiz-Hurtado, G.; Segura, J.; Baigent, C.; Williams, B. Relationship between clinic and ambulatory blood pressure and mortality: An observational cohort study in 59 124 patients. *Lancet* **2023**, *401*, 2041–2050. [CrossRef]
48. Yano, Y.; Hoshide, S.; Tamaki, N.; Nagata, M.; Sasaki, K.; Kanemaru, Y.; Shimada, K.; Kario, K. Efficacy of eplerenone added to renin-angiotensin blockade in elderly hypertensive patients: The Jichi-Eplerenone Treatment (JET) study. *J. Renin-Angiotensin-Aldosterone Syst.* **2011**, *12*, 340–347. [CrossRef]
49. Lu, Z.; Chen, Y.; Li, L.; Wang, G.; Xue, H.; Tang, W. Combination therapy of renin–angiotensin system inhibitors plus calcium channel blockers versus other two-drug combinations for hypertension: A systematic review and meta-analysis. *J. Hum. Hypertens.* **2017**, *31*, 1–13. [CrossRef]
50. Kario, K.; Williams, B. Angiotensin receptor–neprilysin inhibitors for hypertension—hemodynamic effects and relevance to hypertensive heart disease. *Hypertens. Res.* **2022**, *45*, 1097–1110. [CrossRef]
51. Zhang, J.; Zhang, W.; Yan, J.; Ge, Q.; Lu, X.-H.; Chen, S.-X.; Xu, W.-J.; Li, Y.; Li, J.-F.; He, S.-Y.; et al. Efficacy and safety of sacubitril/allisartan for the treatment of primary hypertension: A phase 2 randomized, double-blind study. *Hypertens. Res.* **2023**, *46*, 2024–2032. [CrossRef]
52. Jackson, A.M.; Jhund, P.S.; Anand, I.S.; Düngen, H.-D.; Lam, C.S.P.; Lefkowitz, M.P.; Linssen, G.; Lund, L.H.; Maggioni, A.P.; Pfeffer, M.A.; et al. Sacubitril–valsartan as a treatment for apparent resistant hypertension in patients with heart failure and preserved ejection fraction. *Eur. Heart J.* **2021**, *42*, 3741–3752. [CrossRef]

53. Kario, K.; Okada, K.; Kato, M.; Nishizawa, M.; Yoshida, T.; Asano, T.; Uchiyama, K.; Niijima, Y.; Katsuya, T.; Urata, H.; et al. 24-Hour Blood Pressure-Lowering Effect of an SGLT-2 Inhibitor in Patients with Diabetes and Uncontrolled Nocturnal Hypertension: Results from the Randomized, Placebo-Controlled SACRA Study. *Circulation* **2018**, *139*, 2089–2097. [CrossRef]
54. Zinman, B.; Wanner, C.; Lachin, J.M.; Fitchett, D.; Bluhmki, E.; Hantel, S.; Mattheus, M.; Devins, T.; Johansen, O.E.; Woerle, H.J.; et al. Empagliflozin, Cardiovascular Outcomes, and Mortality in Type 2 Diabetes. *N. Engl. J. Med.* **2015**, *373*, 2117–2128. [CrossRef]
55. Neal, B.; Perkovic, V.; Mahaffey, K.W.; de Zeeuw, D.; Fulcher, G.; Erondu, N.; Shaw, W.; Law, G.; Desai, M.; Matthews, D.R. Canagliflozin and Cardiovascular and Renal Events in Type 2 Diabetes. *N. Engl. J. Med.* **2017**, *377*, 644–657. [CrossRef]
56. Fitchett, D.; Inzucchi, S.E.; Cannon, C.P.; McGuire, D.K.; Scirica, B.M.; Johansen, O.E.; Sambevski, S.; Kaspers, S.; Pfarr, E.; George, J.T.; et al. Empagliflozin Reduced Mortality and Hospitalization for Heart Failure Across the Spectrum of Cardiovascular Risk in the EMPA-REG OUTCOME Trial. *Circulation* **2019**, *139*, 1384–1395. [CrossRef]
57. Wiviott, S.D.; Raz, I.; Bonaca, M.P.; Mosenzon, O.; Kato, E.T.; Cahn, A.; Silverman, M.G.; Zelniker, T.A.; Kuder, J.F.; Murphy, S.A.; et al. Dapagliflozin and Cardiovascular Outcomes in Type 2 Diabetes. *N. Engl. J. Med.* **2019**, *380*, 347–357. [CrossRef]
58. Anker, S.D.; Butler, J.; Filippatos, G.; Ferreira, J.P.; Bocchi, E.; Böhm, M.; Brunner–La Rocca, H.-P.; Choi, D.-J.; Chopra, V.; Chuquiure-Valenzuela, E.; et al. Empagliflozin in Heart Failure with a Preserved Ejection Fraction. *N. Engl. J. Med.* **2021**, *385*, 1451–1461. [CrossRef]
59. Masuda, T.; Nagata, D. Fluid homeostasis induced by sodium-glucose cotransporter 2 inhibitors: Novel insight for better cardio-renal outcomes in chronic kidney disease. *Hypertens. Res.* **2023**, *46*, 1195–1201. [CrossRef]
60. Ye, N.; Jardine, M.J.; Oshima, M.; Hockham, C.; Heerspink, H.J.L.; Agarwal, R.; Bakris, G.; Schutte, A.E.; Arnott, C.; Chang, T.I.; et al. Blood Pressure Effects of Canagliflozin and Clinical Outcomes in Type 2 Diabetes and Chronic Kidney Disease: Insights From the CREDENCE Trial. *Circulation* **2021**, *143*, 1735–1749. [CrossRef]
61. Georgianos, P.I.; Agarwal, R. Ambulatory Blood Pressure Reduction With SGLT-2 Inhibitors: Dose-Response Meta-analysis and Comparative Evaluation With Low-Dose Hydrochlorothiazide. *Diabetes Care* **2019**, *42*, 693–700. [CrossRef]
62. Roy, A.; Naik, N.; Reddy, K.S. Strengths and Limitations of Using the Polypill in Cardiovascular Prevention. *Curr. Cardiol. Rep.* **2017**, *19*, 45. [CrossRef]
63. Yusuf, S.; Pinto, F.J. The polypill: From concept and evidence to implementation. *Lancet* **2022**, *400*, 1661–1663. [CrossRef]
64. Rodgers, A.; Smith, R. The polypill and medicines access: Two decades and counting. *BMJ* **2023**, *382*, p1847. [CrossRef]
65. Melville, S.; Byrd, J.B. Personalized Medicine and the Treatment of Hypertension. *Curr. Hypertens. Rep.* **2019**, *21*, 13. [CrossRef]
66. Hu, Y.; Huerta, J.; Cordella, N.; Mishuris, R.G.; Paschalidis, I.C. Personalized hypertension treatment recommendations by a data-driven model. *BMC Med Informatics Decis. Mak.* **2023**, *23*, 44. [CrossRef]
67. Visco, V.; Izzo, C.; Mancusi, C.; Rispoli, A.; Tedeschi, M.; Virtuoso, N.; Giano, A.; Gioia, R.; Melfi, A.; Serio, B.; et al. Artificial Intelligence in Hypertension Management: An Ace up Your Sleeve. *J. Cardiovasc. Dev. Dis.* **2023**, *10*, 74. [CrossRef]
68. Kario, K.; Hoshide, S.; Mogi, M. Digital Hypertension 2023: Concept, hypothesis, and new technology. *Hypertens. Res.* **2022**, *45*, 1529–1530. [CrossRef]
69. Narita, K.; Hoshide, S.; Ae, R.; Kario, K. Simple predictive score for nocturnal hypertension and masked nocturnal hypertension using home blood pressure monitoring in clinical practice. *J. Hypertens.* **2022**, *40*, 1513–1521. [CrossRef]
70. Byrd, J.B. Personalized medicine and treatment approaches in hypertension: Current perspectives. *Integr. Blood Press. Control.* **2016**, *9*, 59–67. [CrossRef]
71. Rey-García, J.; Townsend, R.R. Renal Denervation: A Review. *Am. J. Kidney Dis.* **2022**, *80*, 527–535. [CrossRef]
72. Barbato, E.; Azizi, M.; Schmieder, R.E.; Lauder, L.; Böhm, M.; Brouwers, S.; Bruno, R.M.; Dudek, D.; Kahan, T.; Kandzari, D.E.; et al. Renal denervation in the management of hypertension in adults. A clinical consensus statement of the ESC Council on Hypertension and the European Association of Percutaneous Cardiovascular Interventions (EAPCI). *Eur. Heart J.* **2023**, *44*, 1313–1330. [CrossRef]
73. Kario, K.; Nomura, A.; Harada, N.; Okura, A.; Nakagawa, K.; Tanigawa, T.; Hida, E. Efficacy of a digital therapeutics system in the management of essential hypertension: The HERB-DH1 pivotal trial. *Eur. Heart J.* **2021**, *42*, 4111–4122. [CrossRef]

Disclaimer/Publisher's Note: The statements, opinions and data contained in all publications are solely those of the individual author(s) and contributor(s) and not of MDPI and/or the editor(s). MDPI and/or the editor(s) disclaim responsibility for any injury to people or property resulting from any ideas, methods, instructions or products referred to in the content.

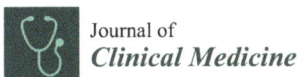
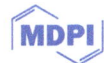

Review

Effects of Different Kinds of Physical Activity on Vascular Function

Francesca Saladini

Cardiology Unit, Cittadella Town Hospital, via Casa di Ricovero 40, 35013 Cittadella, Padova, Italy; saladinifrancesca@gmail.com

Abstract: Regular exercise is one of the main non-pharmacological measures suggested by several guidelines to prevent and treat the development of hypertension and cardiovascular disease through its impact on the vascular system. Routine aerobic training exerts its beneficial effects by means of several mechanisms: decreasing the heart rate and arterial pressure as well as reducing the activation of the sympathetic system and inflammation process without ignoring the important role that it plays in the metabolic profile. Through all these actions, physical training counteracts the arterial stiffening and aging that underlie the development of future cardiovascular events. While the role of aerobic training is undoubted, the effects of resistance training or combined-training exercise on arterial distensibility are still questioned. Moreover, whether different levels of physical activity have a different impact on normotensive and hypertensive subjects is still debated.

Keywords: exercise; aerobic physical activity; arterial stiffness; arterial distensibility; hypertension

Citation: Saladini, F. Effects of Different Kinds of Physical Activity on Vascular Function. *J. Clin. Med.* **2024**, *13*, 152. https://doi.org/10.3390/jcm13010152

Academic Editors: Anna Kabłak-Ziembicka and Christoph Sinning

Received: 29 September 2023
Revised: 26 November 2023
Accepted: 9 December 2023
Published: 27 December 2023

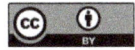

Copyright: © 2023 by the author. Licensee MDPI, Basel, Switzerland. This article is an open access article distributed under the terms and conditions of the Creative Commons Attribution (CC BY) license (https://creativecommons.org/licenses/by/4.0/).

1. Introduction

Physical activity is universally recognized as one of the major non-pharmacological measures to reduce the risk of future cardiovascular events [1,2] and cardiovascular mortality [3]. The importance of physical activity was also confirmed in the latest guidelines released for the management and treatment of arterial hypertension [4], which recommended performing the equivalent of 10 metabolic task-hours per week of recreational physical activity, which corresponds to the suggested 150 min. per week of previous guidelines [5,6], in order to reduce the risk of future hypertension by 6%. The positive effects of exercise are not limited to a mere reduction in blood pressure (BP) values, but it also acts on the metabolic profile and weight reduction [7,8] and also at the microcirculation level, with an improvement in vascular function and structure [9]. However, it is still debated if the favorable effects of exercise are both for aerobic and resistance or combined training, if there are differences in acute and long-term effects and if the entity of the benefit is the same for hypertensive and normotensive patients.

2. Effects of Different Types of Exercise on Arterial Distensibility

Several published papers have highlighted the beneficial role of aerobic training on arterial hypertension [8,10,11] and endothelial function [12,13]. Palatini et al. [8] examined 796 young-to-middle-age untreated hypertensive subjects from the HARVEST study, divided into 153 exercisers and 493 sedentary subjects. As expected, the active subjects presented a lower 24 h BP (78.8 vs. 81.2 mmHg, $p < 0.001$ adjusted for body mass index (BMI), alcohol consumption and smoking habits), diurnal diastolic BP (80.4 vs. 83.3 mmHg, $p < 0.0001$ adjusted for BMI, alcohol consumption and smoking habits) and heart rate (24 h 68.2 ± 0.7 vs. 72.0 ± 0.4 bpm, $p < 0.0001$; diurnal 70.1 ± 0.7 vs. 74.5 ± 0.4 bpm, $p < 0.0001$; nocturnal 59.7 ± 0.7 vs. 62.0 ± 0.4 bpm, $p = 0.004$ adjusted for age, BMI, alcohol intake and smoking habits) in comparison to the sedentary ones. As mentioned above, the efficacy of aerobic exercise for these young patients was due to several components, such as weight loss (BMI among exercisers was 25.2 ± 0.3 vs. 26.2 ± 0.2 kg/m^2, p = 0.002) and also the reduction in the activity of the sympathetic nerve system, as documented by the decrease in urinary norepinephrine at the 24 h urinary collection (norepinephrine/creatinine: 44.2 ± 2.6 μg/24 h vs. 8.9 ± 2.9 μg/24 h, respectively, p = 0.04, as also documented in the subsequent analysis) [14]. As mentioned above, aerobic training has a crucial role in the improvement in arterial function. Again, evidence from the HARVEST study [12] showed the positive impact of regular aerobic exercise during 6 years of follow-up among 366 young-to-middle-age subjects (n = 264 sedentary and n = 102 physically active), as examined through the use of radial applanation tonometry to detect large- and small-artery distensibility, peripheral resistances and the augmentation index. The authors observed that both at the enrolment (Figure 1) and at the final evaluation (Table 1), arterial distensibility parameters were higher for small- and large-artery compliance and lower for peripheral resistances and augmentation indexes among the physically active subjects compared to those who were not active in sports. However, these results only remained statistically significant at the final assessment for small-artery compliance after the inclusion of age and sex in the model [12], for the augmentation index when calculated with one-way repeated-measures ANOVA analysis (p for the interaction of active vs. sedentary × basal versus follow-up was 0.020) and for total peripheral resistance (p for interaction = 0.045) [12]. As documented for the positive effect of aerobic exercise on BP reduction, the mechanisms suggested to be underlying the positive effect of aerobic training on arterial distensibility were again the decreased heart rate of the active subjects (71.2 ± 8.9 bpm) compared to sedentary ones (76.6 ± 9.7 bpm; p < 0.001), which is a well-known, strong component of endothelial function according to previous published data [15–17], and the decrease in activity of the sympathetic nerve system [18], which may counteract the vasoconstriction phenomenon at peripheral sites and inhibit the chronic effect of sympathetic activation on the vascular tree. Also, Vriz et al. [13], in a recently published paper, confirmed the efficacy of aerobic exercise on endothelial function. The authors examined 120 leisure-time exercisers, 120 competitive athletes and 120 sedentary subjects who served as controls, who underwent an echo-tracking ultrasound system to assess carotid artery stiffness by means of the pressure–strain elastic modulus and one-point pulse wave velocity. The pressure–strain elastic modulus was reduced among those who were physically active (both groups) in comparison to those who were not active in sports (p < 0.03), as was the pulse wave velocity (p < 0.02). Moreover, in a multivariate regression analysis, physical activity was discovered to be a significant predictor of both the pressure–strain elastic modulus (p = 0.001) and pulse wave velocity (p < 0.001), even if both the associations were attenuated after the inclusion of heart rate in the model (p = 0.042 and 0.007, respectively). Again, this paper highlighted the important role of physical activity for heart rate as a mediator of the effects on vascular function [13], combined with receding microvascular remodeling, normalization of the capillary density, ameliorating the function of the vascular tree and, finally, counteracting the oxidative stress phenomenon [19–22]. All the evidence mentioned above refers to the efficacy of aerobic training, but what evidence do we have for different kinds of exercise? In the 2018 guidelines for arterial hypertension [5], isometric and resistance training were also recognized to be effective for the reduction in BP levels according to data reported in several randomized clinical trials [23–25], and it was also confirmed in the new guidelines [4]. For example, in the meta-analysis conducted by Cornelissen et al., a significant BP reduction of −3.9 (−6.4; −1.2)/−3.9 (−5.6; −2.2) mm Hg (p < 0.001) was clearly demonstrated, with a larger decrease among those who performed isometric handgrip training: −13.5 (−16.5; −10.5)/−6.1 (−8.3; −3.9) mmHg [23]. With regard to the effects of different exercise programs on vascular function, some evidence came from Ashor et al. [26]. In this meta-analysis involving 42 studies with an overall number of 1627 participants, the authors investigated the role that different types of physical training (aerobic, resistance or combined) had on vascular function, as detected by means of pulse wave velocity and the augmentation index. The authors observed that both parameters were significantly improved by aerobic training (−0.63 m/s, 95% CI:

−0.90, −0.35, $p < 0.01$ for pulse wave velocity; −2.63%, 95% CI: −5.25 to −0.02, $p = 0.05$ for augmentation index), while they were unaffected by resistance training (−0.04 m/s, 95% CI: −0.42, to 0.34, $p = 0.82$ for pulse wave velocity; −1.69%, 95% CI: −4.11 to 0.72, $p = 0.17$ for augmentation index) or combined aerobic/resistance exercise programs (−0.35 m/s, 95% CI: −0.82, 0.12, $p = 0.15$, respectively). These results seem to be in contrast to what was previously observed by Miyachi et al. [27], who found an increase of 14.3% (95% CI 8.5% to 20.1%; 71%; heterogeneity, $p < 0.001$) in stiffness indexes (carotid arterial β stiffness and pulse wave velocity) in comparison with a group of controls, even if this increase seemed to be peculiar to young but not to middle-aged individuals, and of high-intensity resistance training, while resistance training did not affect changes in vascular function. On the opposite side, resistance training performed at a high-intensity level was significantly associated with an increase in stiffness of 11.6% [27]. Moreover, as shown in the meta-analysis conducted by Ashor et al. [26], some studies that investigated some peculiar types of resistance training were included, showing a favorable impact or at least no increase in arterial stiffness such as with lower intensity rather than high intensity training [28], as was also observed by Miyachi et al. [27] with lower-limb rather than upper-limb training [29], eccentric rather than concentric resistance training [30] and the combination of resistance with aerobic training [31]. However, despite the conflicting data regarding the role of combined aerobic and resistance training on vascular function, its proven beneficial effect on the cardio-metabolic system makes resistance training a fundamental adjunct to aerobic physical activity, especially for those individuals with metabolic syndrome [32,33].

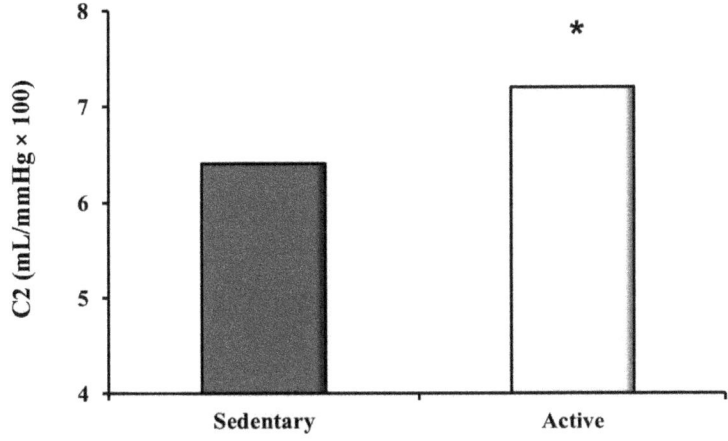

Figure 1. Baseline small-artery compliance in sedentary (n = 264) and active (n = 102) stage I hypertensive subjects from the HARVEST study. Adapted from Saladini F et al. [12]. BMI, body mass index; lifestyle factors: smoking habits, alcohol and coffee consumption and physical activity; parental HT, parental hypertension; SBP, systolic blood pressure; DBP, diastolic blood pressure; CT, total cholesterol; Tg serum triglycerides; HR, heart rate. p * value adjusted for age and sex.

Table 1. Follow-up evaluation of vascular function and hemodynamic indexes in the active verus stage 1 hypertensive participants from the HARVEST study. Adapted from Saladini F et al. [12].

Variables	Sedentary Subjects (n = 110)	Active Subjects (n = 42)	p *
C1, mL/mmHg × 10	16.4 ± 4.5	17.0 ± 4.8	n.s.
C2, mL/mmHg × 100	6.2 ± 2.8	7.9 ± 2.5	0.009
AIx, %	25.8 ± 22.6	14.5 ± 0.24	n.s.
Carotid-radial PWV, m/s	8.8 ± 2.1	9.1 ± 2.2	n.s.
Peripheral resistance, dyne × s × cm^{-5}	1466.0 ± 236	1357.0 ± 228	n.s.
Central SBP, mmHg	120.4 ± 15.0	118.2 ± 10.9	n.s.

Data are presented as mean ± standard deviation. C1, large-artery compliance; C2, small-artery compliance, AIx, augmentation index, PWV, pulse wave velocity; SBP, systolic blood pressure. p * value adjusted for age and sex; n.s., not statistically significant ($p > 0.05$).

3. Effect of Short-Term versus Long-Term Physical Activity on Arterial Distensibility

The positive long-term effect of physical activity on BP reduction and the prevention of target organ damage in hypertensive patients is not questionable. Vriz et al. [34] clearly demonstrated the efficacy of maintaining the same level of aerobic exercise for 3 months on BP levels. They compared 331 male non exercisers, 192 male mild exercisers and 49 male heavy exercisers and found an important reduction in diurnal systolic BP among the subjects who performed physical activity at a high-intensity level in comparison to inactive subjects (135.4 ± 0.6 mmHg among heavy exercisers, 134 ± 0.8 among mild exercisers, 132.2 ± 1.6 mmHg among sedentary subjects; $p < 0.05$ sedentary patients compared to heavy exercisers), demonstrating the beneficial effect of exercise training in reducing BP levels, which persisted through the three months of follow-up, during which the patients went on to perform the same level of exercise [34]. Similarly, in a review article, Cardoso et al. [35] concluded that both single episodes of aerobic training and chronic aerobic training were beneficial in terms of ambulatory BP reduction. In contrast, the beneficial effect of resistance training was demonstrated in the short term but not in the long term [35]. Moreover, long-term physical activity also showed a beneficial effect on hypertension mediated target organ damage [36–40]. Again, data from the HARVEST study [36] demonstrated among 454 untreated stage I hypertensives that regular aerobic physical activity over 8.3 years was associated with a lower left-ventricle mass among exercisers (39.0 ± 7.2 g/m$^{2.7}$) in comparison to sedentary subjects (41.4 ± 9.0 g/m$^{2.7}$; $p = 0.02$). Moreover, an increase in left-ventricular mass among sedentary subjects was detected during the follow-up (1.4 ± 6.5 g/m$^{2.7}$), while no significant progression was observed among the active ones (0.6 ± 7.1 g/m$^{2.7}$; $p = 0.03$). In a multivariate regression analysis, adjusted for several clinical confounders including age, sex, BMI, systolic and diastolic BP, hypertension duration, parental hypertension, follow-up length, smoking habits, coffee and alcohol intake, baseline left-ventricle mass, BP and weight changes during follow-up, aerobic physical training was a negative predictor of the increment in left-ventricular mass (O.R 0.26, 95% CI 0.07–0.09, $p = 0.033$) [36]. According to the literature, several mechanisms have been proposed for the favorable effect of exercise on hypertensive-mediated organ damage. As mentioned above, one of the main determinants is the BP reduction induced by regular physical activity [41,42] followed by the reduction in body weight [43,44], improvement in vascular function and cardiac structure [37] as well as favorable modifications to metabolic parameters such as the increment of insulin sensitivity, a reduction in the activity of the renin–angiotensin–aldosterone system [40,45] and the sympathetic nerve system [7,14]. The efficacy of regular aerobic exercises in the long term was also described at the carotid artery level. Palatini et al. [39] demonstrated that patients who performed regular physical training at the end of a follow-up that lasted 6.5 years showed a reduction in the mean intima-media thickness ($p = 0.01$) at every single site, including the common carotid artery ($p = 0.01$), bulb (however, not significant $p = 0.13$)

and internal carotid artery ($p = 0.05$), as well as in the maximum intima media thickness ($p = 0.006$), again at every single site, including the common carotid artery (however, not significant $p = 0.09$), bulb (again, not reaching the level of statistical significance $p = 0.21$), internal carotid artery ($p = 0.01$), in comparison to sedentary ones. In addition, the authors investigated the role that each single parameter has in the beneficial correlation between exercise and slowing the process of thickening of the intima-media at the carotid artery (Figure 2) and found that the main contributor was the reduction in total cholesterol, arterial pressure, heart rate and BMI [39]. This evidence confirmed the important role of regular physical training in counteracting the arterial stiffening of large vessels, such as the carotid artery, in young-to-middle-aged subjects with stage I hypertension through the important and beneficial modifications that act on the main components of the enhanced risk for cardiovascular disease [39]. The efficacy of long-term of physical activity was also demonstrated at the level of small vessels, confirming the fundamental role of exercise in contrasting the arterial aging phenomenon. This was shown by Saladini F et al. [12], not only at enrolment (Figure 1) but also after 6 years of follow-up (Table 1). Physically active (n = 102) subjects presented better distensibility parameters compared to subjects that did not regularly perform physical training (n = 264). However, the differences at the end of follow-up only reached statistical significance for small-vessel compliance after adjusting for age and gender [12]. The authors also investigated the longitudinal changes in the augmentation index and total peripheral resistances and found a significant time x group interaction (p for active vs. sedentary x baseline versus follow-up was 0.020 and 0.045, respectively [12]). One of the main determinants of the favorable effect of physical training on vascular function is the lower heart rate in trained individuals. According to the literature, the role of heart rate has been controversial for a long time, as previous findings seemed to advocate a cross sectional relationship between heart rate and arterial stiffness. In fact, according to a previous analysis, it was observed that the gradual increment in the heartbeat obtained through the stimulus of a cardiac pacemaker led to a consensual and gradual increment in the velocity of the pressure arterial wave [15,46]. A positive association between heart rate and pulse wave velocity was also found in a longitudinal study, as document by Tomiyama et al. [47] and by Benetos et al. [48], both in patients with normal or increased BP levels. Some clarifications on this issue came from Palatini et al. [49], who investigated the role of heart rate in determining changes in vascular function in the brief term and after several years of follow-up. The authors confirmed the negative cross-sectional correlation (r = −0.407, $p = 0.001$) between office heart rate and augmentation index. However, in the long term, a positive association was found between the ambulatory heart rate and the augmentation index ($p = 0.0006$), central BP ($p = 0.014$) and the amplification of BP from central to peripheral sites ($p = 0.004$) [49], indicating that the decrease in heart rate in the long term had a favorable impact on arterial stiffening, giving an important demonstration as to how regular exercise, through the reduction in the heartbeat in the long term, plays an important role in the decrease in the risk of cardiovascular morbidity and mortality among hypertensive subjects [50–52]. Important mechanisms in microcirculation may also account for the beneficial long-term effects of physical activity on endothelial function. As shown by De Ciuceis et al. [9] in a recent review, physical activity had a crucial role in counteracting vascular remodeling at the level of microcirculation sites among patients with elevated BP levels through the reduction in inflammation and fibrosis and neo angiogenesis, thereby promoting vasodilation and the restoration of the normal activity of the adipose tissue. Due to all these favorable mechanisms, aerobic exercise decreases vascular resistances at peripheral sites and enhances hematic flow in the vessels, preventing the impairment of arterial function.

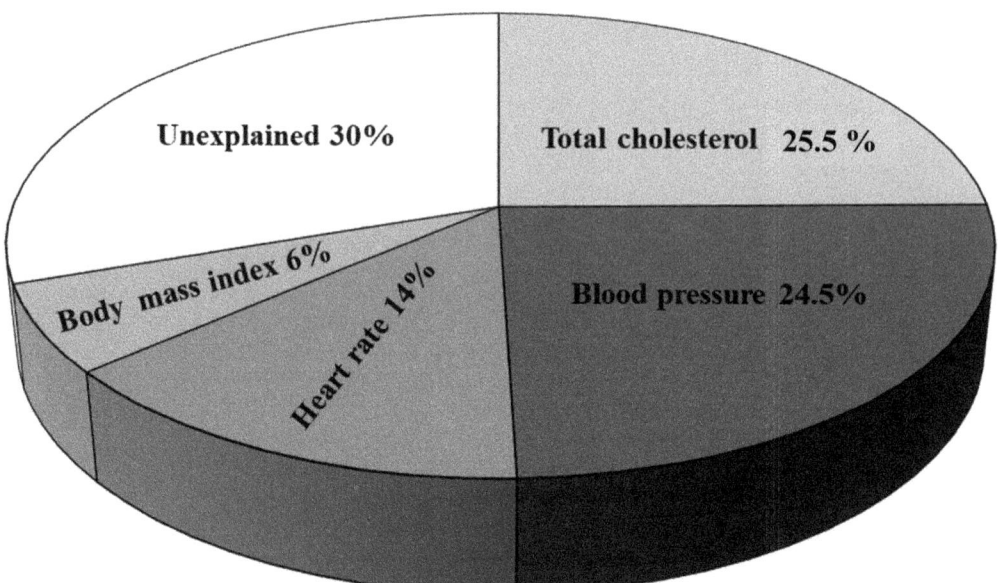

Figure 2. Contributing role that each single parameter exerts in mediating the relationship between thickening of the intima-media at the carotid level and aerobic training. Adapted from Palatini P et al. [39].

4. Effect of Regular Exercise on Vascular Function in Hypertensive and Normotensive Patients

Another debated issue is the potential different effects of regular physical activity in normotensive and hypertensive subjects and the role played by exercise intensity. This topic was explored by Vriz and coworkers [13] in a multifactorial analysis by comparing sedentary subjects with subjects performing leisure physical activity and vigorous exercise who were hypertensive and normotensive. The authors observed a different effect of physical activity according to BP status. A progressive decrease in the pressure–strain elastic modulus ($p = 0.009$) and pulse wave velocity ($p = 0.003$) was found across the different levels of physical activity (sedentariness, leisure activity, competitive sport activity). In contrast, within subjects with high BP levels, reduced values of both the pressure–strain elastic modulus and pulse wave velocity were observed among those who performed leisure-time physical activity, while no beneficial effect was found among those who performed vigorous activity. Moreover, in a two-way ANOVA, a statistically significant association was observed between physical activity level and BP status for the elastic modulus ($p = 0.03$), while the association with the pulse wave velocity did not reach the level of statistical significance ($p = 0.06$). The apparent lack of any effect of strenuous physical activity was explained by an increase in oxidative stress induced by vigorous physical activity in hypertensive subjects, which was in agreement with previous findings [53–56]. This study was in line with previous ones that showed a non-beneficial effect of higher aerobic fitness on the carotid-to-femoral pulse wave velocity among middle-age and older treated hypertensives [57] and no differences for the aortic wave velocity among fit or unfit hypertensive subjects [58].

5. Role of Physical Activity in the Elderly

Another interesting and debated issue is the role of physical activity among elderly subjects. In particular, it is unclear whether regular training at this age may have beneficial effects on vascular function. In older subjects, physiological vascular stiffening due to aging is associated with several comorbidities, including cardiovascular disease, atrial fibrillation, aortic stenosis, ischemic stroke, chronic kidney disease, cognitive impairment, frailty [59,60] and sarcopenia [61]. Whether regular physical activity exerts a positive effect of counteracting the aging process of the vessel wall is poorly known. Some evidence was provided by Vizzi et al. [62], who examined 26 subjects aged from 66 to 92 years performing regular physical activity three times/week. After 8 months, the authors observed no changes in most participants. A mild improvement in their neurodegenerative diseases was found in only two subjects. Similarly, Park et al. [63] observed that a regular program of aquatic exercises, performed in elderly patients with peripheral artery diseases, was useful in reducing the pulse wave velocity and ameliorating exercise capacity, as documented by the improvement in the six-minutes walking test. A beneficial effect of exercise for contrasting vascular stiffening due to aging was also found on top of using pharmacological drugs [64]. Fung et al. [64] examined 478 subjects with a mean age 68.6 years who were non-demented and with a high vascular risk who underwent to two different strategies to preserve cognitive function: drug treatment and/or physical exercise that included mind–body training or strenuous training. Interestingly, both types of exercise, combined with medication (H.R. 2.9 (1.1–7.7) $p = 0.029$ for mind–body training, H.R. 2.4 (1.1–5.3) 0.036 for strenuous exercise), were superior to using medication alone (p = n.s.) in counteracting cognitive decline.

The above findings have important clinical implications suggesting that regular exercise also has a beneficial effect in elderly subjects, as stated in the Guidelines for international exercise recommendations in older adults [65]. These guidelines detail the intensity, frequency and types of exercises suitable for older people, including aerobic exercise as well as balance activities, in order to prevent cardiovascular disease, improve frailty and counteracting cognitive decline [65].

6. Conclusions

Regular exercise training, as suggested by several studies [1,2,4–6], is one of the main non-pharmacological measures to prevent the development of major adverse cardiovascular events due to its favorable impact on heart rate, BP and several components of metabolic syndrome.

Several mechanisms account for these beneficial effects, including the reduction in the activities of the sympathetic nerve system and the renin–angiotensin–aldosterone system and the inflammation process, leading to an improvement in endothelial function and vascular elasticity. The favorable effect of resistance training on endothelial function and large arteries remains somewhat controversial. However, there is evidence showing that this kind of exercise has a positive effect on the metabolic profile (for example, on insulin sensitivity and glucose control [33]), as well as on some measures of endothelial function, such as flow-mediated dilation [66]. These effects make the combination of both aerobic and resistance training the best method for achieving optimal cardiovascular fitness [32]. A clear example of how the different modalities of exercise should be combined in order to obtain the best beneficial effect in terms of cardiovascular protection comes from the meta-analysis conducted by Zhang and co-workers [67]. The authors examined 38 articles involving an overall number of 2089 subjects with cardiovascular disease who underwent aerobic, resistance or combined physical exercise. Each type of exercise led to an improvement in arterial and cardiac functions; aerobic function significantly reduced the aortic systolic pressure and augmentation index, improved pulse wave velocity, cardiac output and the ejection fraction, while resistance training had a beneficial effect on the aortic systolic and diastolic pressure, and combined exercise had a favorable effect on the pulse wave velocity and cardiac output. The authors concluded that a tailored program of different kinds of exercise should be prescribed in order to obtain the maximum beneficial effect on the cardiovascular system.

The favorable effect of intense physical activity seems to be greater among normotensives, while the effect among hypertensives is beneficial only at a lower intensity level. An exercise program should be implemented in all healthy subjects, in particular in those at higher risk of developing hypertension and cardiovascular disease, in order to counteract all micro- and macrovascular complications that may progress to manifesting disease. But exercise, in particular combined exercise [32], should not be denied even to people with overt cardiovascular disease [68], provided it is performed to a light-to-moderate intensity level. However, the major challenge for health care personnel is still to persuade patients to continue with their program of regular training, as the compliance to exercise is very poor [69,70]. Yet, even small repetitions of exercise may counteract the detrimental effects of sedentary behavior [71,72]. In an interesting randomized cross-sectional trial, Fryer and coworkers demonstrated that the simple repetition of a small movement of the leg, such as flexing and extending the feet, after a meal rich in fat, may have an important positive impact on vascular stiffness. Among those subjects who continued to be sedentary for three hours, there was a significant increase in the pulse wave velocity and other indexes of local arterial stiffness, while among those who interrupted the sedentary behavior with 5 min of interval exercises, there was a significant decrease in the augmentation index [71]. Similarly, Horiuchi et al. demonstrated that the interruption of the sitting position by means of leg exercises such as squats [72,73] and or calf raises [73] at twenty-minute intervals had a beneficial impact on arterial stiffness, as mediated by a decrease in blood glucose levels [72].

In conclusion, regular physical exercise, independently of the kind of exercise, has a fundament role in counteracting vascular aging and arterial dysfunction and must be encouraged in every subject in order to prevent future hypertension and cardiovascular events.

Funding: This research received no external funding.

Conflicts of Interest: The author declares no conflicts of interest.

References

1. Fihn, S.D.; Blankenship, J.C.; Alexander, K.P.; Bittl, J.A.; Byrne, J.G.; Fletcher, B.J.; Fonarow, G.C.; Lange, R.A.; Levine, G.N.; Maddox, T.M.; et al. 2014 ACC/AHA/AATS/PCNA/SCAI/STS focused update of the guideline for the diagnosis and management of patients with stable ischemic heart disease: A report of the American College of Cardiology/American Heart Association Task Force on Practice Guidelines, and the American Association for Thoracic Surgery, Preventive Cardiovascular Nurses Association, Society for Cardiovascular Angiography and Interventions, and Society of Thoracic Surgeons. *Circulation* **2014**, *130*, 1749–1767. [PubMed]
2. Visseren, F.L.; Mach, F.; Smulders, Y.M.; Carballo, D.; Koskinas, K.C.; Bäck, M.; Benetos, A.; Biffi, A.; Boavida, J.M.; Capodanno, D.; et al. 2021 ESC Guidelines on cardiovascular disease prevention in clinical practice. *Eur. J. Prev. Cardiol.* **2022**, *29*, 5–115. [CrossRef] [PubMed]
3. Joseph, G.; Marott, J.L.; Torp-Pedersen, C.; Biering-Sørensen, T.; Nielsen, G.; Christensen, A.-E.; Johansen, M.B.; Schnohr, P.; Sogaard, P.; Mogelvang, R. Dose-response association between level of physical activity and mortality in normal, elevated, and high blood pressure. *Hypertension* **2019**, *74*, 1307–1315. [CrossRef] [PubMed]
4. Mancia, G.; Kreutz, R.; Brunström, M.; Burnier, M.; Grassi, G.; Januszewicz, A.; Muiesan, M.L.; Tsioufis, K.; Agabiti-Rosei, E.; Algharably, E.A.E.; et al. 2023 ESH Guidelines for the management of arterial hypertension The Task Force for the management of arterial hypertension of the European Society of Hypertension Endorsed by the European Renal Association (ERA) and the International Society of Hypertension (ISH). *J. Hypertens.* **2023**, *41*, 1874–2071. [PubMed]
5. Mancia, G.; Fagard, R.; Narkiewicz, K.; Rosei, E.A.; Azizi, M.; Burnier, M.; Clement, D.L.; Coca, A.; De Simone, G.; Dominiczak, A.F.; et al. 2018 ESC/ESH Guidelines for the management of arterial hypertension. *Eur. Heart J.* **2018**, *39*, 3021–3104.
6. Whelton, P.K.; Carey, R.M.; Aronow, W.S.; Casey, D.E., Jr.; Collins, K.J.; Dennison Himmelfarb, C.; DePalma, S.M.; Gidding, S.; Jamerson, K.A.; Jones, D.W.; et al. 2017 ACC/AHA/AAPA/ABC/ACPM/AGS/APhA/ASH/ASPC/NMA/PCNA Guideline for the Prevention, Detection, Evaluation, and Management of High Blood Pressure in Adults: A Report of the American College of Cardiology/American Heart Association Task Force on Clinical Practice Guidelines. *Hypertension* **2018**, *71*, 1269–1324. [PubMed]
7. Pekas, E.J.; Shin, J.; Son, W.M.; Headid III, R.J.; Park, S.Y. Habitual Combined Exercise Protects against age-associated decline in vascular function and lipid profiles in elderly postmenopausal women. *Int. J. Environ. Res. Public Health* **2020**, *17*, 3893. [CrossRef] [PubMed]
8. Palatini, P.; Graniero, G.R.; Mormino, P.; Nicolosi, L.; Mos, L.; Visentin, P.; Pessina, A.C. Relation between physical training and ambulatory blood pressure in stage I hypertensive subjects. Results of the HARVEST Trial. Hypertension and Ambulatory Recording Venetia Study. *Circulation* **1994**, *90*, 2870–2876. [CrossRef]
9. De Ciuceis, C.; Rizzoni, D.; Palatini, P. Microcirculation and physical exercise In hypertension. *Hypertension* **2023**, *80*, 730–739. [CrossRef]
10. Cornelissen, V.A.; Buys, R.; Smart, N.A. Endurance exercise beneficially affects ambulatory blood pressure: A systematic review and meta-analysis. *J. Hypertens.* **2013**, *31*, 639–648. [CrossRef]

11. Cornelissen, V.A.; Smart, N.A. Exercise training for blood pressure: A systematic review and meta-analysis. *J. Am. Heart Assoc.* **2013**, *2*, e004473. [CrossRef] [PubMed]
12. Saladini, F.; Benetti, E.; Mos, L.; Mazzer, A.; Casiglia, E.; Palatini, P. Regular physical activity is associated with improved small artery distensibility in young to middle-age stage 1 hypertensives. *Vasc. Med.* **2014**, *19*, 458–464. [CrossRef] [PubMed]
13. Vriz, O.; Mos, L.; Palatini, P. Leisure-time physical activity has a more favourable impact on carotid artery stiffness than vigorous physical activity in hypertensive human beings. *J. Clin. Med.* **2022**, *11*, 5303. [CrossRef] [PubMed]
14. Palatini, P.; Canali, C.; Graniero, G.R.; Rossi, G.; de Toni, R.; Santonastaso, M.; dal Follo, M.; Zanata, G.; Ferrarese, E.; Mormino, P.; et al. Relationship of plasma renin activity with caffeine intake and physical training in mild hypertensive men. HARVEST Study Group. *Eur. J. Epidemiol.* **1996**, *12*, 485–491. [CrossRef] [PubMed]
15. Lantelme, P.; Mestre, C.; Lievre, M.; Gressard, A.; Milon, H. Heart rate: An important confounder of pulse wave velocity assessment. *Hypertension* **2002**, *39*, 1083–1087. [CrossRef]
16. Cunha, R.S.; Pannier, B.; Benetos, A.; Siché, J.-P.; London, G.M.; Mallion, J.M.; Safar, M.E. Association between high heart rate and high arterial rigidity in normotensive and hypertensive subjects. *J. Hypertens.* **1997**, *15*, 1423–1430. [CrossRef] [PubMed]
17. Liang, Y.-L.; Gatzka, C.D.; Du, X.-J.; Cameron, J.D.; Kingwell, B.A. Effects of heart rate on arterial compliance in men. *Clin. Exp. Pharmacol. Physiol.* **1999**, *26*, 342–346. [CrossRef] [PubMed]
18. Wilkinson, I.B.; McEniery, C.M. ARTERIAL Stiffness, endothelial function and novel pharmacological approaches. *Clin. Exp. Pharmacol. Physiol.* **2004**, *31*, 795–799. [CrossRef]
19. Pedralli, M.L.; Marschner, R.A.; Kollet, D.P.; Neto, S.G.; Eibel, B.; Tanaka, H.; Lehnen, A.M. Different exercise training modalities produce similar endothelial function improvements in individuals with prehypertension or hypertension: A randomized clinical trial Exercise, endothelium and blood pressure. *Sci. Rep.* **2020**, *10*, 7628. [CrossRef]
20. Huang, J.; Zhang, H.; Tan, X.; Hu, M.; Shen, B. Exercise restores impaired endothelium-derived hyperpolarizing factor–mediated vasodilation in aged rat aortic arteries via the TRPV4-KCa2.3 signaling complex. *Clin. Interv. Aging* **2019**, *14*, 1579–1587. [CrossRef]
21. Wang, S.; Li, J.; Zhang, C.; Xu, G.; Tang, Z.; Zhang, Z.; Liu, Y.; Wang, Z. Effects of aerobic exercise on the expressions and activities of nitric oxide synthases in the blood vessel endothelium in prediabetes mellitus. *Exp. Ther. Med.* **2019**, *17*, 4205–4212. [CrossRef] [PubMed]
22. Borges, J.P.; Nascimento, A.R.; Lopes, G.O.; Medeiros-Lima, D.J.M.; Coelho, M.P.; Nascimento, P.M.C.; Kopiler, D.A.; Matsuura, C.; Mediano, M.F.F.; Tibirica, E. The impact of exercise frequency upon microvascular endothelium function and oxidative stress among patients with coronary artery disease. *Clin. Physiol. Funct. Imaging* **2018**, *38*, 840–846. [CrossRef] [PubMed]
23. Cornelissen, V.A.; Fagard, R.H.; Coeckelberghs, E.; Vanhees, L. Impact of resistance training on blood pressure and other cardiovascular risk factors: A metaanalysis of randomized, controlled trials. *Hypertension* **2011**, *58*, 950–958. [CrossRef] [PubMed]
24. López-Valenciano, A.; Ruiz-Pérez, I.; Ayala, F.; Sánchez-Meca, J.; Vera-Garcia, F.J. Updated systematic review and meta-analysis on the role of isometric resistance training for resting blood pressure management in adults. *J. Hypertens.* **2019**, *37*, 1320–1333. [CrossRef]
25. Smart, N.A.; Way, D.; Carlson, D.; Millar, P.; McGowan, C.; Swaine, I.; Baross, A.; Howden, R.; Ritti-Dias, R.; Wiles, J.; et al. Effects of isometric resistance training on resting blood pressure: Individual participant data meta-analysis. *J. Hypertens.* **2019**, *37*, 1927–1938. [CrossRef] [PubMed]
26. Ashor, A.W.; Lara, J.; Siervo, M.; Celis-Morales, C.; Mathers, J.C. Effects of exercise modalities on arterial stiffness and wave reflection: A systematic review and meta-analysis of randomized controlled trials. *PLoS ONE* **2014**, *9*, e110034. [CrossRef]
27. Miyachi, M. Effects of resistance training on arterial stiffness: A meta-analysis. *Br. J. Sports Med.* **2013**, *47*, 393–396. [CrossRef]
28. Okamoto, T.; Masuhara, M.; Ikuta, K. Effect of low-intensity resistance training on arterial function. *Eur. J. Appl. Physiol.* **2011**, *111*, 743–748. [CrossRef]
29. Okamoto, T.; Masuhara, M.; Ikuta, K. Upper but not lower limb resistance training increases arterial stiffness in humans. *Eur. J. Appl. Physiol.* **2009**, *107*, 127–134. [CrossRef]
30. Okamoto, T.; Masuhara, M.; Ikuta, K. Effects of muscle contraction timing during resistance training on vascular function. *J. Hum. Hypertens.* **2009**, *23*, 470–478. [CrossRef]
31. Okamoto, T.; Masuhara, M.; Ikuta, K. Combined aerobic and resistance training and vascular function: Effect of aerobic exercise before and after resistance training. *J. Appl. Physiol.* **2007**, *103*, 1655–1661. [CrossRef] [PubMed]
32. Marzolini, S.; Oh, P.I.; Brooks, D. Effect of combined aerobic and resistance training versus aerobic training alone in individuals with coronary artery disease: A meta-analysis. *Eur. J. Prev. Cardiol.* **2012**, *19*, 81–94. [CrossRef]
33. Snowling, N.J.; Hopkins, W.G. Effects of different modes of exercise training on glucose control and risk factors for complications in type 2 diabetic patients: A meta-analysis. *Diabetes Care* **2006**, *29*, 2518–2527. [CrossRef] [PubMed]
34. Vriz, O.; Mos, L.; Frigo, G.; Sanigi, C.; Zanata, G.; Pegoraro, F.; Palatini, P. Effects of physical exercise on clinic and 24-hour ambulatory blood pressure in young subjects with mild hypertension. *J. Sports Med. Phys. Fitness* **2002**, *42*, 83–88. [PubMed]
35. Cardoso, C.G.; Gomides, R.S.; Queiroz, A.C.C.; Pinto, L.G.; Lobo, F.d.S.; Tinucci, T.; Mion, D.; Forjaz, C.L.d.M. Acute and chronic Effects of aerobic and resistance exercise on ambulatory blood pressure. *Clinics* **2010**, *65*, 317–325. [CrossRef] [PubMed]
36. Palatini, P.; Visentin, P.; Dorigatti, F.; Guarnieri, C.; Santonastaso, M.; Cozzio, S.; Pegoraro, F.; Bortolazzi, A.; Vriz, O.; Mos, L. Regular physical activity prevents development of left ventricular hypertrophy in hypertension. *Eur. Heart J.* **2009**, *30*, 225–232. [CrossRef]

37. Sasaki, N.; Matsuura, H.; Kajiyama, G.; Oshima, T. Regular aerobic exercise augments endothelium-dependent vascular relaxation in normotensive as well as hypertensive subjects: Role of endothelium-derived nitric oxide. *Circulation* **1999**, *100*, 1194–1202.
38. Stewart, K.J. Exercise training and the cardiovascular consequences of type 2 diabetes and hypertension: Plausible mechanisms for improving cardiovascular health. *JAMA* **2002**, *288*, 1622–1631. [CrossRef]
39. Palatini, P.; Puato, M.; Rattazzi, M.; Pauletto, P. Effect of regular physical activity on carotid intima-media thickness. Results from a 6-year prospective study in the early stage of hypertension. *Blood Press.* **2011**, *20*, 37–44. [CrossRef]
40. Meyer, A.A.; Kundt, G.; Lenschow, U.; Schuff-Werner, P.; Kienast, W. Improvement of early vascular changes and cardiovascular risk factors in obese children after a six-month exercise program. *J. Am. Coll. Cardiol.* **2006**, *48*, 1865–1870. [CrossRef]
41. Whelton, S.P.; Chin, A.; Xin, X.; He, J. Effect of aerobic exercise on blood pressure: A meta-analysis of randomized controlled trials. *Ann. Intern. Med.* **2002**, *136*, 493–503. [CrossRef] [PubMed]
42. Kelley, G.A.; Kelley, K.A.; Tran, Z.V. Aerobic exercise and resting blood pressure: A meta-analytic review of randomized, controlled trials. *Prev. Cardiol.* **2001**, *4*, 73–80. [CrossRef] [PubMed]
43. MacMahon, S.W.; Wilcken, D.E.; Macdonald, G.J. The effect of weight reduction on left ventricular mass. A randomized controlled trial in young, overweight hypertensive patients. *N. Engl. J. Med.* **1986**, *314*, 334–339. [CrossRef] [PubMed]
44. Himeno, E.; Nishino, K.; Nakashima, Y.; Kuroiwa, A.; Ikeda, M. Weight reduction regresses left ventricular mass regardless of blood pressure level in obese subjects. *Am. Hearth J.* **1996**, *131*, 313–319. [CrossRef] [PubMed]
45. Cornelissen, V.A.; Fagard, R.H. Effects of endurance training on blood pressure, blood pressure–Regulating mechanisms, and cardiovascular risk factors. *Hypertension* **2005**, *46*, 667–675. [CrossRef] [PubMed]
46. Tan, I.; Spronck, B.; Kiat, H.; Barin, E.; Reesink, K.D.; Delhaas, T.; Avolio, A.P.; Butlin, M. Heart rate dependency of large artery stiffness. *Hypertension* **2016**, *68*, 236–242. [CrossRef] [PubMed]
47. Tomiyama, H.; Hashimoto, H.; Tanaka, H.; Matsumoto, C.; Odaira, M.; Yamada, J.; Yoshida, M.; Shiina, K.; Nagata, M.; Yamashina, A. Synergistic relationship between changes in the pulse wave velocity and changes in the heart rate in middle-aged Japanese adults: A prospective study. *J. Hypertens.* **2010**, *28*, 687–694. [CrossRef] [PubMed]
48. Benetos, A.; Adamopoulos, C.; Bureau, J.M.; Temmar, M.; Labat, C.; Bean, K.; Thomas, F.; Pannier, B.; Asmar, R.; Zureik, M.; et al. Determinants of accelerated progression of arterial stiffness in normotensive subjects and in treated hypertensive subjects over a 6-year period. *Circulation* **2002**, *105*, 1202–1207. [CrossRef]
49. Palatini, P.; Saladini, F.; Mos, L.; Fania, C.; Mazzer, A.; Casiglia, E. Low night-time heart rate is longitudinally associated with lower augmentation index and central systolic blood pressure in hypertension. *Eur. J. Appl. Physiol.* **2018**, *118*, 543–550. [CrossRef]
50. Palatini, P.; Thijs, L.; Staessen, J.A.; Fagard, R.H.; Bulpitt, C.J.; Clement, D.L.; de Leeuw, P.W.; Jaaskivi, M.; Leonetti, G.; Nachev, C.; et al. Predictive value of clinic and ambulatory heart rate for mortality in elderly subjects with systolic hypertension. *Arch. Intern. Med.* **2002**, *162*, 2313–2321. [CrossRef]
51. Jouven, X.; Empana, J.-P.; Schwartz, P.J.; Desnos, M.; Courbon, D.; Ducimetière, P. Heart-rate profile during exercise as a predictor of sudden death. *N. Engl. J. Med.* **2005**, *352*, 1951–1958. [CrossRef] [PubMed]
52. Kolloch, R.; Legler, U.F.; Champion, A.; Cooper-DeHoff, R.M.; Handberg, E.; Zhou, Q.; Pepine, C.J. Impact of resting heart rate on outcomes in hypertensive patients with coronary artery disease: Findings from the INternational VErapamil-SR/trandolapril STudy (INVEST). *Eur. Heart J.* **2008**, *29*, 1327–1334. [CrossRef] [PubMed]
53. Dekleva, M.; Lazic, J.S.; Arandjelovic, A.; Mazic, S. Beneficial and harmful effects of exercise in hypertensive patients: The role of oxidative stress. *Hypertens. Res.* **2017**, *40*, 15–20. [CrossRef] [PubMed]
54. Völz, S.; Svedlund, S.; Andersson, B.; Li-Ming, G.; Rundqvist, B. Coronary flow reserve in patients with resistant hypertension. *Clin. Res. Cardiol.* **2017**, *106*, 151–157. [CrossRef] [PubMed]
55. Rizzoni, D.; De Ciuceis, C.; Porteri, E.; Paiardi, S.; Boari, G.E.; Mortini, P.; Cornali, C.; Cenzato, M.; Rodella, L.F.; Borsani, E.; et al. Altered structure of small cerebral arteries in patients with essential hypertension. *J. Hypertens.* **2009**, *27*, 838–845. [CrossRef] [PubMed]
56. Paiardi, S.; Rodella, L.F.; De Ciuceis, C.; Porteri, E.; Boari, G.E.; Rezzani, R.; Rizzardi, N.; Platto, C.; Tiberio, G.A.; Giulini, S.M.; et al. Immunohistochemical evaluation of microvascular rarefaction in hypertensive humans and in spontaneously hypertensive rats. *Clin. Hemorheol. Microcirc.* **2009**, *42*, 259–268. [CrossRef] [PubMed]
57. Pierce, G.L. Aortic Stiffness in Aging and Hypertension: Prevention and Treatment with Habitual Aerobic Exercise. *Curr. Hypertens. Rep.* **2017**, *19*, 90–99. [CrossRef]
58. Kraft, K.A.; Arena, R.; Arrowood, J.A.; Fei, D.-Y. High aerobic capacity does not attenuate aortic stiffness in hypertensive subjects. *Am. Heart J.* **2007**, *154*, 976–982. [CrossRef]
59. Triposkiadis, F.; Xanthopoulos, A.; Lampropoulos, K.; Briasoulis, A.; Sarafidis, P.; Skoularigis, J.; Boudoulas, H. Aortic Stiffness: A Major Risk Factor for Multimorbidity in the Elderly. *J. Clin. Med.* **2023**, *12*, 2321. [CrossRef]
60. Alvarez-Bueno, C.; Cunha, P.G.; Martinez-Vizcaino, V.; Pozuelo-Carrascosa, D.P.; Visier-Alfonso, M.E.; Jimenez-Lopez, E.; Cavero-Redondo, I. Arterial Stiffness and Cognition Among Adults: A Systematic Review and Meta-Analysis of Observational and Longitudinal Studies. *J. Am. Heart Assoc.* **2020**, *9*, e014621. [CrossRef]
61. Zhang, Y.; Miyai, N.; Abe, K.; Utsumi, M.; Uematsu, Y.; Terada, K.; Nakatani, T.; Takeshita, T.; Arita, M. Muscle mass reduction, low muscle strength, and their combination are associated with arterial stiffness in community-dwelling elderly population: The Wakayama Study. *J. Hum. Hypertens.* **2021**, *35*, 446–454. [CrossRef] [PubMed]

62. Vizzi, L.; Padua, E.; D'Amico, A.G.; Tancredi, V.; D'Arcangelo, G.; Cariati, I.; Scimeca, M.; Maugeri, G.; D'Agata, V.; Montorsi, M. Beneficial Effects of Physical Activity on Subjects with Neurodegenerative Disease. *J. Funct. Morphol. Kinesiol.* **2020**, *5*, 94. [CrossRef] [PubMed]
63. Park, S.-Y.; Kwak, Y.-S.; Pekas, E.J. Impacts of aquatic walking on arterial stiffness, exercise tolerance, and physical function in patients with peripheral artery disease: A randomized clinical trial. *J. Appl. Physiol.* **2019**, *127*, 940–949. [CrossRef] [PubMed]
64. Fung, A.W. Effect of physical exercise and medication on enhancing cognitive function in older adults with vascular risk. *Geriatr. Gerontol. Int.* **2020**, *20*, 1067–1071. [CrossRef] [PubMed]
65. Izquierdo, M.; Merchant, R.A.; Morley, J.E.; Anker, S.D.; Aprahamian, I.; Arai, H.; Aubertin-Leheudre, M.; Bernabei, R.; Cadore, E.L.; Cesari, M.; et al. International Exercise Recommendations in Older Adults (ICFSR): Expert Consensus Guidelines. *J. Nutr. Health Aging* **2021**, *25*, 824–853. [CrossRef] [PubMed]
66. Silva, J.K.T.; Menêses, A.L.; Parmenter, B.J.; Ritti-Dias, R.M.; Farah, B.Q. Effects of resistance training on endothelial function: A systematic review and meta-analysis. *Atherosclerosis* **2021**, *333*, 91–99. [CrossRef] [PubMed]
67. Zhang, Y.; Qi, L.; Xu, L.; Sun, X.; Liu, W.; Zhou, S.; van de Vosse, F.; Greenwald, S.E. Effects of exercise modalities on central hemodynamics, arterial stiffness and cardiac function in cardiovascular disease: Systematic review and meta-analysis of randomized controlled trials. *PLoS ONE* **2018**, *13*, e0200829. [CrossRef]
68. Campos, H.O.; Rodrigues, Q.T.; Drummond, L.R.; Lima, P.M.A.; Monteiro, M.d.C.; Wanner, S.P.; Coimbra, C.C. Exercise-based cardiac rehabilitation after myocardial revascularization: A systematic review and meta-analysis. *Rev. Cardiovasc. Med.* **2022**, *23*, 74. [CrossRef]
69. Mora-Rodriguez, R.; Ramirez-Jimenez, M.; Fernandez-Elias, V.E.; de Prada, M.V.G.; Morales-Palomo, F.; Pallares, J.G.; Nelson, R.K.; Ortega, J.F. Effects of aerobic interval training on arterial stiffness and microvascular function in patients with metabolic syndrome. *J. Clin. Hypertens.* **2018**, *20*, 11–18. [CrossRef]
70. Koskinen, J.; Magnussen, C.G.; Taittonen, L.; Räsänen, L.; Mikkilä, V.; Laitinen, T.; Rönnemaa, T.; Kähönen, M.; Viikari, J.S.; Raitakari, O.T.; et al. Arterial structure and function after recovery from the metabolic syndrome: The cardiovascular risk in Young Finns Study. *Circulation* **2010**, *121*, 392–400. [CrossRef]
71. Fryer, S.; Paterson, C.; Turner, L.; Moinuddin, A.; Faulkner, J.; Stoner, L.; Daykin, A.; Stone, K. Localized activity attenuates the combined impact of a high fat meal and prolonged sitting on arterial stiffness: A randomized, controlled cross-over trial. *Front. Physiol.* **2023**, *14*, 1107456. [CrossRef] [PubMed]
72. Horiuchi, M.; Stoner, L. Blood glucose responses are associated with prolonged sitting-induced changes in arterial stiffness: A randomized crossover trial. *Blood Press. Monit.* **2022**, *27*, 345–348. [CrossRef] [PubMed]
73. Horiuchi, M.; Stoner, L. Macrovascular and microvascular responses to prolonged sitting with and without bodyweight exercise interruptions: A randomized cross-over trial. *Vasc Med.* **2022**, *27*, 127–135. [CrossRef] [PubMed]

Disclaimer/Publisher's Note: The statements, opinions and data contained in all publications are solely those of the individual author(s) and contributor(s) and not of MDPI and/or the editor(s). MDPI and/or the editor(s) disclaim responsibility for any injury to people or property resulting from any ideas, methods, instructions or products referred to in the content.

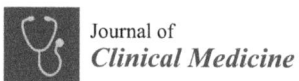

Review

Dietary Salt Restriction and Adherence to the Mediterranean Diet: A Single Way to Reduce Cardiovascular Risk?

Lanfranco D'Elia and Pasquale Strazzullo *

Department of Clinical Medicine and Surgery, "Federico II" University of Naples Medical School, 80131 Naples, Italy; lanfranco.delia@unina.it
* Correspondence: strazzul@unina.it

Abstract: The dietary restriction of salt intake and the adhesion to Mediterranean dietary patterns are among the most recommended lifestyle modifications for the prevention of cardiovascular diseases. A large amount of evidence supports these recommendations; indeed, several studies show that a higher adherence to Mediterranean dietary patterns is associated with a reduced risk of cardiovascular disease. Likewise, findings from observational and clinical studies suggest a causal role of excess salt intake in blood pressure increase, cardiovascular organ damage, and the incidence of cardiovascular diseases. In this context, it is also conceivable that the beneficial effects of these two dietary patterns overlap because Mediterranean dietary patterns are typically characterized by a large consumption of plant-based foods with low sodium content. However, there is little data on this issue, and heterogeneous results are available on the relationship between adherence to salt restriction and to Mediterranean dietary patterns. Thus, this short review focuses on the epidemiological and clinical evidence of the relationship between the adherence to Mediterranean dietary patterns and dietary salt restriction in the context of cardiovascular risk.

Keywords: salt; sodium; Mediterranean dietary pattern; cardiovascular risk; blood pressure

Citation: D'Elia, L.; Strazzullo, P. Dietary Salt Restriction and Adherence to the Mediterranean Diet: A Single Way to Reduce Cardiovascular Risk?. *J. Clin. Med.* 2024, *13*, 486. https://doi.org/10.3390/jcm13020486

Academic Editor: Birna Bjarnason-Wehrens

Received: 4 December 2023
Revised: 8 January 2024
Accepted: 13 January 2024
Published: 16 January 2024

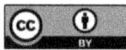

Copyright: © 2024 by the authors. Licensee MDPI, Basel, Switzerland. This article is an open access article distributed under the terms and conditions of the Creative Commons Attribution (CC BY) license (https://creativecommons.org/licenses/by/4.0/).

1. Introduction

Non-communicable diseases (NCDs) and, in particular, cardiovascular diseases (CVD) are the leading causes of death globally [1], and their reduction is a health priority [2]. In turn, high blood pressure (BP) and unhealthy diets are major causes of CVD [1,2].

In this context, the role of dietary salt (i.e., sodium chloride) has been extensively studied in relation to its effects on CVD. In particular, a large body of evidence supports a causal role of excess salt intake in the increase in BP with age, in the development of hypertension [3], and, eventually, in the incidence of CVD [3,4]. Epidemiological evidence regarding the strong relationship between salt intake, BP, and hypertension was provided over 30 years ago [5], and was confirmed thereafter by numerous studies [6,7]. In particular, recent results of the CARDIA study indicated that in a sample of initially normotensive young participants (mean age: 30 years), an average salt consumption of 14 g per day was associated with a 53% higher risk of hypertension than with a consumption of approximately 3 g per day over a 25-year follow-up period [8].

Excess salt intake has detrimental effects on endothelial function, contributes to the salt sensitivity of BP, activates the sympathetic nervous system, and is involved in the inflammatory response, modulating innate and adaptive immunity [9,10]. There is experimental evidence of structural and functional alterations induced by high-salt regimens in the arterial wall above and beyond the effect of high BP [10].

The results of intervention studies are in agreement with observational and experimental data. For instance, robust evidence regarding the effect of changes of dietary salt intake on BP was provided by a seminal study, which showed a significant increment of BP after switching a group of chimpanzees from their habitual low-salt diet to a high-salt diet for six months, and then a switch of BP back to normal when they returned to their usual low-salt regimen [11]. Thereafter, several controlled clinical trials examining the effect of dietary salt intake on BP have been conducted in humans, and their results have been the object of meta-analyses showing a favorable effect of salt intake reduction on BP in different settings (e.g., participants with and without hypertension, diabetic patients, and patients with renal disorders) [12–17].

In addition to the effects on BP, many studies have indicated that elevated salt intake may promote target organ damage and, conversely, several clinical trials have shown that salt restriction leads to an improvement in arterial stiffness [18], urinary albumin excretion [19], central blood pressure [18], and left ventricular mass [20–22].

Given the well-proven relationship between high BP and coronary, cerebrovascular, and renal outcomes, it is expected that salt intake in turn affects the incidence of cardiovascular disorders. Indeed, many longitudinal studies have detected a direct association between salt intake and CVD, and in particular with stroke risk [3,23,24].

Recently, the Mediterranean diet has been recognized as one of the dietary models more in keeping with the model of planetary diet conceived by the EAT–Lancet Commission as a diet for the Anthropocene [25]. The potential beneficial effects of a high level of adhesion to the Mediterranean dietary pattern (MDP) on CVD were hypothesized as early as in the 1950s [26]. That observation has inspired countless studies in which a higher degree of adhesion to the MDP was associated with a reduced risk of all-cause mortality and CVD [27,28]. In this regard, a recent meta-analysis of the effects of seven popular structured dietary patterns has shown that only the MDP substantially reduces all-cause mortality, non-fatal myocardial infarction, and stroke rates [28]. The benefit toward the risk of stroke was also reported by a previous meta-analysis showing that a higher adhesion to the MDP was associated with a lower risk of stroke in both Mediterranean and non-Mediterranean populations, and for both the ischemic and hemorrhagic types of stroke [29]. Likewise, yet another meta-analysis of 16 prospective cohort studies including only women detected a significant association between a higher adherence to the MDP and a lower incidence of total cardiovascular and coronary events, as well as total mortality, and a weaker association between MDP adhesion and the risk of stroke [30]. A very recent observational study, including approximately 2000 middle-aged male and female Greek participants, showed that those who sustained a high degree of adhesion to the MDP over the years had the lowest 20-year CVD risk [31]. In agreement with these results, other prospective cohort studies provided evidence that high adherence to the MDP improves survival in people with a history of CVD [32]. In keeping with the evidence on the relationship between MDP and the risk of cardiovascular events, several studies have also provided evidence of the association between the MDP and numerous cardiovascular risk factors. Thus, adhesion to the MDP was associated with beneficial changes in body weight, waist circumference, BP, insulin resistance, lipid profile, and flow-mediated arteriolar dilation [33]. The favorable effect of the MDP on BP was also found by two meta-analyses that detected a lower average systolic BP in participants with a higher degree of adhesion to the MDP compared to the lower-adhesion group [34,35]. In line with these results are those of another meta-analysis including 58 studies with finding of significantly lower values of waist circumference and serum triglyceride, and higher values of HDL-cholesterol in the high-adhesion MDP individuals [36]. Finally, based on 16 prospective studies, a systematic review found that the greatest adhesion to the MDP was significantly associated with a reduced risk of type 2 diabetes through a non-linear relationship [37].

Given that MDP is characterized by a large consumption of fruits, vegetables, whole grains, legumes, fish, monounsaturated fats (in particular olive oil), and nuts [38], there are many possible biological pathways whereby a variety of substances in the MDP could exert a beneficial role on CVD; for instance, dietary fiber, vitamins, minerals, and polyphenols content may benefit an altered metabolism of glucose and lipids as well as abdominal adiposity, high BP, and cardiovascular organ damage [39]. Based on these considerations, it is conceivable that a lower sodium intake might play a contributory role in the beneficial effects of the MDP, since the sodium content of natural plant-based foods is typically low. Nevertheless, few data are available on this issue and heterogeneous results on the relationship between adherence to salt intake and adherence to the MDP are available [40–45]. Therefore, we carried out a short narrative review focusing on the epidemiological and clinical evidence of the relationship between adhesion to the MDP and dietary salt intake in relation to CVD risk.

2. Epidemiological Evidence

The first strong epidemiological evidence of the direct association between salt intake and BP was provided by the results of the INTERSALT study, showing that the higher the habitual salt intake, the higher the average BP increase with age and the prevalence of hypertension in different populations around the world [5]. The detrimental effect of salt intake on cardiovascular risk was documented by several meta-analyses, in which an unequivocal association was detected with CVD, and in particular with stroke risk. The first of such meta-analyses, including prospective studies of samples of general populations, indicated a direct and significant association between higher salt intake and incidence of CVD [4]. The analysis, including 170,000 participants and more than 11,000 vascular events, showed a 23% greater risk of stroke and a 17% greater risk of total cardiovascular events for an average difference in salt intake of 5 g of salt per day. Further meta-analyses substantially confirmed these trends, despite some differences in the number of studies included in the analyses [3,23].

By the same token, looking at the epidemiological evidence on MDP, a number of prospective studies were carried out on the association between adhesion to the MDP and health outcomes. A recent systematic review has suggested that a high degree of adhesion to the MDP was associated with lower mortality rates in samples of general populations and in patients with previous CVD [27]. In addition, a separate evaluation of six prospective studies indicated that, following MDP, the risk of CVD (i.e., coronary artery disease, stroke, and cardiovascular mortality) decreased; in particular, the reduction in risk ranged from a hazard ratio of 0.44 to 0.71. The association was found when the adhesion to the MDP was expressed both as a continuous and as a dichotomous variable.

Despite this consolidated individual role of low salt intake and MDP adherence in CVD, and the potential synergistic effect of the combination of the two dietary measures, no epidemiological investigation explored this issue. Nevertheless, a few studies tried to assess the relationship between adhesion to the MDP and of the salt content of the diet in this context [40–45] (Table 1).

In a large Spanish population (n = 17,197), a comparison of the mineral content of the MDP and Western dietary patterns was made by a validated semi-quantitative questionnaire with 136 food items [40]. After stratification by quintiles of adhesion to the MDP or to Western dietary patterns, the highest quintile of MDP adhesion was associated with the lowest salt intake after adjustment for total energy intake, with a progressive inverse trend from the first to the last quintile. By contrast, the highest quintile of adhesion to a Western dietary pattern was associated with the highest salt intake, with a progressive direct trend from the first to the last quintile.

As a confirmation that adhesion to the MDP is compatible with a relatively low salt intake, there are the findings of a validated online self-administered questionnaire on an opportunistic large Italian population (n = 11,618), which explored the salt and health-related knowledge and behavior as well as the degree of adhesion to the MDP [42]. The survey indicated that both the degree of knowledge and the behavior regarding salt intake were significantly and positively correlated with the level of MDP adhesion, which suggests that nutritional information and good eating habits tend to go hand in hand. Of note, although the sample showed a decent level of knowledge and behavior regarding salt, remarkable differences in the degree of knowledge were detected in relation to sociodemographic markers, with a low level among adolescents, less educated people, and people with a low level of employment or that were unemployed.

Table 1. Characteristics of the studies reporting the relationship between Mediterranean dietary patterns and salt intake in adult general populations.

First Author (Year) [Ref]	Country	Participants (n)	MDP Adhesion Assessment Method	Salt Intake Assessment	Results
Serra-Majem et al. (2009) [40]	Europe (Spain)	17,197	Semi-quantitative FFQ (136 food items)	Semi-quantitative FFQ (136 food items)	The highest quintile of adhesion to the MDP was associated with the lowest salt intake (adjusted for total energy intake)
Vasara et al. (2017) [41]	Europe (Greece)	252	FFQ (11 food items)	24 h urine collection	No association between degree of adhesion to the MDP and salt intake
Iaccarino Idelson et al. (2020) [42]	Europe (Italy)	11,618	Self-administered questionnaire (4 food items)	Self-administered questionnaire (31 food items)	The level of MDP adhesion was significantly and positively correlated with the degree of knowledge and behavior about salt intake
Malavolti et al. (2021) [43]	Europe (Italy)	719	Semi-quantitative FFQ (EPIC—188 food items)	Semi-quantitative FFQ (EPIC—188 food items)	No association between adhesion to the MDP and salt intake
Moreira et al. (2021) [44]	Europe (Portugal)	1321	Semi-quantitative FFQ (14 food items)	24 h urine collection	In multivariate analysis, salt intake was positively associated with adhesion to the MDP in men. No such association was found in women
Viroli et al. (2021) [45]	Europe (Portugal)	102	Semi-quantitative FFQ (82 food items)	24 h urine collection	No association between adhesion to the MDP and salt intake

FFQ: food frequency questionnaire; MDP: Mediterranean dietary patterns.

On the other hand, other surveys were not in keeping with the above findings. Thus, the results of a study including 719 adults from a Northern Italy community and based on EPIC-FFQ showed that MDP adhesion had little influence on salt intake [43]. However, the assessment of salt intake in this study may have been biased because discretionary salt use was not considered.

A similar trend was also found in surveys that assessed salt intake via 24 h urinary excretion (the gold standard of the salt intake assessment). The results of a cross-sectional survey on a small sample of healthy Greek participants (n = 252) indicated no significant relationship between salt intake and MDP adherence (assessed using an 11-item questionnaire) [41]. Likewise, the results of a study on a small sample of middle-aged Portuguese volunteers (n = 102) showed no association between 24 h urinary sodium excretion and MDP adhesion, even after adjustment for confounding variables. In particular, a high degree of adhesion to the MDP was not associated with a low level of salt intake [45]. In addition, a survey on a sample of older Portuguese participants (n = 1321, ≥65 years) indicated that an excessive salt intake (assessed by 24 h urine excretion) was significantly associated with high adherence to the MDP in men, although with extremely wide confidence intervals (OR = 1.94; 95% CI: 1.03–3.65), while no such association was detected in women (OR = 0.91; 95% CI: 0.62–1.34) [44].

3. Clinical Evidence

Several intervention studies detected a direct effect of salt intake on cardiovascular risk through BP-mediated and BP-independent effects. Among the most robust trials, the TOHP I [46] and TOHP II [47], including patients with pre-hypertension at baseline, showed a significant decrease in BP in the group with salt restriction when compared to the control group. In addition, in the same studies, after 10–15 years of follow-up, a significantly lower risk of CVD was observed in the participants randomized to the salt-reduction group compared to controls [48]. This association was confirmed at the next follow-up, in which a significant linear association between salt intake and mortality was detected [49]. These favorable results of dietary salt restriction on BP were confirmed in several meta-analyses [12,14,17]. In particular, a linear dose–response relationship between the salt intake and the magnitude of the decrease in BP was also detected, with a greater effect in patients with hypertension compared to individuals without hypertension [12]. Intervention studies also support the detrimental effect of excess salt intake on target organ damage, even independently of increases in BP. For instance, the main results of a meta-analysis including 11 randomized controlled trials (RCT) and 431 participants detected a statistically significant effect of reduction in salt intake on arterial stiffness (expressed as carotid–femoral pulse wave velocity): an average weighted reduction of 5.2 g of salt intake per day led to an approximately 3% decrease in arterial stiffness, at least in part independently of the changes in BP [18]. Likewise, a meta-analysis of 23 studies including 516 participants suggested that salt restriction markedly reduces albumin excretion, a risk factor for the development and progression of renal disease [19]. In particular, an average reduction in salt intake (5.4 g of salt per day) was significantly associated with a 32% reduction in urinary albumin excretion. Furthermore, in line with this trend, the results of another meta-analysis showed the effect of salt restriction on central BP parameters (independent cardiovascular risk factors). An analysis including 14 studies and 457 participants, with an intervention time ranging between 1 and 13 weeks, detected that salt restriction led to a significant reduction in central BP parameters (e.g., the augmentation index, central systolic BP, and central pulse pressure) [16].

A milestone of the clinical trials examining the effects of particular dietary patterns on cardiovascular risk, which focused on the role of salt restriction, was the Dietary Approaches to Stop Hypertension (DASH) with sodium restriction trial, in which a reduction in the salt intake of the typical current American diet significantly reduced BP in hypertensive patients on top of other dietary modifications, without clinically apparent adverse effects [50]. Subsequent trials confirmed the DASH-sodium trial's benefit and revealed a greater beneficial effect on BP than during a DASH diet without salt restriction [51,52].

A number of studies were carried out to explore the effect of the MDP, a "natural" dietary pattern, on cardiovascular risk. An interesting and pioneering intervention study was carried out in the Cilento region (a representative place of the MDP in southern Italy), in which 57 non-hospitalized normotensive volunteers underwent a six-week isocaloric dietary intervention with a 70% increase in energy from saturated fatty acids and a corresponding decrease in carbohydrate and mono-unsaturated fat [53]. At the end of this intervention period, BP was significantly increased. After returning to their customary diet (i.e., MDP characterized by olive oil as the main source of fat, high vegetable and fruit consumption, and low animal protein and carbohydrate intake), BP returned to baseline, without changes in body weight throughout the study.

The PREvención con DIeta MEDiterránea (PREDIMED) study, a well-known intervention trial of the MDP including nearly 7500 participants with high cardiovascular risk, evaluated the effects of two MDPs (one with extra-virgin olive oil supplementation and the other with mixed-nuts supplementation) in comparison with a control low-fat diet, without any caloric or salt restriction, on the main CV outcomes [54]. After a median follow-up period of 3.8 years, greater reductions in BP were found for both MDPs compared with the control diet. However, only diastolic BP remained significant after multivariate adjustment.

Recently, a meta-analysis including 35 studies on the effect of the MDP on BP confirmed the beneficial effect of the MDP on BP. In this analysis, the MDP, compared to the usual diet and all other active intervention diets, significantly reduced systolic BP (-1.5 mmHg) and diastolic BP (-0.9 mmHg), in participants with or without hypertension, regardless of baseline BP levels [35]. However, this effect was only confirmed when the MDP was compared to the usual diet, while when compared to all other active intervention diets, the effect was lost.

Although a large number of studies explored the effect of the MDP or salt intake on cardiovascular risk, few intervention studies assessed the effect of salt intake in the context of the MDP and vice versa.

The results of a supplemental analysis of the PREDIMED study supported the add-on beneficial role of salt restriction in the context of the MDP; a decrease in sodium intake to 2300 mg per day was associated with reduced total mortality; by contrast, a positive association was found between an increase in sodium intake to 2300 mg per day and total mortality in a population at high risk of CVD [55]. Hence, in consideration of the study design, reducing sodium intake to 2300 mg/day seems associated with an enhanced beneficial effect of the MDP on CVD in comparison with those who did not reduce sodium intake.

Noteworthily, a recent RCT evaluated the BP effects of a three-month dietary intervention implementing salt restriction either alone or in the context of the MDP and the DASH diet, in adults with high normal BP or grade 1 hypertension [56]. A total of 204 Greek participants were included in the final analysis of the trial, stratified into a control group, a salt-restriction group, a MDP with salt restriction group, and a DASH diet with salt restriction group. The main results of this RCT indicated a greater and significant reduction in the office systolic BP in the MDP with salt restriction group compared to all other study groups (vs. control group: −15.1 mmHg; vs. salt restriction group: −7.5 mmHg; vs. DASH diet with salt restriction group: −3.2 mmHg). However, the MDP with salt restriction and DASH diet with salt restriction groups did not differ concerning the office diastolic BP. In addition, both MDP and DASH diets were more efficient in the reduction of BP than salt restriction alone.

4. Discussion

4.1. Dietary Salt Intake, BP Salt-Sensitivity and Cardiovascular Outcomes

The bulk of evidence provided by experimental, clinical and epidemiological studies supports the concept that excess salt intake has detrimental effects on BP and may promote organ damage mainly due to the rise in BP but also via additional BP-independent mechanisms. Although the majority of subjects experience a decrease in BP upon reduction of salt intake, in particular those with higher BP, there is a substantial inter-individual difference in the degree of the BP response to similar changes in salt intake [57], a phenomenon referred to as BP salt-sensitivity. A number of factors affect BP salt-sensitivity: among these the renin–angiotensin–aldosterone system (RAAS) response to changes in salt intake plays a major role in this regard [58]. In general, at high salt consumption, RAAS activity is suppressed, and this attenuates the tendency towards an increase in BP consequent to the increase in the extracellular fluid volume. However, in some relatively frequent conditions (e.g., obesity and type 2 diabetes), RAAS suppression may be blunted, leading to an increased BP salt-sensitivity. Moreover, activation of the sympathetic nervous system (SNS) may also contribute to the BP salt-sensitivity [59,60].

Many experimental studies showed that high salt consumption may affect arterial structure and function also partly independently of an increase in BP. Indeed, it has been suggested that high salt intake may have unfavorable effects on endothelial activity by increasing the production of transforming growth factor-beta 1 (TGF-b1) [61–63], reducing the bioavailability of nitric oxide (NO) [63], and decreasing the expression of endothelial NO synthase (eNOS) [64]. It has been shown that high endothelial sodium concentration impairs NO production and reduces its cellular plasticity [65]. Likewise, sodium overload may decrease the endothelial glycocalyx sodium barrier and concomitantly increase the endothelial stiffness [65]. The local RAAS may be involved in these events, as high salt intake was associated with increased angiotensin II type 1 receptor (AT1-R) expression in the cardiovascular system [66] and with an increase in AT1-R density in the renal cortex [66,67]. Accordingly, the administration of an AT1-R blocker during salt loading inhibits some detrimental effects mediated by this receptor (e.g., by improving the cardiovascular function and reducing aortic collagen accumulation) [66,68]. Also, chronic inflammation during excess salt intake may contribute to cardiovascular damage [9,69]. Indeed, mechanical stimuli due to high BP lead to a vascular inflammatory response, which involves both innate and adaptive immunity [9,70].

4.2. Benefits, Cost-Effectiveness, and Safety of Moderate Dietary Salt Reduction

Unfortunately, notwithstanding the educational campaigns in favor of salt intake reduction to values below 5 g per day (2 g per day of sodium) based on WHO recommendations, in most countries worldwide the habitual average salt intake largely exceeds this level [71]. To support the benefits of dietary salt reduction, numerous cost-effectiveness analyses indicated that a reduction of dietary salt at the population level is highly cost-effective and cost-saving in reducing CVD [72–74]. Indeed, an analysis of 183 countries found that a government "soft regulation" policy intervention to reduce national sodium consumption by 10% over 10 years was projected to be highly cost-effective (<1 × gross domestic product (GDP) per capita per disability life year (DALY) saved) in most countries [74]. Therefore, hundreds of thousands of deaths, and millions of DALYs, could be avoided each year, at a low cost.

Side effects upon reduction of salt intake to the levels recommended by the WHO are extremely rare in healthy individuals, since homeostatic mechanisms are very effective in maintaining the plasma sodium concentration within a narrow range [75]. On the other hand, more severe chronic restriction and/or the presence of disorders affecting water and electrolyte homeostasis may lead to symptomatic hyponatremia (i.e., a blood sodium level lower than 135 mmol/L), as reported in patients with severe vomiting and/or diarrhea, heart failure, excessive intake of diuretics, kidney disease, polydipsia, and liver cirrhosis [75].

4.3. Association of Low Salt Intake and Adhesion to the MDP

In addition to dietary salt intake reduction, also the benefits of a high degree of adhesion to the MDP are undoubtable. Indeed, a moderate reduction of salt intake and high adhesion to the MDP are both highly recommended lifestyle modifications for the prevention of CVD. In particular, the most recent European Society of Hypertension guidelines indicate both salt reduction and improvement of MDP adhesion as important measures for the prevention and management of hypertension [76]. In addition, the results of a recent trial support a possible synergic effect of these two interventions, inasmuch that MDP with salt restriction provided a greater reduction in systolic BP than either intervention alone in patients with high-normal or grade 1 hypertension [56].

In the natural foods that are prevalent in plant-based diets, such as the MDP, the salt content is low or very low [77]. In spite of this, however, the epidemiological evidence in favor of a direct association between the degree of adhesion to the Mediterranean diet and low habitual salt intake is not unequivocal: a larger use of discretionary salt in cooking and/or at the table and the higher salt content of commercially available processed foods provide a reasonable explanation for these heterogenous results. A recent Italian study supports this explanation, indicating that cereal-based products, including bread, represent a major source of daily non-discretionary salt intake [78].

In a way similar to the case of salt intake reduction, and in spite of the universal recognition of the benefits of plant-based diets such as the Mediterranean diet, the degree of adhesion to this model is still low, as documented by a recent survey of the CREA—Research Centre for Food and Nutrition in Rome, Italy [79]. Indeed, ecological studies in countries of the Mediterranean area indicated a shift in dietary patterns from the 1960s to the 2000s, especially in terms of an increase in animal protein and fat intake and a reduction in fresh plant-based foods [80,81]. This scenario is also supported by the cost of healthy foods (e.g., fresh fruit and vegetables), which may be definitely more expensive compared with processed and ultra-processed foods typical of Western dietary patterns [82]; indeed, a greater prevalence of a lower socioeconomic conditions is associated with a more energy-dense low-quality diet [83]. These unfavorable dietary changes, in turn, contribute to an increase in the incidence of excess body weight and other risk factors for non-communicable chronic diseases, and in particular cardiometabolic disorders, starting from childhood [84,85].

4.4. Conclusions, Limitations of the Study, and Future Perspectives

This short review summarized the benefits of dietary salt reduction and high adhesion to the MDP for cardiometabolic health, and tried to highlight their potential synergistic effects. Nevertheless, it has a few potential limitations, the first of which is the limited data available on the combined effect of these two major dietary preventive measures on CVD risk. We were able to retrieve only few and non-univocal data on the association between the adherence to the MDP and to reduced salt intake. Indeed, whereas a few epidemiological studies reported the expected inverse association between adhesion to the MDP and dietary salt intake [40,42], other studies did not detect any association. Conceivably, the different features of the studies available on this subject, among which the different questionnaires used to evaluate adhesion to the MDP and the different methods adopted for the assessment of habitual salt intake, may have contributed to these heterogeneous results. Therefore, definite conclusions cannot be drawn both for the strength of the combined effect of the two dietary measures on CVD risk and with regard to the association between adhesion to the MDP and salt intake reduction. There is clearly a need to adopt more effective strategies aiming to promote the increase of healthy food availability and of healthy eating patterns, which are key elements of preventive medicine, addressing in particular young people, in order to reduce the persistently high burden of CVD.

Author Contributions: Conceptualization: P.S. and L.D.; writing—original draft preparation, L.D. and P.S.; writing—review and editing, L.D. and P.S.; supervision, P.S. All authors have read and agreed to the published version of the manuscript.

Funding: This research received no external funding.

Conflicts of Interest: The authors declare no conflicts of interest.

References

1. GBD 2019 Risk Factors Collaborators. Global burden of 87 risk factors in 204 countries and territories, 1990–2019: A systematic analysis for the Global Burden of Disease Study 2019. *Lancet* **2020**, *396*, 1223–1249. [CrossRef] [PubMed]
2. GBD 2017 Diet Collaborators. Health effects of dietary risks in 195 countries, 1990–2017: A systematic analysis for the Global Burden of Disease Study 2017. *Lancet* **2019**, *393*, 1958–1972. [CrossRef]
3. Aburto, N.J.; Ziolkovska, A.; Hooper, L.; Elliott, P.; Cappuccio, F.P.; Meerpohl, J.J. Effect of lower sodium intake on health: Systematic review and meta-analyses. *BMJ* **2013**, *346*, f1326. [CrossRef]
4. Strazzullo, P.; D'Elia, L.; Kandala, N.B.; Cappuccio, F.P. Salt intake, stroke, and cardiovascular disease: Meta-analysis of prospective studies. *BMJ* **2009**, *339*, b4567. [CrossRef]
5. Intersalt Cooperative Research Group. Intersalt: An international study of electrolyte excretion and blood pressure. Results for 24–hour urinary sodium and potassium excretion. *BMJ* **1988**, *297*, 319–328. [CrossRef] [PubMed]
6. Zhou, B.; Stamler, J.; Dennis, B.; Moag-Stahlberg, A.; Okuda, N.; Robertson, C.; Zhao, L.; Chan, Q.; Elliott, P.; for the INTERMAP Research Group. Nutrient intakes of middle-aged men and women in China, Japan, United Kingdom, and United States in the late 1990s: The INTERMAP study. *J. Hum. Hypertens.* **2003**, *17*, 623–630. [CrossRef]
7. Khaw, K.T.; Bingham, S.; Welch, A.; Luben, R.; O'Brien, E.; Wareham, N.; Day, N. Blood pressure and urinary sodium in men and women: The Norfolk Cohort of the European Prospective Investigation into Cancer (EPIC-Norfolk). *Am. J. Clin. Nutr.* **2004**, *80*, 1397–1403. [CrossRef]
8. Hisamatsu, T.; Lloyd-Jones, D.M.; Colangelo, L.A.; Liu, K. Urinary sodium and potassium excretions in young adulthood and blood pressure by middle age: The Coronary Artery Risk Development in Young Adults (CARDIA) Study. *J. Hypertens.* **2021**, *39*, 1586–1593. [CrossRef]
9. Miyauchi, H.; Geisberger, S.; Luft, F.C.; Wilck, N.; Stegbauer, J.; Wiig, H.; Dechend, R.; Jantsch, J.; Kleinewietfeld, M.; Kempa, S.; et al. Sodium as an Important Regulator of Immunometabolism. *Hypertension* 2023, *epub ahead of print*. [CrossRef]

10. D'Elia, L.; Strazzullo, P. Isolated systolic hypertension of the young and sodium intake. *Minerva Med.* **2022**, *113*, 788–797. [CrossRef] [PubMed]
11. Denton, D.; Weisinger, R.; Mundy, N.I.; Wickings, E.J.; Dixson, A.; Moisson, P.; Pingard, A.M.; Shade, R.; Carey, D.; Ardaillou, R.; et al. The effect of increased salt intake on blood pressure of chimpanzees. *Nat. Med.* **1995**, *1*, 1009–1016. [CrossRef]
12. Filippini, T.; Malavolti, M.; Whelton, P.K.; Naska, A.; Orsini, N.; Vinceti, M. Blood Pressure Effects of Sodium Reduction: Dose-Response Meta-Analysis of Experimental Studies. *Circulation* **2021**, *143*, 1542–1567. [CrossRef]
13. Ren, J.; Qin, L.; Li, X.; Zhao, R.; Wu, Z.; Ma, Y. Effect of dietary sodium restriction on blood pressure in type 2 diabetes: A meta-analysis of randomized controlled trials. *Nutr. Metab. Cardiovasc. Dis.* **2021**, *31*, 1653–1661. [CrossRef]
14. Huang, L.; Trieu, K.; Yoshimura, S.; Neal, B.; Woodward, M.; Campbell, N.R.C.; Li, Q.; Lackland, D.T.; Leung, A.A.; Anderson, C.A.M.; et al. Effect of dose and duration of reduction in dietary sodium on blood pressure levels: Systematic review and meta-analysis of randomised trials. *BMJ* **2020**, *368*, m315. [CrossRef]
15. Cole, N.I.; Swift, P.A.; He, F.J.; MacGregor, G.A.; Suckling, R.J. The effect of dietary salt on blood pressure in individuals receiving chronic dialysis: A systematic review and meta-analysis of randomised controlled trials. *J. Hum. Hypertens.* **2019**, *33*, 319–326. [CrossRef]
16. D'Elia, L.; La Fata, E.; Giaquinto, A.; Strazzullo, P.; Galletti, F. Effect of dietary salt restriction on central blood pressure: A systematic review and meta-analysis of the intervention studies. *J. Clin. Hypertens.* **2020**, *22*, 814–825. [CrossRef]
17. He, F.J.; Li, J.; Macgregor, G.A. Effect of longer-term modest salt reduction on blood pressure: Cochrane systematic review and meta-analysis of randomized trials. *BMJ* **2013**, *346*, f1325. [CrossRef]
18. D'Elia, L.; Galletti, F.; La Fata, E.; Sabino, P.; Strazzullo, P. Effect of dietary sodium restriction on arterial stiffness: Systematic review and meta-analysis of the randomized controlled trials. *J. Hypertens.* **2018**, *36*, 734–743. [CrossRef]
19. D'Elia, L.; Rossi, G.; Schiano di Cola, M.; Savino, I.; Galletti, F.; Strazzullo, P. Meta-Analysis of the Effect of Dietary Sodium Restriction with or without Concomitant Renin-Angiotensin-Aldosterone System-Inhibiting Treatment on Albuminuria. *Clin. J. Am. Soc. Nephrol.* **2015**, *10*, 1542–1552. [CrossRef]
20. Kupari, M.; Koskinen, P.; Virolainen, J. Correlates of left ventricular mass in a population sample aged 36 to 37 years. Focus on lifestyle and salt intake. *Circulation* **1994**, *89*, 1041–1050. [CrossRef] [PubMed]
21. Schmieder, R.E.; Messerli, F.H.; Garavaglia, G.E.; Nunez, B.D. Dietary salt intake. A determinant of cardiac involvement in essential hypertension. *Circulation* **1988**, *78*, 951–956. [CrossRef] [PubMed]
22. Jula, A.M.; Karanko, H.M. Effects on left ventricular hypertrophy of long-term non-pharmacological treatment with sodium restriction in mild-to-moderate essential hypertension. *Circulation* **1994**, *89*, 1023–1031. [CrossRef]
23. Iacoviello, L.; Bonaccio, M.; Cairella, G.; Catani, M.V.; Costanzo, S.; D'Elia, L.; Giacco, R.; Rendina, D.; Sabino, P.; Savini, I.; et al. Diet and primary prevention of stroke: Systematic review and dietary recommendations by the ad hoc Working Group of the Italian Society of Human Nutrition. *Nutr. Metab. Cardiovasc. Dis.* **2018**, *28*, 309–334. [CrossRef]
24. Jayedi, A.; Ghomashi, F.; Zargar, M.S.; Shab-Bidar, S. Dietary sodium, sodium-to-potassium ratio, and risk of stroke: A systematic review and nonlinear dose-response meta-analysis. *Clin. Nutr.* **2019**, *38*, 1092–1100. [CrossRef]
25. Willett, W.; Rockström, J.; Loken, B.; Springmann, M.; Lang, T.; Vermeulen, S.; Garnett, T.; Tilman, D.; DeClerck, F.; Wood, A.; et al. Food in the Anthropocene: The EAT-Lancet Commission on healthy diets from sustainable food systems. *Lancet* **2019**, *393*, 447–492, Erratum in: *Lancet* **2019**, *393*, 530; Erratum in: *Lancet* **2019**, *393*, 2590; Erratum in: *Lancet* **2020**, *395*, 338; Erratum in: *Lancet* **2020**, *396*, e56. [CrossRef]
26. Keys, A. Mediterranean diet and public health: Personal reflections. *Am. J. Clin. Nutr.* **1995**, *61* (Suppl. 6), 1321S–1323S. [CrossRef]
27. Laffond, A.; Rivera-Picón, C.; Rodríguez-Muñoz, P.M.; Juárez-Vela, R.; Ruiz de Viñaspre-Hernández, R.; Navas-Echazarreta, N.; Sánchez-González, J.L. Mediterranean Diet for Primary and Secondary Prevention of Cardiovascular Disease and Mortality: An Updated Systematic Review. *Nutrients* **2023**, *15*, 3356. [CrossRef]
28. Karam, G.; Agarwal, A.; Sadeghirad, B.; Jalink, M.; Hitchcock, C.L.; Ge, L.; Kiflen, R.; Ahmed, W.; Zea, A.M.; Milenkovic, J.; et al. Comparison of seven popular structured dietary programmes and risk of mortality and major cardiovascular events in patients at increased cardiovascular risk: Systematic review and network meta-analysis. *BMJ* **2023**, *380*, e072003. [CrossRef]
29. Chen, G.C.; Neelakantan, N.; Martín-Calvo, N.; Koh, W.P.; Yuan, J.M.; Bonaccio, M.; Iacoviello, L.; Martínez-González, M.A.; Qin, L.Q.; van Dam, R.M. Adherence to the Mediterranean diet and risk of stroke and stroke subtypes. *Eur. J. Epidemiol.* **2019**, *34*, 337–349. [CrossRef] [PubMed]
30. Pant, A.; Gribbin, S.; McIntyre, D.; Trivedi, R.; Marschner, S.; Laranjo, L.; Mamas, M.A.; Flood, V.; Chow, C.K.; Zaman, S. Primary prevention of cardiovascular disease in women with a Mediterranean diet: Systematic review and meta-analysis. *Heart* **2023**, *109*, 1208–1215. [CrossRef] [PubMed]
31. Georgoulis, M.; Damigou, E.; Chrysohoou, C.; Barkas, F.; Anastasiou, G.; Kravvariti, E.; Tsioufis, C.; Liberopoulos, E.; Sfikakis, P.P.; Pitsavos, C.; et al. Mediterranean diet trajectories and 20-year incidence of cardiovascular disease: The ATTICA cohort study (2002-2022). *Nutr. Metab. Cardiovasc. Dis.* **2024**, *34*, 153–166. [CrossRef] [PubMed]
32. Tang, C.; Wang, X.; Qin, L.Q.; Dong, J.Y. Mediterranean Diet and Mortality in People with Cardiovascular Disease: A Meta-Analysis of Prospective Cohort Studies. *Nutrients* **2021**, *13*, 2623. [CrossRef] [PubMed]
33. Papadaki, A.; Nolen-Doerr, E.; Mantzoros, C.S. The Effect of the Mediterranean Diet on Metabolic Health: A Systematic Review and Meta-Analysis of Controlled Trials in Adults. *Nutrients* **2020**, *12*, 3342. [CrossRef]

34. Bakaloudi, D.R.; Chrysoula, L.; Leonida, I.; Kotzakioulafi, E.; Theodoridis, X.; Chourdakis, M. Impact of the level of adherence to the Mediterranean Diet on blood pressure: A systematic review and meta-analysis of observational studies. *Clin. Nutr.* **2021**, *40*, 5771–5780. [CrossRef] [PubMed]
35. Filippou, C.D.; Thomopoulos, C.G.; Kouremeti, M.M.; Sotiropoulou, L.I.; Nihoyannopoulos, P.I.; Tousoulis, D.M.; Tsioufis, C.P. Mediterranean diet and blood pressure reduction in adults with and without hypertension: A systematic review and meta-analysis of randomized controlled trials. *Clin. Nutr.* **2021**, *40*, 3191–3200. [CrossRef]
36. Bakaloudi, D.R.; Chrysoula, L.; Kotzakioulafi, E.; Theodoridis, X.; Chourdakis, M. Impact of the Level of Adherence to Mediterranean Diet on the Parameters of Metabolic Syndrome: A Systematic Review and Meta-Analysis of Observational Studies. *Nutrients* **2021**, *13*, 1514. [CrossRef] [PubMed]
37. Sarsangi, P.; Salehi-Abargouei, A.; Ebrahimpour-Koujan, S.; Esmaillzadeh, A. Association between Adherence to the Mediterranean Diet and Risk of Type 2 Diabetes: An Updated Systematic Review and Dose-Response Meta-Analysis of Prospective Cohort Studies. *Adv. Nutr.* **2022**, *13*, 1787–1798. [CrossRef]
38. Widmer, R.J.; Flammer, A.J.; Lerman, L.O.; Lerman, A. The Mediterranean Diet, its Components, and Cardiovascular Disease. *Am. J. Med.* **2015**, *128*, 229–238. [CrossRef]
39. Farias-Pereira, R.; Zuk, J.B.; Khavaran, H. Plant bioactive compounds from Mediterranean diet improve risk factors for metabolic syndrome. *Int. J. Food Sci. Nutr.* **2023**, *74*, 403–423. [CrossRef]
40. Serra-Majem, L.; Bes-Rastrollo, M.; Román-Viñas, B.; Pfrimer, K.; Sánchez-Villegas, A.; Martínez-González, M.A. Dietary patterns and nutritional adequacy in a Mediterranean country. *Br. J. Nutr.* **2009**, *101* (Suppl. 2), S21–S28. [CrossRef]
41. Vasara, E.; Marakis, G.; Breda, J.; Skepastianos, P.; Hassapidou, M.; Kafatos, A.; Rodopaios, N.; Koulouri, A.A.; Cappuccio, F.P. Sodium and Potassium Intake in Healthy Adults in Thessaloniki Greater Metropolitan Area-The Salt Intake in Northern Greece (SING) Study. *Nutrients* **2017**, *9*, 417. [CrossRef]
42. Iaccarino Idelson, P.; D'Elia, L.; Cairella, G.; Sabino, P.; Scalfi, L.; Fabbri, A.; Galletti, F.; Garbagnati, F.; Lionetti, L.; Paolella, G.; et al. Salt and Health: Survey on Knowledge and Salt Intake Related Behaviour in Italy. *Nutrients.* **2020**, *12*, 279. [CrossRef]
43. Malavolti, M.; Naska, A.; Fairweather-Tait, S.J.; Malagoli, C.; Vescovi, L.; Marchesi, C.; Vinceti, M.; Filippini, T. Sodium and Potassium Content of Foods Consumed in an Italian Population and the Impact of Adherence to a Mediterranean Diet on Their Intake. *Nutrients* **2021**, *13*, 2681. [CrossRef]
44. Moreira, S.; Moreira, P.; Sousa, A.S.; Guerra, R.S.; Afonso, C.; Santos, A.; Borges, N.; Amaral, T.F.; Padrão, P. Urinary Sodium Excretion and Adherence to the Mediterranean Diet in Older Adults. *Nutrients* **2021**, *14*, 61. [CrossRef]
45. Viroli, G.; Gonçalves, C.; Pinho, O.; Silva-Santos, T.; Padrão, P.; Moreira, P. High Adherence to Mediterranean Diet Is Not Associated with an Improved Sodium and Potassium Intake. *Nutrients* **2021**, *13*, 4151. [CrossRef]
46. TOHP I. The effects of non-pharmacologic interventions on blood pressure of persons with high normal levels. Results of the Trials of Hypertension Prevention, Phase I. *JAMA* **1992**, *267*, 1213–1220.
47. TOHP II. Effects of weight loss and sodium reduction intervention on blood pressure and hypertension incidence in overweight people with high-normal blood pressure. The Trials of Hypertension Prevention, phase II. *Arch. Intern. Med.* **1997**, *157*, 657–667.
48. Cook, N.R.; Cutler, J.A.; Obarzanek, E.; Buring, J.E.; Rexrode, K.M.; Kumanyika, S.K.; Appel, L.J.; Whelton, P.K. Long term effects of dietary sodium reduction on cardiovascular disease outcomes: Observational follow-up of the trials of hypertension prevention (TOHP). *BMJ* **2007**, *334*, 885–888. [CrossRef]
49. Cook, N.R.; Appel, L.J.; Whelton, P.K. Sodium Intake and All-Cause Mortality Over 20 Years in the Trials of Hypertension Prevention. *J. Am. Coll. Cardiol.* **2016**, *68*, 1609–1617. [CrossRef] [PubMed]
50. Svetkey, L.P.; Sacks, F.M.; Obarzanek, E.; Vollmer, W.M.; Appel, L.J.; Lin, P.H.; Karanja, N.M.; Harsha, D.W.; Bray, G.A.; Aickin, M.; et al. The DASH Diet, Sodium Intake and Blood Pressure Trial (DASH-sodium): Rationale and design. DASH-Sodium Collaborative Research Group. *J. Am. Diet Assoc.* **1999**, *99* (Suppl. 8), S96–S104. [CrossRef] [PubMed]
51. Appel, L.J.; Moore, T.J.; Obarzanek, E.; Vollmer, W.M.; Svetkey, L.P.; Sacks, F.M.; Bray, G.A.; Vogt, T.M.; Cutler, J.A.; Windhauser, M.M.; et al. A clinical trial of the effects of dietary patterns on blood pressure. DASH Collaborative Research Group. *N. Engl. J. Med.* **1997**, *336*, 1117–1124. [CrossRef] [PubMed]
52. Sacks, F.M.; Svetkey, L.P.; Vollmer, W.M.; Appel, L.J.; Bray, G.A.; Harsha, D.; Obarzanek, E.; Conlin, P.R.; Miller, E.R.; Simons-Morton, D.G.; et al. Effects on blood pressure of reduced dietary sodium and the dietary approaches to stop hypertension (DASH) diet. DASH-sodium collaborative research group. *N. Engl. J. Med.* **2001**, *344*, 3–10. [CrossRef]
53. Strazzullo, P.; Ferro-Luzzi, A.; Siani, A.; Scaccini, C.; Sette, S.; Catasta, G.; Mancini, M. Changing the Mediterranean diet: Effects on blood pressure. *J. Hypertens.* **1986**, *4*, 407–412. [CrossRef]
54. Toledo, E.; Hu, F.B.; Estruch, R.; Buil-Cosiales, P.; Corella, D.; Salas-Salvadó, J.; Covas, M.I.; Arós, F.; Gómez-Gracia, E.; Fiol, M.; et al. Effect of the Mediterranean diet on blood pressure in the PREDIMED trial: Results from a randomized controlled trial. *BMC Med.* **2013**, *11*, 207. [CrossRef]
55. Merino, J.; Guasch-Ferré, M.; A Martínez-González, M.; Corella, D.; Estruch, R.; Fitó, M.; Ros, E.; Arós, F.; Bulló, M.; Gómez-Gracia, E.; et al. Is complying with the recommendations of sodium intake beneficial for health in individuals at high cardiovascular risk? Findings from the PREDIMED study. *Am. J. Clin. Nutr.* **2015**, *101*, 440–448. [CrossRef]
56. Filippou, C.; Thomopoulos, C.; Konstantinidis, D.; Siafi, E.; Tatakis, F.; Manta, E.; Drogkaris, S.; Polyzos, D.; Kyriazopoulos, K.; Grigoriou, K.; et al. DASH vs. Mediterranean diet on a salt restriction background in adults with high normal blood pressure or grade 1 hypertension: A randomized controlled trial. *Clin. Nutr.* **2023**, *42*, 1807–1816. [CrossRef]

57. Strazzullo, P.; Galletti, F.; Dessì-Fulgheri, P.; Ferri, C.; Glorioso, N.; Malatino, L.; Mantero, F.; Manunta, P.; Semplicini, A.; Ghiadoni, L.; et al. Prediction and consistency of blood pressure salt-sensitivity as assessed by a rapid volume expansion and contraction protocol. Salt-Sensitivity Study Group of the Italian Society of Hypertension. *J. Nephrol.* **2000**, *13*, 46–53.
58. Hall, J.E. Control of sodium excretion by angiotensin II: Intrarenal mechanisms and blood pressure regulation. *Am. J. Physiol.* **1986**, *250*, R960–R972. [CrossRef]
59. Laffer, C.L.; Bolterman, R.J.; Romero, J.C.; Elijovich, F. Effect of salt on isoprostanes in salt-sensitive essential hypertension. *Hypertension* **2006**, *47*, 434–440. [CrossRef]
60. Elijovich, F.; Laffer, C.L.; Amador, E.; Gavras, H.; Bresnaham, M.R.; Schiffrin, E.L. Regulation of plasma endothelin by salt in salt-sensitive hypertension. *Circulation* **2001**, *103*, 263–268. [CrossRef]
61. Ying, W.-Z.; Sanders, P.W. Dietary salt increases endothelial nitric oxide synthase and TGF-b1 in rat aortic endothelium. *Am. J. Physiol.* **1999**, *277 Pt 2*, H1293–H1298. [PubMed]
62. Ying, W.-Z.; Sanders, P.W. Dietary salt modulates renal production of transforming growth factor-b in rats. *Am. J. Physiol.* **1998**, *274 Pt 2*, F635–F641. [CrossRef]
63. Matsuoka, H.; Itoh, S.; Kimoto, M.; Kohno, K.; Tamai, O.; Wada, Y.; Yasukawa, H.; Iwami, G.; Okuda, S.; Imaizumi, T. Asymmetrical dimethylarginine, an endogenous nitric oxide synthase inhibitor, in experimental hypertension. *Hypertension* **1997**, *29 Pt 2*, 242–247. [CrossRef] [PubMed]
64. Ni, Z.; Vaziri, N.D. Effect of salt loading on nitric oxide synthase expression in normotensive rats. *Am. J. Hypertens.* **2001**, *14*, 155–163. [CrossRef] [PubMed]
65. Oberleithner, H.; Peters, W.; Kusche-Vihrog, K.; Korte, S.; Schillers, H.; Kliche, K.; Oberleithner, K. Salt overload damages the glycocalyx sodium barrier of vascular endothelium. *Pflug. Arch.* **2011**, *462*, 519–528. [CrossRef]
66. Nickenig, G.; Strehlow, K.; Roeling, J.; Zolk, O.; Knorr, A.; Bohm, M. Salt induces vascular AT1 receptor overexpression in vitro and in vivo. *Hypertension* **1998**, *31*, 1272–1277. [CrossRef] [PubMed]
67. Frohlich, E.D. The salt conundrum: A hypothesis. *Hypertension* **2007**, *50*, 161–166. [CrossRef]
68. Matavelli, L.C.; Zhou, X.; Varagic, J.; Susic, D.; Frohlich, E.D. Salt loading produces severe renal hemodynamic dysfunction inde pendent of arterial pressure in spontaneously hypertensive rats. *Am. J. Physiol. Heart Circ. Physiol.* **2007**, *292*, H814–H819. [CrossRef]
69. Zanoli, L.; Briet, M.; Empana, J.P.; Cunha, P.G.; Mäki-Petäjä, K.M.; Protogerou, A.D.; Tedgui, A.; Touyz, R.M.; Schiffrin, E.L.; Spronck, B.; et al. Vascular consequences of inflammation: A position statement from the ESH Working Group on Vascular Structure and Function and the ARTERY Society. *J. Hypertens.* **2020**, *38*, 1682–1698. [CrossRef]
70. Ait-Oufella, H.; Sage, A.P.; Mallat, Z.; Tedgui, A. Adaptive (T and B cells) immunity and control by dendritic cells in atherosclerosis. *Circ. Res.* **2014**, *114*, 1640–1660. [CrossRef]
71. World Health Organization. *Guideline: Sodium Intake for Adults and Children*; World Health Organization: Geneva, Switzerland, 2012.
72. Bibbins-Domingo, K.; Chertow, G.M.; Coxson, P.G.; Moran, A.; Lightwood, J.M.; Pletcher, M.J.; Goldman, L. Projected effect of dietary salt reductions on future cardiovascular disease. *N. Engl. J. Med.* **2010**, *362*, 590–599. [CrossRef]
73. Smith-Spangler, C.M.; Juusola, J.L.; Enns, E.A.; Owens, D.K.; Garber, A.M. Population strategies to decrease sodium intake and the burden of cardiovascular disease: A cost-effectiveness analysis. *Ann. Intern. Med.* **2010**, *152*, W170–W173. [CrossRef] [PubMed]
74. Webb, M.; Fahimi, S.; Singh, G.M.; Khatibzadeh, S.; Micha, R.; Powles, J.; Mozaffarian, D. Cost effectiveness of a government supported policy strategy to decrease sodium intake: Global analysis across 183 nations. *BMJ* **2017**, *356*, i6699. [CrossRef]
75. Palmer, B.F. Hyponatremia in the intensive care unit. *Semin. Nephrol.* **2009**, *29*, 257–270. [CrossRef] [PubMed]
76. Mancia, G.; Kreutz, R.; Brunström, M.; Burnier, M.; Grassi, G.; Januszewicz, A.; Muiesan, M.L.; Tsioufis, K.; Agabiti-Rosei, E.; Algharably, E.A.E.; et al. 2023 ESH Guidelines for the management of arterial hypertension The Task Force for the management of arterial hypertension of the European Society of Hypertension Endorsed by the International Society of Hypertension (ISH) and the European Renal Association (ERA). *J. Hypertens.* **2023**, *41*, 1874–2071. [CrossRef]
77. Bull, N.L.; Buss, D.H. Contribution of foods to sodium intakes. *Proc. Nutr. Soc.* **1990**, *39*, 40A.
78. Vici, G.; Rosi, A.; Angelino, D.; Polzonetti, V.; Scazzina, F.; Pellegrini, N.; Martini, D. on behalf of the SINU Young Working Group. Salt content of prepacked cereal-based products and their potential contribution to salt intake of the italian adult population: Results from a simulation study. *Nutr. Metab. Cardiovasc. Dis.* **2023**; *in press*. [CrossRef]
79. Aureli, V.; Rossi, L. Nutrition Knowledge as a Driver of Adherence to the Mediterranean Diet in Italy. *Front. Nutr.* **2022**, *9*, 804865. [CrossRef] [PubMed]
80. Noah, A.; Truswell, S. Commodities consumed in Italy, Greece and other Mediterranean countries compared with Australia in 1960s and 1990s. *Asia Pac. J. Clin. Nutr.* **2003**, *12*, 23–29. [PubMed]
81. Garcia-Closas, R.; Berenguer, A.; González, C.A. Changes in food supply in Mediterranean countries from 1961 to 2001. *Public Health Nutr.* **2006**, *9*, 53–60. [CrossRef]
82. Lopez, C.N.; Martinez-Gonzalez, M.A.; Sanchez-Villegas, A.; Alonso, A.; Pimenta, A.M.; Bes-Rastrollo, M. Costs of Mediterranean and western dietary patterns in a Spanish cohort and their relationship with prospective weight change. *J. Epidemiol. Community Health* **2009**, *63*, 920–927. [CrossRef]

83. Aggarwal, A.; Monsivais, P.; Cook, A.J.; Drewnowski, A. Does diet cost mediate the relation between socioeconomic position and diet quality? *Eur. J. Clin. Nutr.* **2011**, *65*, 1059–1066. [CrossRef]
84. Buckland, G.; Bach, A.; Serra-Majem, L. Obesity and the Mediterranean diet: A systematic review of observational and intervention studies. *Obes. Rev.* **2008**, *9*, 582–593. [CrossRef]
85. Shrewsbury, V.; Wardle, J. Socioeconomic status and adiposity in childhood: A systematic review of cross-sectional studies 1990–2005. *Obesity* **2008**, *16*, 275–284. [CrossRef]

Disclaimer/Publisher's Note: The statements, opinions and data contained in all publications are solely those of the individual author(s) and contributor(s) and not of MDPI and/or the editor(s). MDPI and/or the editor(s) disclaim responsibility for any injury to people or property resulting from any ideas, methods, instructions or products referred to in the content.

MDPI AG
Grosspeteranlage 5
4052 Basel
Switzerland
Tel.: +41 61 683 77 34

Journal of Clinical Medicine Editorial Office
E-mail: jcm@mdpi.com
www.mdpi.com/journal/jcm

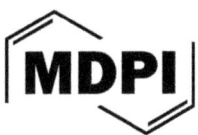

Disclaimer/Publisher's Note: The statements, opinions and data contained in all publications are solely those of the individual author(s) and contributor(s) and not of MDPI and/or the editor(s). MDPI and/or the editor(s) disclaim responsibility for any injury to people or property resulting from any ideas, methods, instructions or products referred to in the content.

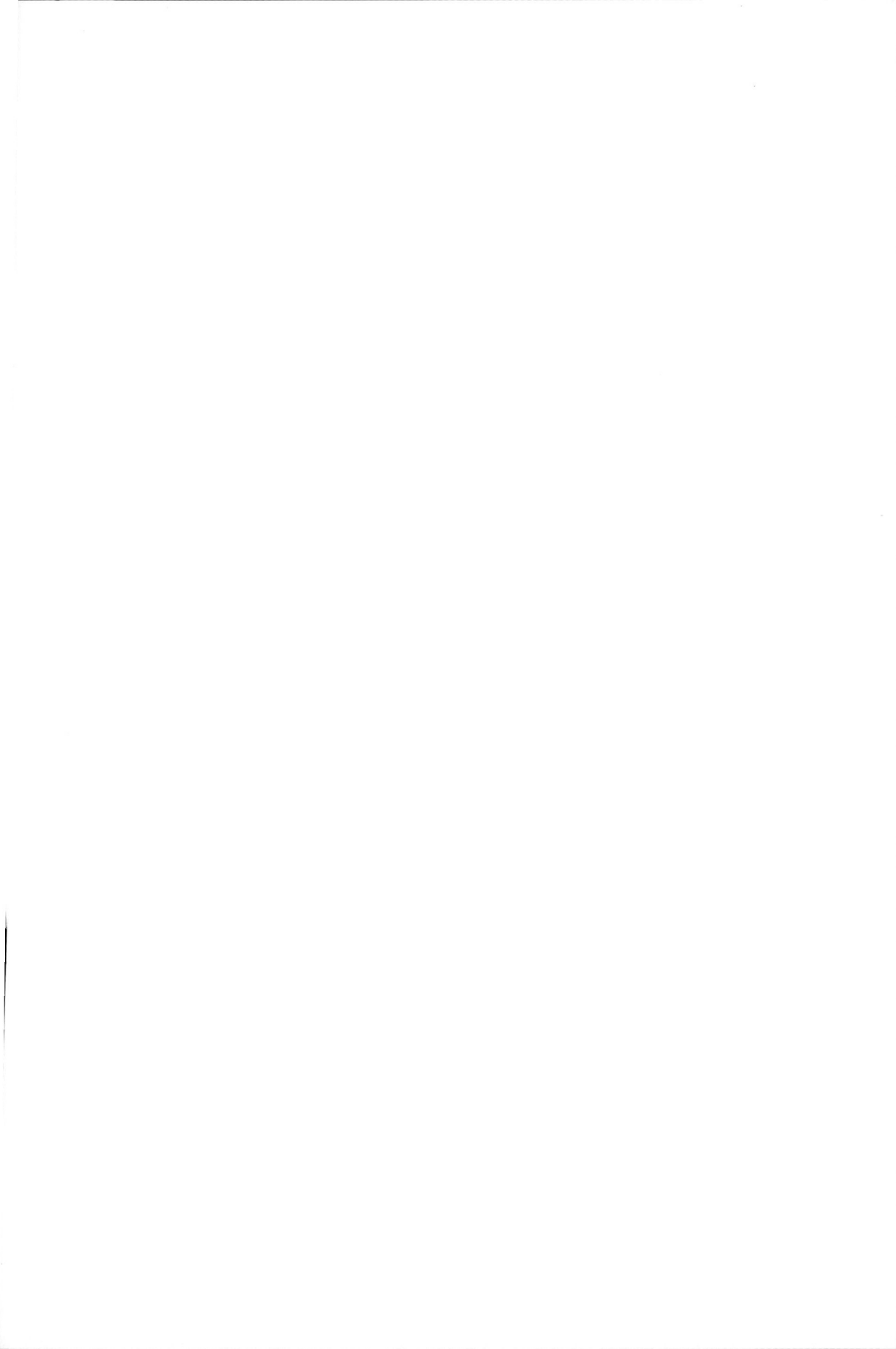

www.ingramcontent.com/pod-product-compliance
Lightning Source LLC
LaVergne TN
LVHW070614100526
838202LV00012B/646